Physical Examination of
the Musculoskeletal System

Physical Examination of the Musculoskeletal System

Melvin Post, M.D.
Professor of Orthopaedic Surgery
Rush-Presbyterian-St. Luke's Hospital and Medical Center
Chairman, Department of Orthopaedic Surgery
Michael Reese Hospital and Medical Center
Chicago, Illinois

YEAR BOOK MEDICAL PUBLISHERS, INC.
Chicago • London • Boca Raton

2   3   4   5   6   7   8   9   0   Y   B   90,   89,   88

Library of Congress Cataloging-in-Publication Data

Physical examination of the musculoskeletal system.

  Includes bibliographies and index.
  1. Orthopedia—Diagnosis.   2. Musculoskeletal
system—Diseases—Diagnosis.   3. Physical diagnosis.
I. Post, Melvin, 1928-   . [DNLM: 1. Bone Diseases—
diagnosis.   2. Joint Diseases—diagnosis.   3. Musculoskeletal System.   4. Physical Examination. WE 141 P578]
RD734.P48   1986   616.7'0754   86-9119
ISBN 0-8151-6744-X

Sponsoring Editor: James D. Ryan, Jr.
Manager, Copyediting Services: Frances M. Perveiler
Production Project Manager: Etta Worthington
Proofroom Supervisor: Shirley E. Taylor

*To the physician
whose greatest worth is as a diagnostician*

Contributors

Lorin M. Brown, M.D.
Director of Pediatric Orthopaedic Surgery
Michael Reese Hospital and Medical Center
Chicago, Illinois

James H. Dobyns, M.D.
Professor of Orthopaedics
Mayo Medical School
Consultant in Orthopaedics and Surgery of the Hand
Mayo Foundation
Rochester, Minnesota

Jorge O. Galante, M.D.
Professor and Chairman of Orthopaedic Surgery
Rush-Presbyterian-St. Luke's Hospital and Medical Center
Chicago, Illinois

Michael Jablon, M.D.
Director of Hand Surgery
Michael Reese Hospital and Medical Center
Chicago, Illinois

Kenneth A. Johnson, M.D.
Consultant, Orthopaedic Surgery
Director of Foot Service
Mayo Clinic
Associate Professor, Orthopaedic Surgery
Mayo Graduate School of Medicine
Rochester, Minnesota

Harold E. Kleinert, M.D.
Clinical Professor of Surgery
University of Louisville School of Medicine
Louisville, Kentucky

Glenn C. Landon, M.D.
Assistant Professor of Orthopaedic Surgery
Baylor College of Medicine
Houston, Texas

Ronald L. Linscheid, M.D.
Professor of Orthopaedic Surgery
Mayo Medical School
Consultant in Orthopaedic Surgery and Surgery of the Hand
Mayo Clinic
Rochester, Minnesota

Bernard F. Morrey, M.D.
Associate Professor in Orthopaedic Surgery
Mayo Medical School
Consultant in Orthopaedic Surgery
Mayo Clinic
Rochester, Minnesota

Melvin Post, M.D.
Professor of Orthopaedic Surgery
Rush-Presbyterian-St. Luke's Hospital and Medical Center
Chairman, Department of Orthopaedic Surgery
Michael Reese Hospital and Medical Center
Chicago, Illinois

Robert B. Salter, M.D.
Professor and Chairman of Orthopaedic Surgery
Hospital for Sick Children
Toronto, Ontario, Canada

W. John Sharrard, M.D., Ch.M., F.R.C.S.
Senior Orthopaedic Surgeon
Royal Hallamshire Hospital and Children's Hospital
Sheffield, England

Manmohan Singh, M.D.
Assistant Professor of Orthopaedics
Rush Medical College
Director of Foot and Ankle Service
Department of Orthopaedic Surgery
Michael Reese Hospital and Medical Center
Chicago, Illinois

Russell F. Warren, M.D.
Associate Professor of Orthopaedic Surgery
Cornell Medical College
Director of Sports Medicine
Hospital for Special Surgery
New York, New York

Foreword

Dr. Melvin Post has fulfilled a definite need in creating this modern book entitled *Physical Examination of the Musculoskeletal System.* A distinguished group of clinicians has contributed to this book. The chapter on history taking and the general medical examination, by Dr. Post himself, is written with painstaking care. It includes all the essential eponyms and is filled with reminders about the psychological and emotional aspects of pain. A physician especially qualified in the field, Dr. Post covers the physical examination of the shoulder girdle, and provides a useful tabulation of the importance of understanding the origins, insertions, functions, paralysis, and special tests of the shoulder girdle muscle action.

Bernard F. Morrey outlines the physical examination of the elbow, with an important presentation of associated joint involvement and assessment. The chapter by Ronald L. Linscheid and James H. Dobyns on physical diagnosis of the wrist is noteworthy in its discussion of interrelationships, signs, and symptoms of normal and pathological processes of bone, nerve, tendons, and ligaments, etc.

Michael Jablon and Harold E. Kleinert present a succinct system of examination of the hand that includes postural deformities and even fingernail features. The chapter entitled "Physical Examination of the Spine," with its close association with abnormalities of the shoulder, is written by Dr. Post; he provides a useful, handy reference table of nerves (normal and abnormal functions) and special tests for each. The tabulation is continued through his chapter on physical examination of the thoracic and lumbar spine, with a strong emphasis on the neurological basis of orthopedic tests.

Glenn C. Landon and Jorge O. Galante contribute an up-to-date system of examination of the range of motion of the hip joint in health and disease, and conclude with the principles of evaluation of a patient with a total hip arthroplasty. Lorin M. Brown and W. John Sharrard outline the principles of the lower extremities of the child from the foot up, and Dr. Brown and Robert Salter provide essential information about examinations of the lower extremities of the child from the hip down.

Russell F. Warren provides a compendium of the old and the new procedures of the examination of the knee, equipped with all the new terminology and tests for ligament instability. Manmohan Singh and Kenneth A. Johnson admirably record the steps in the examination of the adult, compared with the child, foot and ankle, and offer classification of pes planus, metatarsalgia, and the dysvascular foot, which is useful for students and experienced clinicians.

This book is written for the handy bookshelves in the clinic examining rooms, doctors' offices, and every student's library. In the United States, patients are generally pleased to see a doctor reach for a book and read something interesting to them about the condition under consideration. There are enough of both eponymic and noneponymic names to make every test easy to locate, with the definitions brief and easy to read. While operations may come and go, the knowledge of physical diagnosis in this book should be here to stay.

MARSHALL R. URIST, M.D.
PROFESSOR OF SURGERY (ORTHOPEDICS)
UNIVERSITY OF CALIFORNIA, LOS ANGELES
LOS ANGELES, CALIFORNIA

Preface

The cornerstone of clinical medicine was founded on a system of inquiry and observation. An accurate diagnosis is established by using this method of investigation. It is accomplished by taking a history and performing a physical examination. Although modern technology and new radiologic methods have added immeasurably to the armamentarium of the physician, it is the history and physical examination that still stand as the basis of an effective medical evaluation. This is the most objective method for diagnosing disease. However, it requires superior communicative skills and presumes the correct use of one's senses and judgment. It is fundamental in the training of a clinician.

With the advent of modern technology and the need to learn a large amount of new information that has truly expanded the horizons of the physician, it is unfortunate there has been less emphasis on traditional methods of medical school education and the basic sciences, with the result that the clinician is in real danger of losing a high degree of diagnostic acumen.

The technique of history taking is well known and the principles of physical examination have not changed. But there is a need to emphasize the necessity of performing a careful examination and to reinterpret this examination in the light of modern medicine. Why? Because the difference between those who follow the principles of a careful medical evaluation and those who believe it is an unnecessary burden is the difference between the physician who is an educated, thoughtful physician-scientist and another who is merely a clever technician.

This book reviews the principles of physical diagnosis as it relates to the musculoskeletal system. It is not intended as a text dealing with a general medical evaluation alone. It does stress that a complete history and physical examination are often needed in order to correctly evaluate diseases affecting the musculoskeletal system. A distinguished group of physicians have attempted to stress the primary importance of the history and the physical examination in diagnosing disease. Standardized descriptive definitions and methods of determining muscle power and motions are used throughout the book.

I wish to express my gratitude to Ms. June Pedigo, who illustrated much of the text, and to Mr. Daniel J. Doody and the editorial staff of Year Book Medical Publishers who supported and helped to make this book possible.

MELVIN POST, M.D.

Contents

CHAPTER 1

General Medical Examination

Melvin Post, M.D.

History Taking

A systematic method of taking a history and performing a thorough physical examination will enable the physician to establish an initial data base. When this initial body of knowledge about the patient is accurately collected, a problem list may be developed from which plans and progress notes can be integrated. A patient's problem may affect an individual's physical or emotional health. The following outline is one of many that is suggested as one way of performing a general medical evaluation.

Chief complaint
Present illness
Past history
    Childhood illness
    Adult illness
    Operations
    Drug sensitivity and allergic reactions
Systemic review
    General
    Head
    Eyes
    Nose
    Throat
    Neck
    Respiratory
    Cardiovascular
    Gastrointestinal
    Genitourinary
    Metabolic and endocrine
    Lymphatic
    Musculoskeletal
    Hematopoietic

Neuropsychiatric
Social history
Family history
Physical examination
  General appearance and mental status
  Skin
  Lymphatics
  Head and neck
  Eyes
  Ears
  Nose
  Throat and mouth
  Teeth
  Chest and lungs
  Cardiovascular
  Abdomen
  Hernia
  Genitalia
  Rectum
  Musculoskeletal
    Back–spine
    Extremities
  Neurologic
Admission laboratory data
Initial diagnosis
Problem list
  Date entered
  Date resolved

Interview

When patients believe they are ill or complain of acute pain, for example, they seek the help of a physician. Successful treatment of any condition begins with an accurate history. The interview is an art that must be learned and constantly practiced. The physician must be articulate and conversant with individuals in every walk of life. This will determine how the physician will proceed with the medical evaluation and how the patient eventually will be treated. During the initial meeting the physician must gain the confidence of the patient from the outset.

At the initial meeting, the physician must listen carefully to the complaint(s) of the patient and to the answers of his guided questions, and at the same time comprehend and assess the information that is gathered. An attempt should be made to place a priority on the importance of the patient's answers. Only when all the facts or symptoms are obtained and fully understood in their correct sequence should the physical examination be undertaken. Some patients are more easily upset than others and may be less clear about their problem(s). In any event, they should not be hurried. It may be necessary to interview the patient a second or third time to gather all the essential information that will allow a true understanding of the problem. If the patient is a deaf mute it is essential to take the time, however long, to determine the complaints of the patient. If the patient is confused or speaks another language a friend or relative may be needed to help with the interview. Thus, a history can be obtained that will permit an early classification of a disease state, if it exists, and to clearly understand the individual relative to the history so that correct treatment decisions can be made. The examining physician must realize that it is often necessary to obtain a complete history, reviewing all medical systems, before the interview is complete because such symptoms and findings may relate to these systems as well as the musculoskeletal system. It is far better to overinterview than accept an inadequate history.

If the complaint(s) are few and localized the history can be abbreviated. For example, the patient who states he has cut his thumb has a clear-cut history. But are there any allergies to drugs, or any other disease states that may affect treatment? Was tetanus immunization once received, and if so, when? While a complete history and physical examination may not be needed, enough of an adequate history and examination is required in order to render optimum treatment. However, a patient who complains of a persistent or a radiating pain about a joint requires a more complete examination. The inexperienced physician is less likely to omit important points of the examination if there is adherence to a systematic method of history taking relative not only to the chief complaint(s) but also to other systems possibly affected that may shed additional information on the problem. The chief complaint may cross many lines of specialization and it is the educated physician who will appreciate the importance of a detailed examination. Whether it be local or the result of a distant abnormality, the purpose of the examination, especially by one who is an initiate, is to gain experience in recognizing a disturbance in form and function regardless of the involved system(s). Every illness ordinarily evokes an emotional response in a patient. The questioner must be astute in recognizing the patient's reaction, whether verbal or by gesture. An individual may deny an illness or may have a different threshold of pain than another with the same disease state. Having understood the patient's problem and the disease process, the physician must begin to react to the patient in an appropriate manner, to explain to the patient the disease or problem, and what must be done to solve the problem, including any alternative treatment. Only after this is accomplished should a specific treatment be selected that is best for the individual. The physician should remain objective and at the same time inform the patient, so that the patient can make an intelligent choice about his care. In other words, the patient or guardian should be a part of the decision-making process whenever possible.

The history consists of the chief complaint(s) and present illness, which should be documented in a chronological order. This is followed by the past history, which itemizes all medical conditions in the life of the patient before the present event. During this interview, the physician has a golden opportunity to put the patient at ease, and to establish a genuine physician-patient relationship.

If after preliminary questioning about a particular system significant information is obtained, more detailed questions may be asked. It will permit the pieces of a puzzle to form a clear picture of the problem. As many questions are asked as are needed to clarify a given symptom. Even the age and sex of the patient can be significant. If a patient complains of thigh pain, for example, its specific location, character, frequency, duration, variation, aggravation, distribution or radiation, intensity, and course should be determined. Was the pain caused by trauma, and if so what was the kind and degree of trauma? Was the pain increased or relieved by specific motions, stress, or activity? There are varying kinds of pain that may relate to a neurologic condition, or a peripheral nerve, muscle, or joint. During the interview, the physician should make an effort to determine the origin of the pain. Accordingly, a thorough knowledge of anatomy and physiology is key to an interpretation of the complaint(s). If a specific injury was sustained, was it recent or old? How did it happen, when and where, and what were the movements of the body parts or the objects extraneous to the body when the accident occurred? Only after as much information as possible about the present complaint(s) has been obtained should a history about other systems be sought.

A review of systems should include a general statement about the patient's health, including any changes in appetite or well-being, or a denial by the patient of fever, chills, or night sweats, for example.

Questions are asked about the head, ear, nose, throat, neck, and even the skin. Have there been headaches? Were there rashes, pigment changes, pruritus, raised skin areas, or any character change at all in the skin? Has bleeding from the nose been present? Have there been recurring sore throats, hoarseness, or difficulty in swallowing? Has the patient noticed masses, stiffness, or changes in the range of motion in the neck?

Concerning the respiratory system, questions should include the presence of cough, the sputum, hemoptysis, dyspnea, pain, and wheezing. Regarding the cardiovascular system, questions should be asked about pain, dyspnea, orthopnea, syncope, fatigue, edema, palpitations, cramps, and paresthesias, and even about changes in the color of hands and feet. The abdomen and its contents, including the genitourinary organs, are related to diverse questions about the tongue and mouth, dysphagia, appetite, weight loss, bowel habits, stools, jaundice, vomiting, pain, micturition, dysuria, retention, and hematuria. Questions related to the functioning of the metabolic and endocrine systems should concern weight, hair distribution, growth, and development. A detailed menstrual history should be included. A lymphatic review should be sought and the patient questioned about any lumps or bumps. Questions about the musculoskeletal system should include queries about pain, stiffness, swelling, buckling, or the locking of a joint. Has there been an increasing deformity, and if so, for how long and under what circumstances? These same general questions should also relate to the spine. Questions concerning the nervous system should be asked about headaches, vision, diplopia, hearing, tinnitus, vertigo, taste, smell, speech, changes in consciousness, syncope, convulsions, involuntary movements, weakness, paresthesias, and sphincter control. Inquiries about the blood should include questions about skin color, bleeding of any nature, bruising, and swelling. In addition, psychiatric questions about insomnia, altered behavior, recent changes in the person's life, and emotional stresses may impart important information.

Once a review of the present history is obtained, the past history should be completed by obtaining a social and family history. It may follow at this point or can be obtained after the present illness. A data base about childhood illnesses, which should include questions about whether or not there was jaundice at birth, blood transfusions, or when the child first sat, walked and talked, can have great significance. All immunizations, allergies, and injuries, and all medical, surgical, and obstetric treatments should be recorded.

A history about specific medications of any nature and all adverse reactions should be sought. A personal and social history including occupation(s), diet, smoking, alcohol habits, recreations, travel to distant areas and other countries, work and family habits, and relationships may be important. A family history about parents, grandparents, siblings, and other family members documenting disease states, deaths, and illnesses can be important.

It should be borne in mind that if the surgeon is to correctly diagnose a condition, all systems must be scrutinized. Once the history is completed, the physician should put the patient at ease by further explaining what will occur during the examination.

Physical Examination

The patient should undress and put on a loose gown that allows the physician to examine the entire body if necessary, while respecting the modesty and dignity of the individual. In fact, the physical examination requires the use of the physician's senses to permit inspection, palpation, percussion, smell, and auscultation, for example, in bruits. The height, weight, temperature, and blood pressure, both standing and recumbent, if possible, should be recorded initially, as well as a general statement given by the examiner on the appearance of the patient, the degree of apparent illness, and whether or not the patient is in pain. If there is serious trauma, a statement regarding the clinical appearance of shock should be recorded. Thereafter, the nutritional status and any obvious deformities should be noted. A general description of the skin, including texture, scars, elasticity, and pigmentation, should be recorded, along with observations about palpation of the subcutaneous tissue. Specific gait patterns and movements of the extremities can be reserved for the more detailed regional examination of the musculoskeletal system.

Next in order of the general evaluation is the appearance of the head, face, mouth and teeth, and ears; special attention should be made to record any deviation from the norm. The appearance and even the expression of the eyes, as well as other facial expressions, is a source of important data. Exophthalmos, pallor, redness, or jaundice of the eyes should be observed. A general examination of the neck, including the thyroid, should be made.

A general examination of the hands, feet, and nails should be performed. In addition, a general examination of lymph nodes in the cervical, supraclavicular, axillary, epitrochlear, abdominal, inguinal, and femoral regions should be performed. If it is germane, the breasts should be examined even in a male patient. A notation of any lumps and bumps should be recorded. Finally, in this part of the examination, the general color of the extremities, particularly of the distal parts, and any evidence of edema and its degree should be recorded. Differences in each side should be noted.

Following this part of the general evaluation, the various systems may be examined. Although the patient is usually examined from the right side, the physician may use any comfortable position that will increase the number of findings.

In examining the respiratory system, the type of breathing, the presence of cyanosis, or clubbing of the fingers, and the appearance of the sputum should be noted. During inspection, the shape of the chest and any abnormalities of its movements should be recorded. Palpation will permit the physician to determine the position of the trachea, detect the apex beat, chest movements, and any areas of tenderness or fremitus. Similarly, percussion will allow the determination of the location of the upper border of liver dullness, other areas of dullness, or the area of cardiac dullness. Auscultation provides information concerning the breath and voice sounds, or any adventitious sounds.

Examination of the cardiovascular system should include palpation and recording of the pulses bilaterally, for the temporal, carotid, radial, brachial, femoral, popliteal, dorsal pedal, and posterior tibial arteries. The character, rate, and rhythm of the pulses should be described. During inspection, any deformities, dilated vessels, or abnormal pulses should be recorded. Palpation will give the location and character of the apex beat, or other impulses and thrills. Cardiac dullness or other dullness is determined during percussion. Auscultation at the four heart valves will give important information about the rate, character, note, and type of sound heard, as well as about murmurs, or other sounds such as friction sounds.

Inspection of the abdomen should include observation of the teeth, tongue, gums, scars, distension, veins, hernias (abdominal wall, femoral, inguinal, and incisional), discoloration, masses, movement, and feces. The various organs (liver, spleen, kidneys, stomach, bowel, and bladder) or other masses are examined by palpation and percussion, and their sizes, positions, areas of tenderness or any other abnormalities noted. Even auscultation for bruits, bowel sounds, or lack of such sounds is important, and when indicated, a rectal examination of the anus and a digital examination can provide useful information about any masses in the rectum or enlargement of the prostate, including masses palpated through the rectum.

An examination of the metabolic and endocrine systems should describe the appearance of the body habitus, the size and relative proportions, and positions of the limbs and trunk. A description should be given of any pigmentation, hair distribution, and its quality, as well as for any lumps over the body and their distribution. Secondary sexual characteristics as well as an examination of the penis, testes, and spermatic cord, inspection of the vulva, and digital examination of the vagina, cervix, uterus, and ovaries should be obtained if needed. In this age of specialization, physicians better versed in these specific regions are often called in for consultation, such as for a gynecologic consultation.

Muscle Examination

Table 1–1 shows the numerical system for grading the power of muscles during muscle testing.[1] If an examiner understands this method of grading he will be able to establish the power grade of a muscle and recognize any changes from the initial examination. This will enable the examiner to differentiate organic disease from psychogenic illness. If a more objective analysis is desired thereafter the strength of the muscle group can be tested by using a dynamometer instrument. For example, hand grasp or pinch strength may be so measured.

A numerical value of 5 represents normal muscle power, while a decreasing grade indicates that power is correspondingly decreased. A plus (+) or minus (−) assignment of each numerical rating can better refine the power grade of a muscle. The examiner should not rely on this method of measuring muscle strength alone but must examine the muscle fully since a grade of 5 is consistent

TABLE 1–1.

Classification of Muscle Grading

GRADE*	PERCENT	MUSCLE STRENGTH
0 = Zero	0	No evidence of contractility
1 = Trace	10	Evidence of slight contractility, no joint motion with gravity eliminated
2 = Poor	25	Complete range of motion with gravity eliminated
3 = Fair	50	Complete range of motion against gravity
4 = Good	75	Complete range of motion against gravity with some resistance
5 = Normal	100	Complete range of motion against gravity with full resistance

* Increments of each number may be expressed as a plus or minus for a given grade.

with a significant amount of muscle atrophy. This is possible because the residual strength of muscles in individuals who are well developed can give a false numerical rating. In older people and in patients recently operated upon, care should be exercised in stressing a part during muscle testing for fear of causing iatrogenic injury. Muscles with nearly normal strength can be tested by having the subject attempt to move the part in the direction against applied resistance or by having the subject hold the part with the muscle contracted while the examiner attempts to move the part against the usual muscle pull. If the muscle is weak and the patient unable to move the muscle against gravity, it should be tested with gravity eliminated. Finally, if the part is too weak for movement, muscle contraction can be determined by palpation of the tendon. Whenever possible, the same examiner should perform the examination again.

A description of the power grade of the muscle, and its endurance, rapidity, and dexterity should be noted. Muscles should be gently palpated for evidence of tenderness and any evidence of contractions, especially when a part fails to move. In addition, the examiner must determine whether or not there is muscle spasm, a muscle contracture of an individual muscle or muscle group, or relative weakness of a muscle because of myositis or even a local phlebitis that may prevent the muscle from fully contracting due to pain.

Muscles should be inspected and observed for fasciculation and spasms (tetanus). The terms fasciculation and fibrillation are often confused. Fasciculations are small local contractions of muscles that are visible through the skin. They represent a discharge of a number of muscle cells that are innervated by a single motor axon. Fibrillations represent small, local involuntary muscle contractions that are invisible beneath the skin. They result from spontaneous activation of single muscle cells. Conversely, tremors are involuntary movements in which opposing muscle groups contract in such a way as to cause rhythmic or alternating movements of the joint. The normal degree of tension in the muscle (tonus) must also be assessed. Rigidity refers to an increase in muscular tonus wherein resistance is maintained during passive movements and without collapse of the muscle. Spasticity refers to a muscle tonus where there may be a collapse of the muscle during testing. Comparisons of active and passive ranges of motions are important in muscle testing in that active motion requires muscle strength with a grade of at least 3.

Before there can be reliable testing of muscle strength, the examiner must also know whether or not there is nerve paralysis causing the muscle weakness. It follows that an effective neurologic examination is an integral part of the musculoskeletal examination. If the strength of muscles about a joint cannot be adequately tested the examiner must also know whether or not the joint is normal or diseased because a diseased joint, for example, an arthritic joint, may preclude adequate muscle strength testing due to a mechanical block. During the recording of a muscle grade if there is a suggestion of muscle atrophy, especially when comparing each side, the circumferences of an extremity should be measured at specific levels by taking a consistent point above or below a fixed or reference point. For example, the circumferences of the legs can be measured by arbitrarily measuring 10 cm below the tibial tubercles, which allows a comparison in the muscles of the legs of an individual.

During the examination the patient should be comfortable and rested, and a comparison of the muscles of the contralateral side recorded. Notations about the shape and contour of the part, and the consistency and quality of a muscle should be made. The actions of multiple muscles may combine to produce the same movement. Thus, it is necessary to observe and palpate the muscle and its tendon, thereby eliminating the possibility that neighboring muscles are acting. It is equally important to know the position of a part before testing muscle strength. For example, the true strength of the flexors of the fingers may be affected if muscle testing occurs while the wrist is flexed. Another example occurs when an examiner is uncertain the scapula is actively fixed against the chest cage while testing for deltoid muscle power.

Joint Motions

The accepted method for testing joint motion(s) is based upon the principle of the neutral zero, first described by Cave and Roberts.[2] This method was approved in 1964 by the Orthopaedic Associations of the English-speaking world. It is simple, reliable and reproducible. Most important, it permits comparisons to be made. Motion testing of various joints of each region of the body will be described in detail in subsequent chapters. In principle, the starting position is 0° and not 180°. Thus, full extension of the elbow is 0° and not 180°. In a pathologic state, the starting point may be other than 0°. In any event, the specific range of motion should be given for each position, indicating abduction, adduction, flexion, and varus position for a given part. Moreover, data should be recorded for passive and active ranges of motion. In many instances both types of measurement may provide important information.

The general principles of measuring motion as defined by Cave and Roberts[2] may be summarized as follows: "(1) All motion should be measured by degrees from a neutral point of zero; (2) the neutral points from which the motion is measured must be defined; (3) it is always worthwhile to mention the comparative motions in the joint of the opposite limb; (4) angles should be measured with a goniometer or a protractor; (5) motions of joints above and below the affected part should be measured." The specific motions of each region of the body will be described in their respective chapters.

Musculoskeletal System

The musculoskeletal system is to the orthopedic surgeon what the cardiovascular system is to the cardiologist. But a disease state knows no boundaries. It is often necessary to have the details of the complete examination that allows for a

TABLE 1–2.
Standard Orthopedic Definitions for Positions and Deviations

TERMS	DEFINITION
Abduction	To draw away or deviate from the midline of the body
Adduction	To deviate or draw toward the midline of the body
Eversion	Turning outward
Extension	The act of straightening; when the part distal to a joint extends it straightens
External rotation	Rotary motion in the transverse plane away from the midline
Flexion	The act or condition of being bent; when a joint is flexed the part distal to the joint bends
Internal rotation	Rotary motion in the transverse plane toward the midline
Inversion	Turning inward
Kyphosis	An increased rounding of the normal thoracic curve of the spine
Lordosis	The anterior concavity in the curvature of the lumbar and cervical spines when viewed from the side
Pronation	Assuming a prone position is applied to the foot, it refers to a combination of eversion and abduction movements resulting in a lowering of the medial margin of the foot
Supination	The act of assuming a supine position; applied to the foot it refers to a raising of the medial margin of the foot, applied to the palm of the hand it refers to a turning of the palm upward
Varus*	Refers to deviation of a part or portion of an extremity distal to a joint away from the midline of the body
Valgus*	Refers to deviation of a part or portion of the extremity distal to a joint toward the midline of the body

* Valgus and varus are often used in the vernacular to describe the deformity of a fracture site wherein the part distal to a fracture is away or toward the midline of the body, respectively.

correlation of the findings of various interrelated systems. The specific medical evaluations of each major region of the musculoskeletal system will be given in the text to follow. Standard definitions that describe positions and deviations of a part are given in Table 1–2.

Once the standardized methods for measuring the grade of muscle strengths and joint motions are mastered an examination of the musculoskeletal system may be undertaken. An examination of this system may start with a general inspection of the entire body. For example, during the early part of the general medical evaluation, the finding of gouty tophi may be noted in the external ears, feet, and hands, and may have important implications in a patient who has complaints of pain about his joints and associated findings. The general movement of major joints and a comparison of each side should be noted. Even the manner in which a person stands or holds the extremity should be noted and could be important. The general contour and length of the extremity in relationship to the torso may be significant. The warmth of a joint and any swelling or tenderness should be recorded. Specific points about a joint where a mass may be palpated should be described and illustrated if this will help clarify the description. Joints should be tested for stability.

Nervous System

No examination of the musculoskeletal system is complete without a thorough evaluation of the nervous system. The two systems are probably more often interdependent than any other medical system in diseases treated by the orthopedic surgeon.

The kind of speech should be reported. Is there dysphasia or dysarthria? If positive findings exist, mention should be made as to the presence of auditory, visual, or tactile agnosia. Here too, reference to spine motion, especially cervical spine motion, in relationship to any neurologic changes should be made. The examiner should be certain that during any portion of the medical examination that harm is not done. For example, when a patient has a suspected fracture of the cervical spine, movement of the neck must be avoided. This is one of the few times the examiner must rely on excellent roentgenograms of the cervical spine before examination in order to establish a precise diagnosis of an injured part when there is such an injury. If indicated, an examination of the cranial and peripheral nervous system should be made.

If a patient is unconscious, confused, or drowsy, the diagnostic skill of the surgeon is exceptionally important. The unconscious patient cannot relate a history or follow commands. A confused individual is disoriented, while a drowsy patient can respond to verbal stimuli and has a semblance of consciousness. The very young child or infant also falls into this category in the sense that a history cannot be communicated directly, and so the surgeon must rely on others for this portion of the examination. In this event, certain essential tests may be needed, such as computered axial tomography for a space-occupying lesion.

It is important to bear in mind at all times the segmental supply of the muscles being examined and their peripheral nerve supply. Similarly, it is very useful to know the sensory dermatomes of the skin (Fig 1–1). Superficial sensation is tested with a pin while deep pain may be tested by squeezing the muscles of the limb. Vibration and cortical sensation should be tested if it is needed. Two-point discrimination tests the ability of the patient to discriminate between two points or a single point. It should be recalled that the spinal cord is shorter than the vertebral column. It actually terminates at the first lumbar vertebral level. The C8 spinal segment is opposite the seventh vertebra, and L5 spinal segment exits the foramen between the L-4–L-5 vertebrae.

The tendon reflexes are involuntary contractions of a muscle in response to a brisk tap on a tendon. The reflexes can be divided into deep and superficial reflexes. For example, a deep tendon reflex such as the knee jerk depends upon the reflex contraction of the quadriceps and its segmental innervation of L3-4 supplied by the femoral nerve. A reflex may be absent and is termed 0; diminished, or rated as 1; average as 2; exaggerated as 3; or show clonus for a rating of 4. The reflexes of both sides of the body should be tested. If a reflex is difficult to elicit the test can often still be performed by using reinforcement. In the lower extremity, a Jendrassik maneuver is used when the patient holds the hands together by cupping and locking the fingers of both hands and pulling in opposite directions. For the upper extremity, the same type of reinforcement may be achieved by clenching the opposite hand not being examined or by biting hard. Abnormal reflexes such as the Babinski should be considered if there is any suspicion of an upper motor neuron lesion. Primitive reflexes are normally demonstrated in early infancy and their absence early or manifestation at a later time can be of clinical significance. The Moro reflex is present at birth until several months of age. It may be absent on one side in the presence of a lower motor neuron lesion. If it persists after 6 months of age, it may indicate cerebral

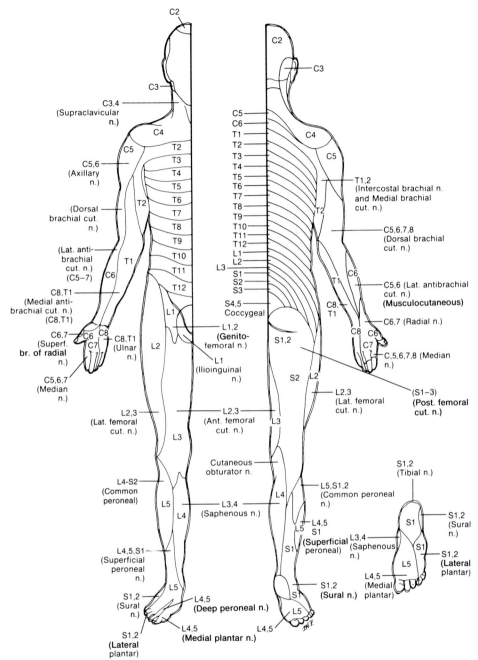

FIG 1–1. Dermatomes and common sensory and peripheral nerves.

disease. A brachial plexus palsy or even a fractured clavicle at birth may show an absent test.

Once the initial data base has been established and all pertinent problems are listed, the examiner may record his impression(s) and prepare a preliminary diagnosis with accompanying differential diagnoses given in order of priority. Plans may be formulated to confirm the diagnosis. It may require a variety of laboratory and roentgenographic tests. The examiner must always keep in mind if any illness was missed or if a part of the examination was unnecessary. In addition, he should decide if other data were needed to screen for a missed illness and what other data were helpful in identifying or managing a disease entity already described.[3]

Once diagnostic studies have refined the problem (history, physical examination, and laboratory data) treatment may be instituted. The patient should be included in the management decisions.

Finally, appropriate progress notes should represent what has happened with the problem. The notes should include subjective and objective information, such as pertinent laboratory data. They should also state the examiner's analysis of the information and any treatment changes and the reasons for any change.

References

1. Post M: *The Shoulder: Surgical and Nonsurgical Management.* Philadelphia, Lea & Febiger, 1978.
2. Cave EF, Roberts SM: A method for measuring and recording joint function. *J Bone Joint Surg* 1936; 34:455.
3. Sandlow LJ, Bashook PG: *Problem Oriented Medical Records.* Chicago, Michael Reese Hospital and Medical Center, 1978.

CHAPTER 2

Physical Examination of the Shoulder Girdle

Melvin Post, M.D.

A carefully developed history and thorough physical examination of the shoulder permit an early, accurate diagnosis. This is especially important for the shoulder region because pain, for example, can seriously impair the function of the entire upper extremity. Thus, the history and physical examination of the shoulder should at least encompass an examination of those areas of the upper extremity that may be germane to the presenting problem. The findings of the opposite extremity should be compared.

If there is a single localized complaint of pain in the anterolateral aspect of the shoulder, indicating a diagnosis of a bursitis, a more complete history and physical examination can be avoided when the physician is confident this is the only cause of pain. When a patient complains of radiating pain about the shoulder a more exacting examination is needed. The physician must gather enough information and findings to recognize a dysfunction in the shoulder or at a distant site. It is important to pinpoint an abnormality of a disease process and relate it to an anatomical part and its function. Each symptom should be fully explored and an attempt made to unify them into one disease process or more than one if it exists.

The age of the patient, his occupation, the side of dominance, and his specific job requirements, as well as his educational level are important to know. Even with a well-documented diagnosis and excellent treatment, the patient may need retraining for another type of job. What is done to a patient can affect his future function and the kind of work that is possible.

Four moving parts comprise the shoulder girdle and determine its movement. They constitute the "scapulothoracic articulation," and the glenohumeral, the acromioclavicular, and sternoclavicular joints. They are all interdependent, and a decrease in the function of one certainly affects the others. Together, they work as one harmonious unit, and any defect in one will affect the whole. The shoulder girdle is more dependent on its muscles, ligaments, and surrounding soft tissue than almost any other anatomical region in the body. During the examination, the physician must constantly integrate the findings so as to minimize missing any clues that will help to establish a diagnosis. To do this, the physician must trust his findings by practicing the art and techniques of physical examination.

Inspection

The examination starts with a general inspection of the thorax, the spine, and the shoulder girdle. The general appearance of the skin, general nourishment, posture, and attitude of the extremities should be noted. The size and shape of scars or stretch marks, for example, along with any skin discoloration or other evidence of skin injury should be recorded. Changes in the contour of the shoulder girdle and muscle development or atrophy of the surrounding tissues should also be recorded, recalling that the state of the musculature and subcutaneous tissues is influenced by the general nutrition of the patient. In healthy athletic-type individuals good muscle development is apparent, whereas in the undernourished patient there may be wasting of the muscles and subcutaneous tissues. For example, atrophy of the muscles about the shoulder in a boy may suggest muscle disease such as muscular dystrophy (Fig 2–1).

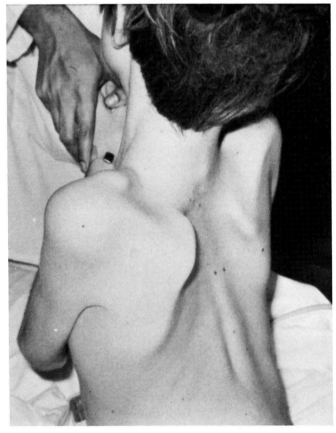

FIG 2–1. 14-year-old boy with classic muscular dystrophy is shown with severe wasting of shoulder girdle muscles. Note winging of scapulae. Right shoulder girdle musculature is wasted to the extent that shoulder girdle causes elevation of the scapula above chin level. This is termed "loose shoulder."

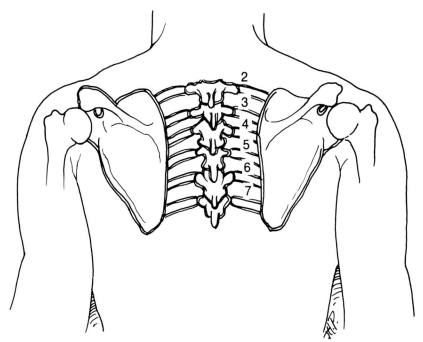

FIG 2–2. Normal position of the scapulae are shown. Superior angle rests opposite second rib while inferior angle lies slightly below seventh rib.

A comparison of findings of both sides of the body is important when viewing the general body contour. Are the scapulae similarly positioned on the torso (Fig 2–2), or are the hand and rest of the upper extremity abnormal in any way (Fig 2–3)? Are there obvious contractures or muscle tears (Fig 2–4)? Are the upper extremities suspended from the torso in a normal manner? Are there any obvious raised areas or enlarged areas or bumps (Fig 2–5)?

Is there a normal rounding of the shoulders, or abnormal depressions in the skin or in the areas above and below the clavicle? Check for swelling or a depression about the acromioclavicular or sternoclavicular joints, especially when there has been a history of trauma. Obesity may obscure the underlying anatomy. If symmetry is lost, is it due to atrophy, or a disruption of the anatomy of the underlying parts, or a combination of both? Is there a chronic dislocation leading to a loss of the normal contour, rather than deltoid atrophy, for example (Fig 2–6)? In addition, the shoulder girdle should be viewed from behind. The position of the scapulae, and the presence or absence of a kyphosis or scoliosis should be observed. Normally, the scapulae rest in a position between the second and seventh ribs with the scapulae vertebral borders located 5 cm from the spinous processes (see Fig 2–2). Any deviation from this "normal position" is considered to be abnormal. Thus, the presence of scoliosis may give the false impression of winging of the scapulae (Fig 2–7).

An important aspect of the inspection is to note the motions of the shoulder. Are they complete, natural, harmonious, smooth, jerky, incomplete, or obviously painful? Does the whole shoulder girdle move as an integrated unit?

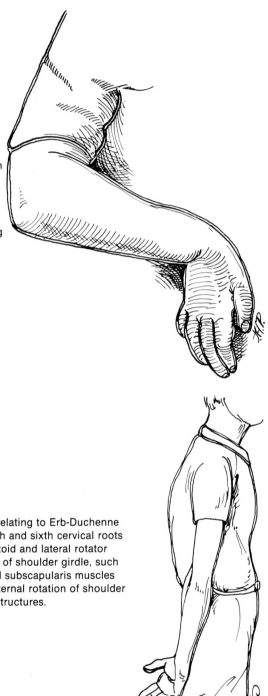

FIG 2–3. Classic example of the "porter's tip" hand is shown. It is associated with a lesion in upper trunk of brachial plexus that produces adduction and medial rotation of humerus. Dysfunction of biceps results in an inability to flex elbow or supinate forearm, thereby allowing forearm to remain extended and pronated with palm facing backward and outward. Musculature of hand remains unaffected.

FIG 2–4. Hand and upper extremity relating to Erb-Duchenne palsy is shown. In this condition the fifth and sixth cervical roots are involved. There is a paralysis of deltoid and lateral rotator muscles of humerus and other muscles of shoulder girdle, such as the supraspinatus, infraspinatus, and subscapularis muscles with an inability to abduct arm. Note internal rotation of shoulder relating to a contracture of soft tissue structures.

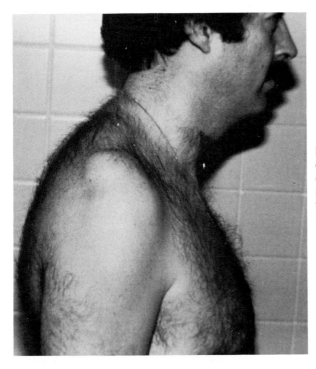

FIG 2–5. Large ganglion cyst arose from right acromioclavicular joint and was not painful. It could be transluminated with a narrow beamed light source.

Palpation

Both the patient and the examiner should be comfortable, either seated in a chair, on the edge of a table, or in the standing position. It is helpful for the examiner to know the underlying anatomy, especially as it applies to anatomical landmarks. Palpation should be performed from the front, side, and back of the patient, again comparing both sides. All scars and their extent and consistency should be recorded. Even a so-called well-healed scar may reveal a disruption of muscle edges or defect if deeply but prudently palpated. Is there tenderness of an ordinary scar or of a keloid? Skin temperature should be determined. Is the skin hyperelastic, or thinned, especially at the site of a previous cortisone injection? Palpation of the subcutaneous tissue, muscles, and the joint capsule may provide important information. For example a snapping sensation over the proximal portion of the long head of the biceps during the testing of motions may suggest a subluxation of the tendon from its groove. Specific bony parts and their prominence should be palpated. These include the whole contour of the acromion, the tuberosities, the coracoid and the acromioclavicular and sternoclavicular joints, the scapular spine, and their relationships to other close structures such as the spine. Palpation of the suprasternal notch should not be neglected.

Palpation of the usual hard rigid superior surface of the shoulder may reveal a movable portion that may be related to a congenital os acromiale, which may not be apparent on ordinary roentgen films. The greater tuberosity of the humerus may be palpated while the arm is in slight internal rotation or in a neutral anatomical position. It is located just beneath the anterolateral edge of the acromion, and in asthenic individuals, a slight depression may be felt between the acromion and, in heavily muscled individuals, greater tuberosity that may not be palpated.

The bicipital groove is positioned just anteriorly and medially beyond the greater tuberosity. The depression of this groove lies between the slightly raised edges of the greater and lesser tuberosities. The peaks of their walls are readily palpated with the arm in neutral position. The groove may be more easily palpated with the thumb while the elbow is flexed as the arm is rotated inward or outward (Fig 2–8). This maneuver should be performed carefully in patients with inflammation of the synovial membrane that encompasses the long head of the biceps since severe pain may be produced.

With the arm in neutral position, immediately beyond the lesser tuberosity lies the coracoid process. The coracoid tip lies 2.5 cm below the clavicle. The clavicle lies just beneath the skin, and in thin individuals, a good portion of its contour is easily discerned. The convex middle and inner third of the clavicle can be palpated slightly superior to and occasionally slightly anterior to the manubrium. A careful examination can determine the presence of an anterior or

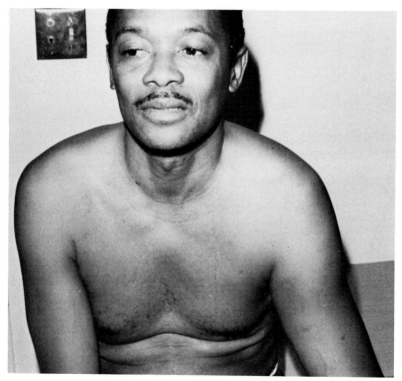

FIG 2–6. An adult male sustained an anterior dislocated left shoulder many months before with involvement of the axillary nerve. The shoulder remained anteriorly dislocated. Deltoid function was very poor. Note loss of contour in left shoulder associated with flattening of contour.

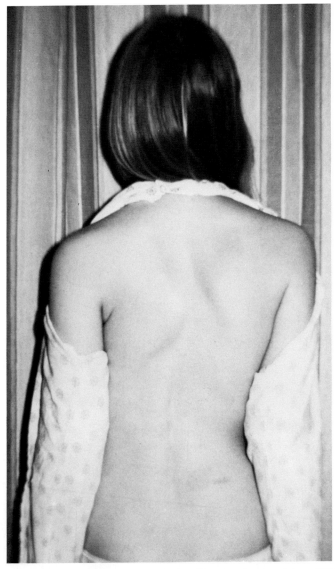

FIG 2-7. Teenage girl with idiopathic scoliosis with normal musculature gave the false impression that there was winging of scapula. When spine was treated and straightened, scapula aligned in a normal position on chest cage.

posterior sternoclavicular dislocation. An anterior dislocation may be manifested as a raised firm bony area superiorly or anterosuperiorly above the top of the manubrium sternum, which shows as an asymmetry when compared with the opposite side. A posterior dislocation will present as a definite anterior depression. The examiner should take care not to depress the medial end of the clavicle too firmly since the symptoms and findings of such a dislocation may be exacer-

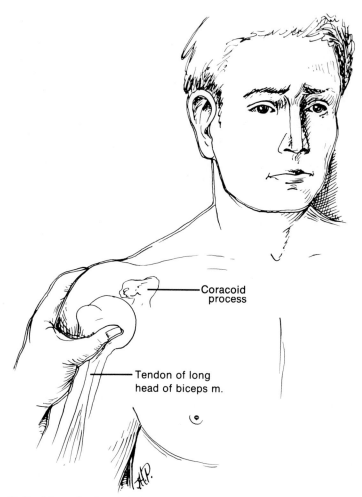

FIG 2–8. Method for palpating the biceps groove containing long head of biceps is shown.

bated. When the sternoclavicular area is severely swollen, a depression can be hidden. In such cases the use of a computed tomographic scan will determine a correct diagnosis.

The examiner may then move his fingers laterally along the clavicle to the acromioclavicular joint. The cylindrical shape of the clavicle blends into a flattened shape near its lateral third of the clavicle, and is prominent laterally. The distal end of the clavicle is raised slightly above the acromion with which it articulates and can be palpated.

The patient should be asked to actively or passively elevate and circumduct the arm. During these maneuvers, the examiner should palpate the shoulder at its various joints for grating, grinding, and crepitus.

The examiner can easily palpate the posterior edge of the acromion. This is the key to locating the scapular spine. When the fingers are moved medially from this point, the scapular spine is palpated. The superomedial angle of the scapula is located at the medial end of the scapular spine, and can be difficult to feel in obese and heavily muscled people. Above the scapular spine is the prominent hollow, the supraspinatus fossa, and the fossa, while below the spine lies the infraspinatus fossa. These fossae are prominent in patients with significant muscle atrophy (Fig 2–9).

The vertebral border of the scapula is easily palpated. It lies 5 cm lateral to the tips of the spinous processes. The superior border is positioned at the level of T-3. The inferior tip of the scapula lies at the level of T-7 (see Fig 2–2).

Palpation of the Deep Tissues

The examiner must have a comprehensive knowledge of anatomy and the spatial relationships of the deep structures if maximum meaning is to be gained from the palpation method. It is essential to differentiate normal from abnormal structures and masses and their sizes as well as shapes, and depressions or structures that are absent. Specific tender areas should be described and related to anatomical structures. For example, a nontender mass overlying the acromio-clavicular joint may be present as a ganglion mass (see Fig 2–5). In thin individuals, this type of pathologic entity may be transilluminated with a narrow-beamed light source. A tender area overlying the intertubercular groove of the humerus may be palpated, and may represent bicipital tendinitis or a rupture of the long head of the biceps if this structure is absent from its groove.

Palpation of the muscles may disclose tenderness. This part of the examination should be gentle. Prudent squeezing and excessive compression should be avoided. The muscles should be palpated bilaterally, and tone, consistency, size,

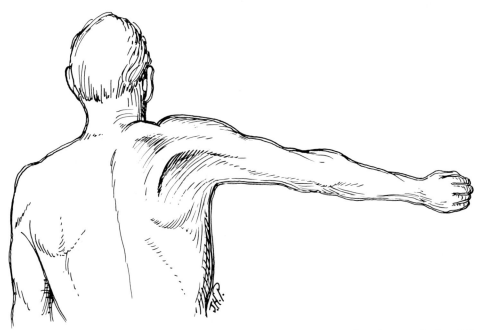

FIG 2–9. Inspection of posterior right shoulder demonstrates atrophy of supraspinatus and infraspinatus muscles. Fossae containing these muscles are depressed.

and shape should be determined. The patient should be asked to contract specific muscles. In this event, either by inspection or palpation alone or in combination, defects or abnormal masses may be felt. Muscle atony secondary to acute denervation recognized by flabbiness and a rubbery or woody sensation on palpation suggests muscular dystrophy or polymyositis.

Prolonged immobilization of muscle in a shortened position for weeks or months causes the development of atrophy and contracture of skeletal muscle. This condition may be permanent or reversible, and can be determined by careful, passive motion testing of related joints. Contractures are most often found in the adductors and internal rotators of the shoulder. Normally, if the patient is able to place the hands behind the neck, with the elbow flat on a table or against a wall, there is no contracture of the pectoral muscles. Similarly, if the patient can elevate his arm, place the hand behind his head, and touch the opposite side of the neck and can place the hand behind the back, there is full external and internal rotation of the shoulder and no rotator muscle contracture (Fig 2–10,A–D). Thus, the examination should attempt to differentiate contracture, muscle spasm, and mechanical obstruction, all of which may be present and limit joint motion. Pretreatment differentiation will certainly alter management and help decide what end result can be achieved. For example, if an advanced, chronic internal rotation contracture of the shoulder is too severe, the surgeon may elect to perform a derotation osteotomy of the humerus rather than radical soft tissue releases.

During testing of the various articulations of the shoulder girdle, including the glenohumeral, acromioclavicular, sternoclavicular, and scapulothoracic articulations, the palpation of any subluxations and any grating or grinding sensations should be noted. Loose joints associated with relaxed capsules may be easily overlooked. The palpation of peripheral pulses in the upper extremity may provide information relating to a diagnosis of thoracic outlet syndrome (Fig 2–11).

Percussion

Tenderness to palpation can provide useful information in diagnosing disease. For example, tenderness elicited by deep palpation of the suprascapular notch may point to a diagnosis of entrapment of the suprascapular nerve when the history points to this condition. Local points of osseous tenderness can also suggest occult fractures that may not at first be evident on initial roentgenograms. In this case the use of bone scanning techniques can be useful.

Auscultation

When there has been a history of injury, and other findings exist—such as an increasing mass about the shoulder—the use of a stethoscope may detect an audible bruit indicating an aneurysm. This may be confirmed by arteriography. A condition of true aneurysm after an injury should not be confused with bruits that may be heard in patients with renal disease who have arteriovenous shunts surgically created in the upper extremities for use in renal dialysis.

Muscle Strength

The examiner must differentiate individual muscles and muscle groups and learn to grade them effectively. Slipshod and hurried techniques often will lead

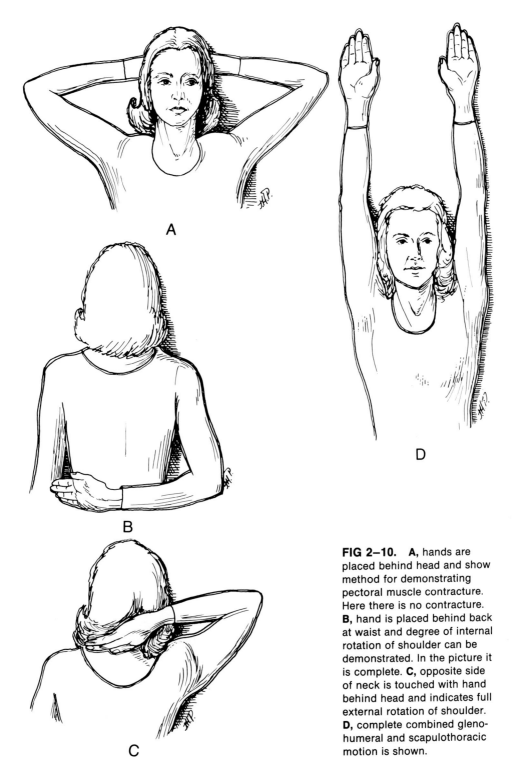

FIG 2–10. **A,** hands are placed behind head and show method for demonstrating pectoral muscle contracture. Here there is no contracture. **B,** hand is placed behind back at waist and degree of internal rotation of shoulder can be demonstrated. In the picture it is complete. **C,** opposite side of neck is touched with hand behind head and indicates full external rotation of shoulder. **D,** complete combined glenohumeral and scapulothoracic motion is shown.

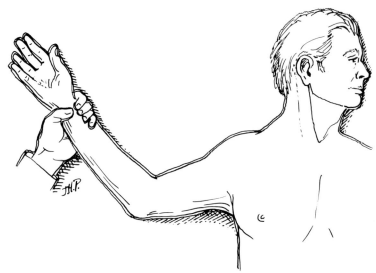

FIG 2–11. Adson's test for thoracic outlet syndrome is shown. While radial pulse is palpated, arm is abducted and patient asked to turn head in opposite direction, taking a deep breath and holding it. If pulse disappears, test is positive. It does not mean that patient has a true compression of a vessel, requiring surgical treatment.

to missed diagnoses. For example, a patient may complain of an inability to raise the arm and convey the impression that it is related to muscle weakness when in fact, it may be associated with joint stiffness. Trick motions may also allow the arm to be actively raised, giving the impression that a muscle is contracting normally when it is not. A record of meaningful observations permits the easy differentiation of psychogenic conditions and a progression of disease states. It has already been pointed out in Chapter 1 that when muscles are in spasm, during contracture of muscle groups, pain caused by muscle disease or other local factors must be differentiated, which may prevent the full contraction of the muscle. Nerve involvement also may prevent a complete testing of muscle strength.

Nowhere in the body is the action of multiple muscles affected by gravity more than in the shoulder. During the testing of muscle strength about the shoulder the examiner should observe and palpate the muscle and its tendon so as to eliminate the action of neighboring muscles. It is important to observe whether or not the scapula is anchored in position before testing muscle strengths about the shoulder. For example, the examiner may mistake serratus anterior or trapezius weakness for a loss in deltoid strength (Fig 2–12). Alternatively, in the presence of a weak deltoid, the scapula can actively rotate, giving the impression that abduction power of the arm is strong. Thus, careful testing will permit the surgeon to distinguish weakness of the muscles that stabilize the scapula, including the trapezius and serratus anterior, from other muscles, such as weakness of the deltoid. A weak serratus anterior permits the shoulder girdle to be passively lifted so that the tip of the acromion can be positioned at a level opposite the patient's chin. This condition is termed "loose shoulder" as observed in patients with Duchenne's muscular dystrophy (see Fig 2–1).

Table 2–1 shows the important muscles about the shoulder girdle, their actions and nerve supply, the effect of paralysis, and the tests used to determine abnormalities.

Winging of the Scapula

The actions of the trapezius and serratus anterior muscles are essential to keep the scapula in a normal position on its chest wall. Other muscles, such as the rhomboids, also aid in stabilizing the scapula and help keep it in position against the thorax. Paralysis of the serratus anterior or trapezius leads to winging.

Trapezius paralysis causes the scapula to be displaced downward and outward (Fig 2–13). The upper portion of the scapula is dislocated away from the midline. When winging results from serratus anterior weakness, the scapula is displaced inward and upward (Fig 2–14). The inferior angle of the scapula in this case approaches the spine (see Fig 2–14).

There are various degrees of weakness that result in a corresponding winging of the scapula. In less pronounced cases of serratus anterior weakness, winging of the scapula is noted when the patient attempts to raise the arm in forward flexion (Fig 2–15). Scapula winging is more obvious as the arm is raised against resistance, whereas with complete paralysis of the serratus the scapula cannot be fixed to the thorax, making it difficult for the patient to elevate the arm, which is

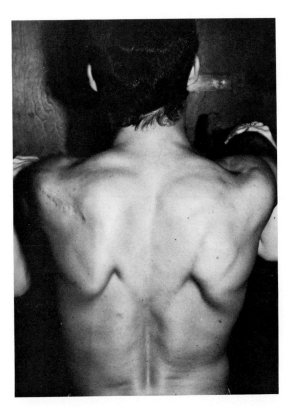

FIG 2–12. A 28-year-old man was surgically treated for "recurring posterior dislocation of his shoulder" that had not been adequately documented. He complained of weakness about his left shoulder and an inability to lift heavy objects. Note mild winging of his left scapula relating to serratus anterior weakness that was permanent. This related to his complaints rather than any intrinsic pathology within the left glenohumeral joint.

TABLE 2–1.

Muscles Controlling Shoulder Actions*

MUSCLE	NERVES	NORMAL FUNCTION(S)	PARALYSIS	TEST(S)
Trapezius	Spinal accessory and C3–C4	Upper fibers elevate lateral clavicle and scapula; lower fibers brace and press scapula to the thorax	Winging of the scapula; scapula is displaced downward and laterally; superior angle is farther away from vertebral column than inferior angle; scapula bracing, overhead motion, and shoulder elevation are impaired	Patient shrugs shoulders against resistance; abducts arm against resistance; braces shoulder by backward movement and adduction of scapula
Serratus anterior	Long thoracic and C5–C7	Draws scapula forward keeping it closely applied to the thorax; when shoulder girdle is fixed, muscle acts as an accessory muscle of respiration	Winging of the scapula, especially the inferior angle, with limited forward movement of the shoulder; elevation of the arm above the head is impaired, and on raising the arm from the side the scapula fails to rotate; scapula is displaced upward and inward	Patient thrusts outstretched arm against wall or against resistance by examiner; abduction of the arm causes little winging, showing an important difference from the effect of trapezius paralysis
Latissimus dorsi	Thoracodorsal and C6–C8	Adducts arm by pulling it backward and medially rotates it; upper fibers cause slight bracing and elevation of shoulder, whereas lower fibers depress	No gross changes at rest	Downward and backward movement against resistance is applied under patient's elbow resulting in brisk contraction that can be palpated at inferior angle of scapula when patient coughs
Teres major	Thoracodorsal (lower subscapular) and C6–C7	Action is same as for latissimus dorsi	Joint capsule cannot be adequately tightened; humeral head fixation inadequate when carrying heavy objects; adduction can be satisfactorily performed by pectoralis major and latissimus dorsi	Same as for latissimus dorsi; muscle is palpable at lower lateral border of scapula
Rhomboids	Dorsal scapular and C4–C5	Weak adductors and elevators of shoulder girdle; with serratus anterior and trape-	Impression between vertebral border of scapula and chest wall is deepened, disappear-	Patient holds hand on hip, arm back and medial while examiner attempts to force elbow

Muscle	Nerve and roots	Action	Effect of paralysis	Test
		zius, rhomboids draw scapula to the thorax and brace scapula	ing with arm raising	laterally and forward, palpating muscle bellies during test
Levator scapulae	Dorsal scapular, C3–C5, and direct branches from third and fourth cervical nerves	Elevates shoulder girdle and moves it forward; assists in rotation of the scapula like the rhomboids; when shoulder is lowered, acromioclavicular joint is fixed, it flexes cervical spine laterally	Isolated paralysis has not been documented	Same as for rhomboids
Sternocleido-mastoid	Spinal accessory and branches from cervical plexus	Tilts head toward shoulder of same side and turns face toward the opposite side; accessory muscle of respiration.	Impairment of rotation of the head; head tilted toward unaffected side and the chin is turned toward the affected side; no important loss of shoulder function	Turn patient's head to one side and then to other side, with resistance over the opposite temporal area
Subclavius	Nerve to subclavius and C5–C6	Braces sternal end of clavicle against sternum	Isolated paralysis has not been observed	None
Deltoid	Axillary and C5–C6	Raises arm to horizontal; anterior fibers adduct humerus, acromial fibers abduct and posterior fibers extend arm	Weakness of abduction but still possible by rotation of the scapula by serratus anterior and trapezius if humeral head is fixed in the glenoid cavity	With patient's arm abducted to 90°, the examiner resists upward movement
Subscapularis	Subscapular and C5–C7	Medial rotation of humerus; inferior fibers adduct humerus	Scapula remains in its normal position; isolated paralysis causes little weakness of rotation	With elbow at side and flexed 90°, the patient resists examiner's attempt to force hand laterally
Supraspinatus	Suprascapular and C4–C6	Elevates humerus in antero-lateral direction; aids in rotating scapula in sagittal plane; pulls head of humerus upward	Isolated paralysis causes little change in position of shoulder at rest; associated with deltoid paralysis, the shoulder joint space will widen	Abduct arm against resistance (but this is occasionally difficult since trapezius overlies supraspinatus)
Infraspinatus	Suprascapular and C4–C6	Lateral rotation of humerus and adduction of humerus	No visible change in position of shoulder; paralysis of both muscles together causes loss of external rotation, whereas paralysis of one muscle makes external rotation difficult	With elbow at side and flexed to 90°, patient resists examiner's attempt to push hand medially toward abdomen
Teres minor	Axillary and C4–C6	Scapula rotates about a vertical axis		

TABLE 2–1. *Continued*

MUSCLE	NERVES	NORMAL FUNCTION(S)	PARALYSIS	TEST(S)
Pectoralis major	Medial and lateral pectoral and C5–T1	Medial rotation and adduction of humerus; elevates acromial end of clavicle and scapula by contraction of upper fibers; depresses clavicle via lower fibers and depresses head of humerus; clavicular portion assists in flexion of arm	Shoulder is elevated and depression of arm weakened; poor adduction; internal rotation of humerus unaffected while subscapularis is intact	With arm in front of body, patient resists attempt by examiner to force it laterally; two portions of muscle are visible and palpable
Pectoralis minor	Medial pectoral and C6–C8	Draws acromial end of clavicle forward and depresses it; assists serratus anterior in drawing scapula forward	No important loss of function if paralysis is isolated	Isolated testing difficult
Coracobrachialis	Musculocutaneous and C5–C6	Assists in fixing humeral head in glenoid cavity; rotates scapula slightly and flexes humerus	Isolated paralysis rare; subluxation of shoulder will occur if adduction of the abducted arm is attempted against resistance, even if long head of triceps is functioning normally	Isolated testing difficult
Biceps brachii	Musculocutaneous	Most important function is flexion and supination of forearm	Flexion of forearm is weakened but no significant loss of function in shoulder	Flexion of supinated forearm against resistance
Triceps brachii	Radial and C6–C8	Extends forearm; long head extends the humerus at shoulder joint and in fixing the head of the humerus and is a weak adductor of the humerus	Loss of extension of the elbow against resistance; loss of long head, if associated with coracobrachialis paralysis, causes subluxation of the shoulder; deltoid can extend arm independently	With forearm in varying positions of flexion, patient resists effort of examiner to flex forearm further

* From Post M: Muscles of the shoulder girdle, their nerve innervations, principal actions and effect of paralysis, in Post M (ed): *The Shoulder: Surgical and Nonsurgical Management*. Philadelphia, Lea & Febiger, 1978, chap 2, pp 14–15. Used by permission.

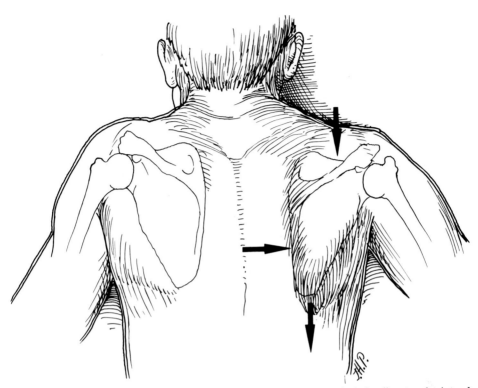

FIG 2–13. Position of right scapula is shown with trapezius paralysis leading to winging of shoulder blade. Scapula is displaced downward and outward. Upper portion of scapula is dislocated away from midline.

made worse when there is weakness of both the serratus and trapezius muscles. Winging is greatly exaggerated if more than one of the major muscles is affected. The greater the degree of winging secondary to an increasing paralysis of muscle groups that stabilize the scapua, the greater is the disability of the shoulder. It should be recalled that other conditions may mimic winging of the scapula (Fig 2–16, A and B).

Latissimus Dorsi

When testing the strength of the latissimus dorsi, a cough reflex causes the muscle to contract and is especially noted in very thin individuals. In hysterical paralysis, palpation of the muscle may give the false impression of weakness or paralysis when the patient is asked to press downward against the examiner's hand, whereas during active coughing the muscle is felt to contract quite well.

Deltoid

Movement of the arm to the horizontal and frontal planes is carried out by the deltoid. The second half of movement from the horizontal plane upward is carried out mainly by the upper fibers of the trapezius aided by the serratus anterior. The trapezius may compensate in some measure for a paralyzed deltoid within the first half of this movement. In deltoid paralysis, the second

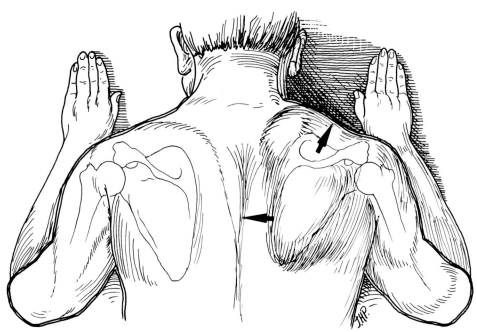

FIG 2–14. Position of right scapula is shown with paralysis of serratus anterior muscle. Here scapula is displaced inward and upward. Inferior angle of scapula approaches spine.

component of overhead motion comes into play from the beginning, and confines overhead active movement to 45°, as it relates to glenohumeral motion alone when the scapula is fixed in its normal anatomical position on the chest wall (Fig 2–17). When testing deltoid muscle power, both the anterior deltoid and middle deltoid portions of the muscle should be examined, especially if the patient has had an injury or previous surgery. The anterior deltoid is tested by asking the patient to actively flex the arm forward against resistance; the middle deltoid portion of the muscle mass is similarly examined by resisting lateral elevation of the arm (Fig 2–18).

Joint Motion

The shoulder joint constitutes the most complex motions in the body. The shallow glenoid and the surrounding musculature make it possible for the observed wide range of motion. Figure 2–19 shows the three planes of motion of the shoulder that are possible. It is the combination of motions throughout these planes that make the measurement of shoulder joint motion difficult.

With the upper extremity in anatomical position, the starting position is 0° rather than 180°. In pathologic states, the starting points may be other than zero. All motions are recorded with three numbers. Motions that lead away from the body are recorded first on the left side of the starting position, 0°, and motions that lead toward the body are recorded to the right side of the centrally positioned neutral 0° starting point.

In all cases of fixed positions two numbers are recorded, the position in the given plane and the neutral 0° starting point. When the value of the fixed joint position is away from the midline, it is recorded to the left of the 0° starting point. If the value of the fixed joint position is toward the midline, it is placed on the right of the 0° starting point. Figure 2–19 shows the sagittal, frontal, and transverse planes. All rotations are recorded as R, and not in the planes in which they occur. Table 2–2 gives the accepted terminology and normal ranges of motions at the shoulder joint. It is important to differentiate glenohumeral from scapulothoracic motion. Whenever possible, motion should be tested with the patient erect, which will allow testing of the greatest possible range of motion. Figure 2–20 demonstrates the method of measuring motions at the shoulder joint. The sum of the components makes up the combined glenohumeral and scapulothoracic motions.

Horizontal flexion is motion of the arm in the horizontal plane anterior to the frontal (coronal) plane across the body, and is measured from 0° to 135°. Horizontal extension is the horizontal motion posterior to the frontal (coronal) plane of the body and measures 0° to 30° (see Fig 2–20, A). Abduction is motion upward and away from the body and measures 0° to 180°, and adduction is the

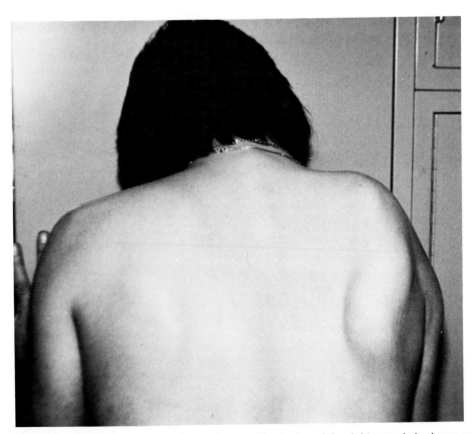

FIG 2–15. Severe serratus anterior weakness with winging of the right scapula is shown as the patient presses against the wall in front.

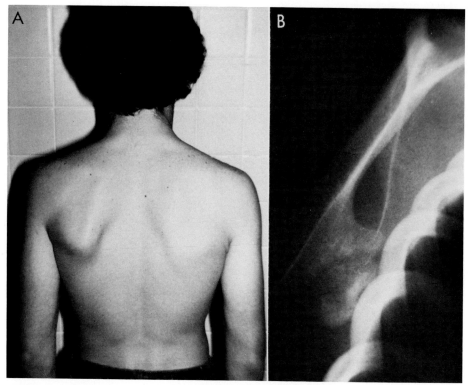

FIG 2–16. **A,** left scapula appears to be winged and relates to serratus anterior weakness. In fact, there was no weakness of any muscles in the shoulder girdle. **B,** cause of appearance of the winging of the left scapula was due to an osteochondroma on undersurface at inferior angle of the scapula. When this was removed, the scapula rested in a normal position. (From Post M: Muscles of the shoulder girdle, their nerve innervations, principle actions and effect of paralysis, in Post M (ed): *The Shoulder: Surgical and Nonsurgical Management*, ed 2. Philadelphia, Lea & Febiger, chap 22, in press. Used by permission.)

opposite motion of the arm, toward the midline of the body and beyond, and measures 0° to 75° (see Fig 2–20, B).

Forward flexion is the forward and upward motion of the arm in the sagittal plane of the body and measures 0° to 180°. Backward extension is the upward motion of the arm in the posterior sagittal plane and measures 0° to 50° (see Fig 2–20, C). Combined glenohumeral and scapulothoracic motion entails the rotation of the scapula (see Fig 2–20, D). Shoulder elevation and depression are measured in degrees (see Fig 2–20, E). Forward flexion and backward extension of the shoulder girdle are measured in degrees from a neutral 0° starting point. They measure motion of the scapula and clavicle (see Fig 2–20, F). Inward and outward rotation are recorded with the arm at the side (see Figs 2–20, G and 2–21). Rotation is also measured with the arm abducted 90° (see Fig 2–20, H).

Comparison measurements at the shoulder can be more readily made if each examination is recorded by directly charting motions on diagrammed charting sheets of paper or cardboard. This method allows accurate and easy determina-

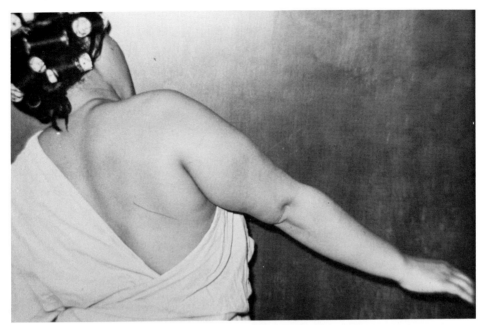

FIG 2–17. An adult female was shot in the right shoulder girdle causing a permanent palsy of right axillary nerve. Patient lost her ability to abduct arm because deltoid was paralyzed.

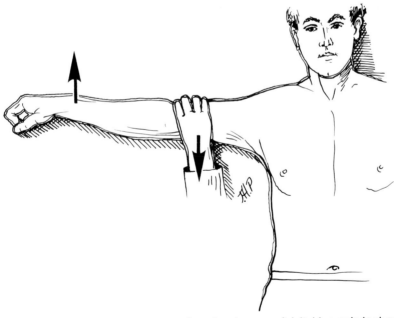

FIG 2–18. Method for testing strength and endurance of deltoid muscle is shown.

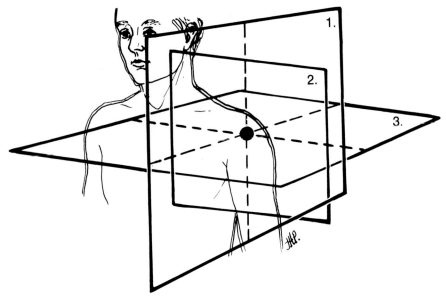

FIG 2–19. The three planes of the shoulder are shown: (1) sagittal; (2) frontal, and (3) transverse.

tion of motions at the shoulder. Table 2–2 shows the average ranges of shoulder motions.

In 1983, the American Shoulder and Elbow Surgeons organization adopted a basic shoulder evaluation form that can be used to record motions and evaluate pain in a practical manner (Fig 2–22). While examining for both active and

TABLE 2–2.

Shoulder Motions*

TERMINOLOGY OF MOTION	PLANE OF MEASUREMENT	AVERAGE RANGE OF MOTION, °	COMMON NAME
Backward extension	Sagittal	50–0–180	Posterior elevation
Forward flexion			Anterior elevation
Abduction	Frontal	180–0–75	Lateral elevation–
Adduction			Medial elevation†
Horizontal extension	Transverse	30–0–135	None
Horizontal flexion			
With arm at side	—	65–0–80	Rotation
External rotation			
Internal rotation			
With arm in 90° abduc-			
tion (lateral elevation)	—	90–0–70	Rotation
External rotation			
Internal rotation			

* From Post M: Normal motions of the shoulder, in Post M (ed): *The Shoulder: Surgical and Nonsurgical Management.* Philadelphia, Lea & Febiger, 1978, chap 2, p 19. Used by permission.
† In coronal plane neutral to trunk.

passive ranges of motion, the examiner should observe the patient to determine if there is pain and whether or not there is a harmonious, smooth range of motion involving the entire shoulder girdle. Ordinarily, when a complete range of painless active motion is obtained there is no need to test further. Occasionally, passive testing will determine whether there is any grinding or grating sensation to palpation and associated discomfort that may not be apparent on active testing of the motion. The rhythm of motion in each shoulder should be compared with the opposite side to determine any differences.

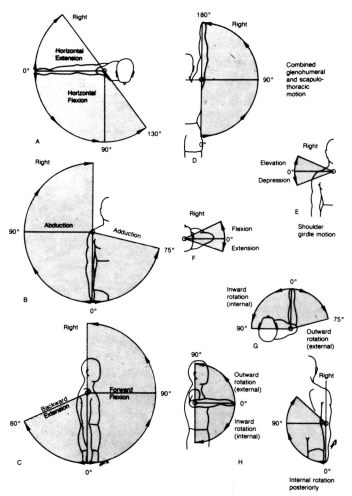

FIG 2–20. Method of measuring motions at shoulder joint are shown. (From Post M (ed): *The Shoulder: Surgical and Nonsurgical Management.* Philadelphia, Lea & Febiger, 1978. Reproduced by permission.

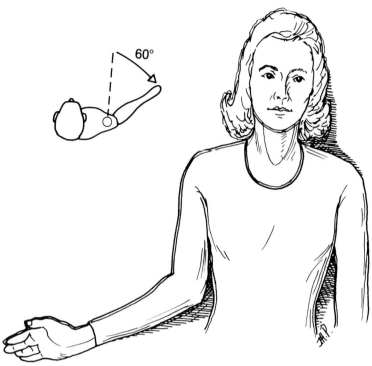

FIG 2–21. External rotation may be recorded with elbow at side either in erect or recumbent positions.

Muscle and Tendon Ruptures

Rupture of the Long Head of the Biceps

Before the long head of the biceps ruptures it may be involved in a disease process that causes localized pain and prevents normal shoulder function. The most accurate sign for bicipital tendinitis of the long head of the biceps is pain obtained on deep palpation of the bicipital groove (see Fig 2–8). The long head of the biceps tendon does not move passively in its groove when the biceps muscle contracts. Rather, the humeral head acts as a trochlea that moves beneath the long head of the biceps tendon. Thus, there is minimal excursion of the tendon during rotation movements. Several tests can be used to help diagnose this condition. These are predicated on the absence or loss of the normal functions of the biceps muscle. These include flexion of the forearm on the arm, as an aid in supination of the forearm if the radius is pronated, and elevation of the arm. If the forearm is fixed, the biceps can act to elevate the shoulder, thereby acting on the arm.

Diagnosis

The chief complaint of the patient with acute biceps rupture (Figs 2–23 and 2–24, A and B) is pain over the anterior shoulder in conditions relating to

American Shoulder and Elbow Surgeons
Basic Shoulder Evaluation Form

Shoulder: R/L

Name _____ Hospital no. _____

Date of Examination: _____

(Circle choice)
I. Pain: (5=none, 4=slight, 3=after unusual activity, 2=moderate, 1=marked,
           0=complete disability, and NA=not available) _____
II. Motion
    A. Patient sitting (enter motion or NA if not measured):
        1. Active total elevation of arm: _____ degrees*
        2. Passive internal rotation:
           (Circle segment of posterior anatomy reached by thumb)
           (Enter NA if reach restricted by limited elbow flexion)
           1=Less than trochanter   8=L2   15=T7
           2=Trochanter   9=L1   16=T6
           3=Gluteal   10=T12   17=T5
           4=Sacrum   11=T11   18=T4
           5=L5   12=T10   19=T3
           6=L4   13=T9   20=T2
           7=L3   14=T8   21=T1
        3. Active external rotation with arm at side: _____ degrees
        4. Passive external rotation at 90° abduction: _____ degrees
           (enter "NA" if cannot achieve 90° of abduction)
    B. Patient supine:
        1. Passive total elevation of arm: _____ degrees*
        2. Passive external rotation with arm at side: _____ degrees

* Total elevation of the arm is measured by viewing the patient from the side and using a
goniometer to determine the angle between the *arm* and the *thorax*.

III. Strength (5=normal, 4=good, 3=fair, 2=poor, 1=trace, 0=paralysis, and
              NA=not available) (Enter numbers below)
    A. Anterior deltoid _____
    B. Middle deltoid _____
    C. External rotation _____
    D. Internal rotation _____
IV. Stability (5=normal, 4=apprehension, 3=rare subluxation, 2=recurrent subluxation,
              1=recurrent dislocation, 0=fixed dislocation, and NA=not available)
              (Enter numbers below)
    A. Anterior _____
    B. Posterior _____
    C. Inferior _____
V. Function (4=normal, 3=mild compromise, 2=difficulty, 1=with aid, 0=unable, and
            NA=not available) (Enter numbers below)
    A. Use back pocket (if male); fasten bra (if female) _____
    B. Perineal care _____
    C. Wash opposite axilla _____
    D. Eat with utensil _____
    E. Comb hair _____
    F. Use hand with arm at shoulder level _____
    G. Carry 10 to 15 lb with arm at side _____
    H. Dress _____
    I. Sleep on affected side _____
    J. Pulling _____
    K. Use hand overhead _____ _____
    L. Throwing _____
    M. Lifting _____
    N. Do usual work _____ (Specify type of work) _____
    O. Do usual sport _____ (Specify sport) _____
VI. Patient Response:
    (Circle choice)
    (3=Much better, 2=Better, 1=Same, 0=Worse, and NA=Not available/applicable)

Completed by: _____

FIG 2–22.   Practical basic shoulder evaluation form approved by the American Shoulder
and Elbow Surgeons for evaluating pain and function in shoulder is shown.

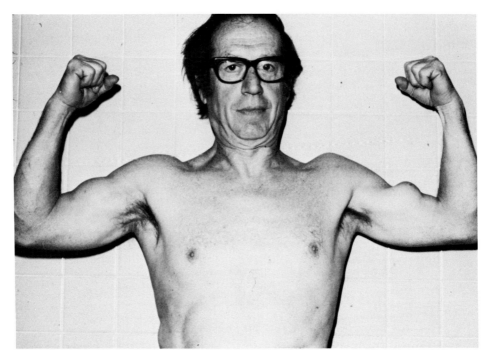

FIG 2–23. Adult male tore long head of left biceps muscle. Note retraction of muscle belly distally and "bunching" of muscle.

tendinitis or rupture. The onset of pain with tendinitis may be acute or insidious. In young adults, a history of excessive use of the shoulder, such as in playing tennis, is often given as a cause of the pain. The patient can frequently isolate the discomfort and may place the hand over the whole front of the shoulder to indicate an area of pain. The one constant feature in pinpointing the diagnosis is mild to severe tenderness along the intertubercular groove. The absence of

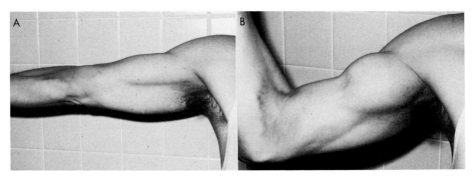

FIG 2–24. **A,** adult male shows no apparent pathology when right arm is extended. **B,** when the patient is asked to contract the biceps, note retraction of muscle belly proximally, indicating tear of distal biceps tendon. Ecchymosis is noted about cubital fossa.

tenderness suggests that another diagnosis is likely. In a vast majority of patients there is a normal range of shoulder motion.

Three signs are often associated with these conditions. These are Yergason's supination sign, in which a positive response indicates wear and tear of the long head of the biceps or synovitis of its sheath; Ludington's sign, in which a positive result indicates rupture; and Heuter's sign, in which flexion of a pronated forearm is more energetic when the biceps is tense than when the forearm is supinated. This last sign is absent with biceps tendon disruption. Another test for this condition is termed Speed's test. The patient anteriorly elevates the shoulder against resistance while extending the elbow and supinating the forearm. A positive test result occurs when pain is limited to the bicipital groove. The aforementioned tests are not pathognomonic but suggest a disease state in the region of the bicipital groove.

Yergason's Sign

The patient's elbow is flexed to 90° with the forearm pronated. While the examiner holds the patient's wrist so as not to resist supination, he then directs that active supination be made against resistance (Fig 2–25). Pain localized to the bicipital groove suggests a disease state of the long head of the biceps as, for example, synovitis of the tendon sheath.

Ludington's Sign

With the patient's fingers interlocked on top of his head and the arms abducted, the biceps muscle is actively contracted. Active disease within the bicipital groove may cause pain (Fig 2–26).

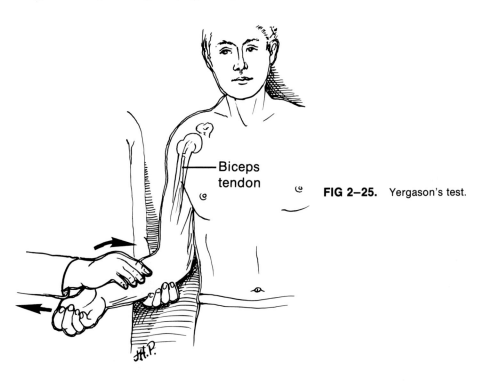

Biceps tendon

FIG 2–25. Yergason's test.

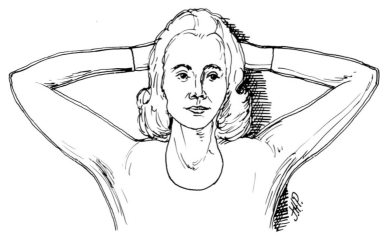

FIG 2–26. Ludington's sign.

Positive test results for both Yergason's and Ludington's signs are more likely to be positive in the acute stage of disease. In tendon rupture or advanced degeneration, pain may be minimal.

Heuter's Sign

Forearm flexion in pronation is more energetic when the biceps muscle is tense than when the forearm is in supination. In pronation, the radius crosses the ulna so that in flexion the radius is supported and is directed into flexion with only slight exertion. With flexion of the forearm, the biceps contracts and its muscle belly swells. Flexion of the forearm in pronation is accomplished primarily by the brachialis muscle, the biceps remaining soft and flabby. However, in forcible movements the biceps also contracts during flexion of the pronated forearm, but forcible forearm flexion in supination causes a striking difference in biceps muscle contraction. Thus, a contraction of the biceps in pronation always causes a movement of supination immediately afterward. With biceps tendon disruption this sign is absent.

Rupture of the biceps tendon or its muscle is the result of muscle action in the older adult. Less forceful contraction is needed to rupture the long head of the biceps, for example, than in the younger adult patient. In the former case, degenerative pathologic changes in the tendon permit relatively easy rupture. There may be no history or only a slight history of trauma, whereas in a younger patient a history of acute trauma and perhaps violent trauma is often elicited. Such a history may include the lifting of very heavy objects. The sudden contracture of the biceps muscle against an asynchronous movement may cause such a tendon rupture.

In the elderly patient, long-standing attrition of the tendon may lead to elongation of the tendon and eventual complete rupture. The biceps brachii may rupture at any place along its course depending on the force and mechanism of injury. There is a greater wear on a flattened long head of the proximal portion as it passes from its groove over the articular surface of the humeral head, thereby explaining why it is much more involved in rupture.

Most patients report a sudden "snap" that occurs in the act of lifting light or heavy objects. Occasionally, the older patient cannot recall any history of injury and may feel only mild to considerable pain over the muscle structure. They complain of a "bunching up" of the muscle with attempted contraction and discoloration about the arm in the acute stage of rupture. The patient may complain of some weakness in the arm, although the patient is usually more disturbed merely by inability to contract the muscle. Thus, bunching of the muscle belly is the most common finding. If the long head of the biceps is ruptured, the bunching of the muscle is distal (see Fig 2–23), whereas rupture of the distal biceps brachii tendon causes the contracted belly of the biceps muscle to appear high above the crease of the elbow (see Fig 2–24). In the latter case, occasionally, the distal biceps tendon is intact and the biceps brachii muscle fibers alone are torn and pulled upward.

Subluxation of the Biceps Tendon

Subluxation or dislocation of the long head of the biceps may be confused with tendinitis and even rupture. It is not as common in the young adult as in the older patient. There may be a history of a definite and severe wrenching injury followed by a disability. The very young patient often complains of a painful snap in the shoulder as in the throwing of an object. Tenderness over the anterior aspect of the shoulder is present and may be associated with an acute swelling over the anterior aspect of the shoulder. Limitation of motion and loss of strength and forward flexion and abduction are characteristic.

To elicit a positive test result for subluxation of the long head of the biceps the patient is asked to hold a 5-lb weight in each hand and then bring the extended arms overhead, holding them in extreme external rotation. As the examiner places the fingers on the long head of the biceps, the patient lowers the arm to the side in the coronal plane. As the arm reaches 110° to 90°, there may be an audible snap that is associated with a sharp pain. Longitudinal axial roentgenogram views of the intertubercular groove may show an abnormal shallow groove.

Rupture of the Pectoralis Major Tendon

The most common symptom is a sudden sharp pain in the arm and shoulder as the injury occurs. Occasionally, the patient describes a snapping sensation in the shoulder. Frequently, swelling and ecchymosis result over the site of rupture. If the swelling is not massive, a groove or depression may be palpated (Fig 2–27, A and B). With attempted contraction, pain is increased and there is weakness in adduction and internal rotation. A visible bulge of torn muscle may be seen during the contraction. If the diagnosis is in doubt, the normal pectoralis shadow will not be visible on xeroradiograms.

Rupture of the Triceps

Rupture of the triceps brachii is uncommon. When rupture does occur a depression of sulcus may be palpated or seen in the triceps contour. With complete rupture of the triceps tendon, active extension is lost (Fig 2–28).

Deltoid Rupture

Rupture of the deltoid is rare. The findings may be confused with congenital deficiencies of the deltoid when there is no history of trauma, and there are actual defects in the deltoid muscle mass and associated weakness in abduction

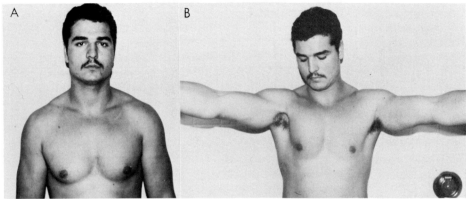

FIG 2–27. **A,** weightlifter complained of weakness during certain motions and especially adduction of his shoulder. **B,** when asked to contract the pectoral major muscle, an obvious defect was noted that related to a recent injury during weight lifting. There was a partial tear of the pectoralis major. (From Post M: Muscles of the shoulder girdle, their nerve innervations, principle actions and effect of paralysis, in Post M (ed): *The Shoulder: Surgical and Nonsurgical Management,* ed 2. Philadelphia, Lea & Febiger, chap 14, in press. Used by permission.)

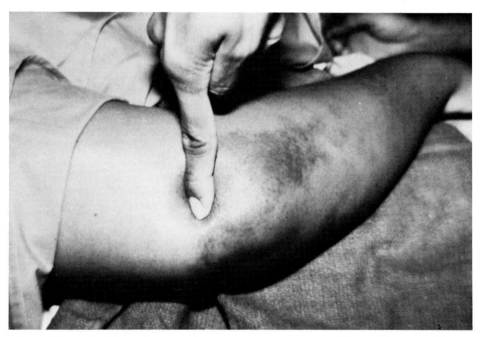

FIG 2–28. Complete rupture of the distal triceps with avulsion of the tendon from the olecranon resulted in the patient's inability to actively extend the elbow. Note the depression defect in the triceps structure. Ecchymosis about the elbow and forearm is shown two days after injury. (From Post M: Muscles of the shoulder girdle, their nerve innervations, principle actions and effect of paralysis, in Post M (ed): *The Shoulder: Surgical and Nonsurgical Management,* ed 2. Philadelphia, Lea & Febiger, chap 14, in press. Used by permission.)

power of the arm. In true rupture, the anterior or middle deltoid can be involved. It is caused by a sudden and violent resistance against the forward flexed or laterally elevated arm (Fig 2–29).

Rotator Cuff Tear

Abduction of the arm is initiated by supraspinatus action and its activity continues throughout the entire range of abduction. The rotator muscles and their tendons create a fixed fulcrum by holding the humeral head against the shallow glenoid while the deltoid muscle exerts its action.

Diagnosis

Patients who sustain symptomatic rotator cuff tears are usually in their later years of life. Many are older than 50 years and frequently give a history of recurrent attacks of shoulder pain most often on the dominant side. Occasionally, the patient relates a history of an acute trauma from a fall. There may be a history of chronic persistent or recurring attacks of pain without a specific history of injury. The pain may be worse at night and awaken the patient from a sound sleep.

Especially after trauma and an acute rupture, the patient can experience pain that increases hours later and gives a feeling of weakness with an inability to abduct the arm at all. Even with very large rotator cuff tears a patient may still have the ability to actively and fully abduct the arm into the overhead position. However, abductor and external rotator muscle weakness may be very significant (Fig 2–30, A and B).

Dawbarn described a sign in which a tender point is present over the greater tuberosity. This sign may be associated with fracture, bursitis, and rupture of the supraspinatus tendon. It occurs when a tender point disappears during full abduction after the painful spot is carried beneath the protective arch of the acromion. The presence of crepitus is not pathognomonic of a tear but is frequently present. External rotator and deltoid muscle testing will demonstrate weakness in these groups of muscles in varying degrees.

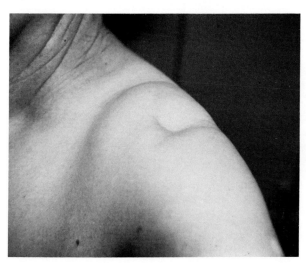

FIG 2–29. Patient complained of inability to lift heavy objects with his left shoulder. He had sustained severe pulling injury few years before. Note defect in lateral deltoid at its origin at acromion. There was weakness on testing active abduction motion.

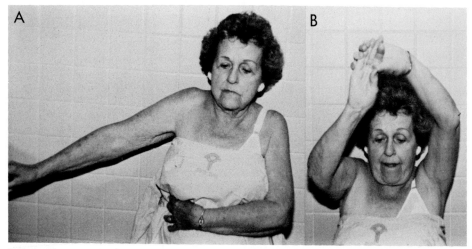

FIG 2–30. **A,** patient had failed rotator cuff surgery. There was massive tear that could not be repaired. There was poor abduction and forward flexion. **B,** patient could passively elevate her arm.

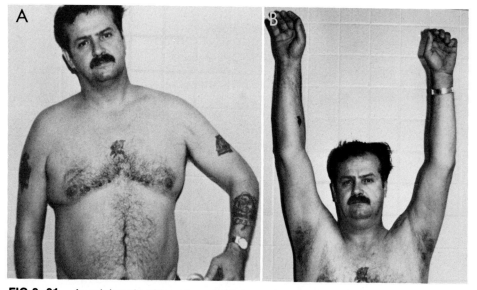

FIG 2–31. An adult male with a severe impingement syndrome of his left shoulder is shown; he could actively forward flex and elevate his arm 40°. Pain prevented him from going beyond this point. A highly positive impingement sign was present. When the left subacromial space was injected with 10 ml of 1% of lidocaine, patient had complete active elevation of his shoulder and full strength in all muscle groups. (From Post M: *The Shoulder: Surgical and Nonsurgical Treatment,* ed 2. Philadelphia, Lea & Febiger, in press. Used by permission.)

The impingement sign causes localized shoulder pain when the arm is forcibly forward flexed or laterally elevated against the anteroinferior edge of the acromion (Fig 2–31). An impingement sign may also result from impingement against the coracoacromial ligament. It is usually evident when the arm is elevated at least 90° to 100°, or may be observed with elevation significantly beyond this range. An impingement can occur when the greater tuberosity is forced against the coracoacromial ligament, and thus, the arm should be internally rotated while forward flexing the arm. A positive sign can be seen when the extrascapular subacromial soft tissue is inflamed or there is an incipient rotator cuff tear. A grade I impingement relates to fewer or less severe complaints of pain and findings, while a grade II impingement is more severe. A grade III impingement is usually associated with a rotator cuff tear. The injection of 10 ml of 1% lidocaine into the subacromial space may relieve all pain and permit a full range of active painless motion. This is confirmation of a positive impingement test.

Although rotator cuff tear and the associated symptoms and findings are common, if not suspected, it occasionally may be confused with a diagnosis of a paralytic brachial neuritis.

Plain films of the shoulder may show a severe superior subluxation of the humeral head. When the interval between the undersurface of the acromion and superior portion of the humeral head is less than 7 mm, a tear of the rotator cuff is suggested. The sine qua non for a full-thickness rotator cuff rupture is a positive arthrogram when it shows a leakage of dye outside the normal space of the capsule. The amount of dye that is leaked cannot be correlated with the extent of the tear.

Dislocation, Subluxation, and Instability

Nowhere in the body is the treatment of joint dislocations, subluxations, and instability more dependent on a precise diagnosis than in the shoulder. Dislocation is defined as a complete loss of the continuity of the joint surfaces. Subluxation refers to a partial or incomplete loss of the normal contact of the articular surfaces of the glenohumeral joint. Instability is an unsteadiness in the fixation of the fulcrum between the humeral head and its glenoid. The last condition is a type of subluxation that is described by the patient as the joint "coming out or apart," and there is a normal translational movement of the humeral articular surface on the glenoid that is excessive. The labrum may or may not be torn in each of these conditions.

History

An accurate history is essential in order to correctly diagnose the specific condition. It should include the age at onset of the first dislocation or subluxation. Have other members of the family had a similar history? Was the first or subsequent dislocation or subluxation associated with significant trauma and was the incident atraumatic and voluntary? The examiner should carefully assess the mechanism of dislocation or subluxation, as well as the position of the extremity immediately afterwards. Was there a spontaneous relocation or was any manipulation needed for each episode? How many recurrences have occurred? Were they spontaneous or voluntary? Were they multidirectional and if so, in what directions? Were both shoulders involved? Can the episodes be caused at will or by the mere contraction of the shoulder girdle muscles? How was each dislocation or subluxation treated? What was the pain level, if any, for each episode? Was there any subsequent disability? Are other joints in any of the extremities lax or hypermobile? Has the patient ever experienced a convulsion? Has the patient been under emotional stress, psychiatric treatment, or have behavioral problems been noted?

Physical Findings

With an acute anterior dislocation there is a loss of contour manifested by flattening of the lateral contour of the shoulder. The patient is in obvious pain with a traumatic dislocation (Fig 2–32) and holds the arm still in slight abduction. The examiner should test for neurologic deficit, especially when it involves an injury to the axillary nerve. In this case there may be hypesthesia over the lateral aspect of the shoulder correlating to the C5 dermatome. In posterior dislocations, an anterior depression of the skin surface is ordinarily noted while a bulge may be observed posteriorly that is caused by the projection of the humeral head beyond its posterior glenoid (Fig 2–33). Here the arm is held in slight adduction and internal rotation. With inferior subluxation (Fig 2–34, A) or dislocation there may be a loss of a contour circumferentially, both anteriorly, laterally, and posteriorly with a flattening of the deltoid.

When a patient has previously experienced pain associated with dislocation or subluxation, "apprehension" may be apparent and the patient may guard against testing motions for fear that the shoulder will "come out of socket" and cause pain or discomfort (Fig 2–35). While testing for apprehension, the proxi-

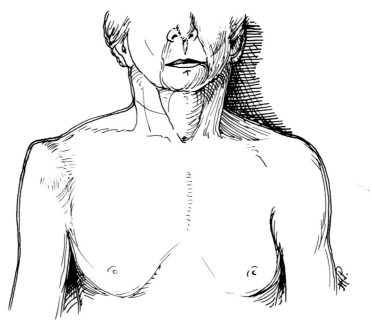

FIG 2–32. Patient with an anterior dislocation shows flattening of lateral contour of shoulder. Arm is held in slight abduction.

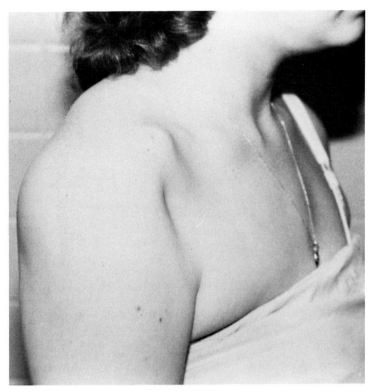

FIG 2–33. Patient with congenital voluntary posterior recurring subluxation of right shoulder is shown. This young woman had had this condition since age 7 years. Note depression in anterior shoulder and bulging mass in posterior aspect of the shoulder girdle relating to the posterior dislocation of the humeral head. She could spontaneously dislocate or reduce the shoulder merely by contracting her muscles. (From Post M: Muscles of the shoulder girdle, their nerve innervations, principle actions and effect of paralysis, in Post M (ed): *The Shoulder: Surgical and Nonsurgical Management,* ed 2. Philadelphia, Lea & Febiger, chap 2, in press. Used by permission.)

mal humerus is passively abducted and externally rotated (Fig 2–36). An apprehensive appearance of pain or discomfort appears on the face of the patient as he anticipates a subluxation or perhaps dislocation of the humeral head anteriorly from its glenoid. Similarly, a positive apprehension test may also be present with posterior instability when the arm is forward flexed, adducted, and internally rotated. There may be a facial expression of great discomfort or pain. The test is performed with the patient supine so as to obtain maximum muscle relaxation but can be done in the erect sitting position. The humerus is stressed in various positions of abduction and external rotation with anterior dislocation. An attempt is made to lever the shoulder from its normal position on the glenoid face. This should be done prudently when excessive looseness of the ligaments and capsule is present. The examiner may determine that there is an obvious abnormal translational movement of the humeral head on its glenoid space and the diagnosis may become obvious. In a true case of dislocation the humeral head may lock in an abnormal position so that a manipulation by the examiner is

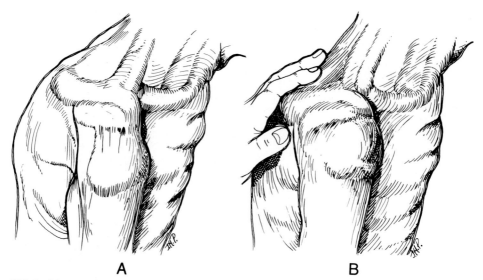

FIG 2–34. **A,** patient who had sustained a stroke had paralysis of the shoulder girdle muscles and multidirectional instability of the joint. Note obvious inferior subluxation in illustration and depression circumferentially in deltoid muscle mass. **B,** when elbow is supported by a hand or sling subluxation disappears and contour becomes normal.

required to relocate the humeral head upon its glenoid. Most important, it is essential to differentiate the direction of the dislocation, subluxation, or instability and to determine if the condition is multidirectional for in each case the treatment is different.

Neurologic Examination

Pain and loss of function in the shoulder may relate to a distant cause and not to a localized problem. Part of the neurologic examination includes a thorough evaluation of the muscle strength about the shoulder. Weakness of specific muscle groups, including the external rotator muscles and deltoid, may relate to a significant tear in the rotator cuff or perhaps a neurologic cause (Figs 2–34, A and B, and 2–37). In addition to muscle strength testing, sensory sensation, and deep and superficial tendon reflexes should be examined. The examiner should compare any loss in sensation in the upper extremity bilaterally and relate the dermatome(s) involved in the neurologic deficit (see Fig 2–11). From these data, a neurologic level of the pathologic lesion can be assessed and the specific nerves involved in the pathology can be pinpointed. For example, following an anterior shoulder dislocation hypesthesia may be present over the lateral aspect of the upper arm, as determined by testing lightly with multiple pinpricks and comparing with the opposite shoulder. The surgeon should evaluate any central nervous system dysfunction and attempt to relate it to pathology whether it be in the peripheral nerve or the spinal cord.

An impingement upon the spinal cord produces pyramidal tract signs in the lower extremities and in the areas in the upper limbs innervated by nerve seg-

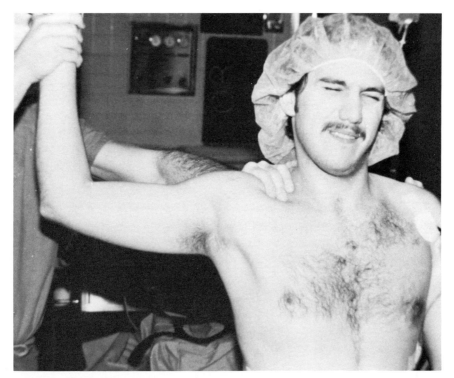

FIG 2–35. Positive apprehension test in patient with a recurring anterior subluxation is shown. He complained of instability in his shoulder. The patient experienced discomfort just before the shoulder actually subluxated. (From Post M: Muscles of the shoulder girdle, their nerve innervations, principle actions and effect of paralysis, in Post M (ed): *The Shoulder: Surgical and Nonsurgical Management,* ed 2. Philadelphia, Lea & Febiger, chap 20, in press. Used by permission.)

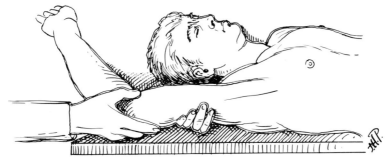

FIG 2–36. Apprehension test may be performed with patient in supine position as shown.

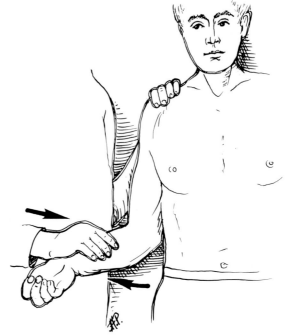

FIG 2–37. Method for testing strength in external rotator muscles of shoulder is shown.

ments below the level of the lesion. Deep tendon reflexes will be hyperactive in the legs and produce increased tone, clonus, and bilateral Babinski's signs. Because of posterior column involvement, flexion of the neck may produce paresthesias into the arms and down the back (Lhermitte's sign). This is a typical example of how pain in the shoulder may relate to a disease process that is distant and refers pain to the shoulder.

Herpes zoster infection has an affinity for the dorsal root ganglia and produces a characteristic vesicular skin rash that follows along the nerve root distribution. Thus, involvement of the spinal assessory nerve may cause winging of the scapula and is usually associated with severe pain.

Nerve Root Dysfunction

Conditions such as spinal cord tumors, cervical spondylosis, cervical disk disease, and viral infections, including herpes zoster infection that involves the dorsal root ganglia, may cause unilateral or bilateral symptoms and findings referable to the shoulder. The physical examination for these conditions is reviewed in Chapter 6, Physical Examination of the Cervical Spine.

Dysfunction of Peripheral Nerves

The brachial plexus traverses the shoulder girdle region and may be subjected to various disease states, including open injuries, malignant tumors, such as a Pancoast tumor, and various other traumatic and idiopathic conditions all of which may cause pain or loss of function, not only in the shoulder girdle but in the entire upper extremity.

Brachial Plexus Neuritis

Brachial plexus neuritis is a disease of unknown etiology that is usually associated with early pain and is localized to the shoulder and lateral aspect of the upper arm. Pain is increased by movement of the arm(s) at the shoulder but not by neck movement. Considerable localized muscle tenderness may also be present. The opposite shoulder can also be involved by weakness and paralysis of muscle groups in addition to pain. Sensory loss is usually minimal.

Suprascapular Nerve Entrapment

The suprascapular nerve passes beneath the suprascapular ligament. It may be injured by a fracture, a direct blow to the shoulder, encroachment of the notch because of intrinsic or extrinsic reasons or its cause may be unknown.

The diagnosis of suprascapular nerve entrapment is made by exclusion and is based not only on the history but also on the abnormal findings of electrodiagnosis. The hallmark of suprascapular nerve entrapment is pain that is deep and poorly delineated.

In severe cases of neuropathy, atrophy and weakness of the supraspinatus and infraspinatus may be noted. Occasionally, certain scapular motions may be painful. Adduction of the extended arm across the body tenses the nerve so that pain may be increased. Thumb pressure over the region of the suprascapular notch may increase the level of the pain and cause severe tenderness.

Paralyses Due to Birth Injury

Birth injury may cause paralysis of muscles about the upper extremity. In Erb-Duchenne palsy, by far the most common type, C5 and C6 nerve roots are injured. The abductor and external rotator muscles can remain partially or completely paralyzed and allow the arm to lie in an attitude of internal rotation and adduction. Weakness or complete paralysis may persist in the deltoid, the short rotators of the shoulder, the biceps, supinator, and occasionally, the serratus anterior and coracobrachialis. With growth, anterior joint capsule contracture involving the subscapularis, the pectoralis major, and the fascial coverings result. After age 5 years, in the more severe cases, posterior subluxation of the humeral head may occur from the unopposed pull of the contracted unparalyzed latissimus dorsi teres major, and subscapularis muscles.

Whole Arm Palsy (Erb-Duchenne-Klumpke)

Whole arm paralysis occurs when the nerve roots extending from C5 through C8 and possibly T1 are involved. In this type, anisocoria and narrowing of the palpebral fissure are not uncommon. Paralysis of extensive muscle groups in the entire upper extremity is severe and the entire upper extremity may remain flaccid. The scapula may be winged.

Lower arm paralysis (Klumpke's) occurs when C7 and C8 nerve roots are injured and results in weakness of the muscles of the wrist and finger flexors, as well as the intrinsic hand muscles in lower arm palsy, and is the least common type. With sensory deficits there may be severe or little sensory loss. The terminal part of the Moro reflex may be normal, with an inability of the digits to spread and the thumb and index digits to flex (Fig 2–38). A grasping reflex is lost.

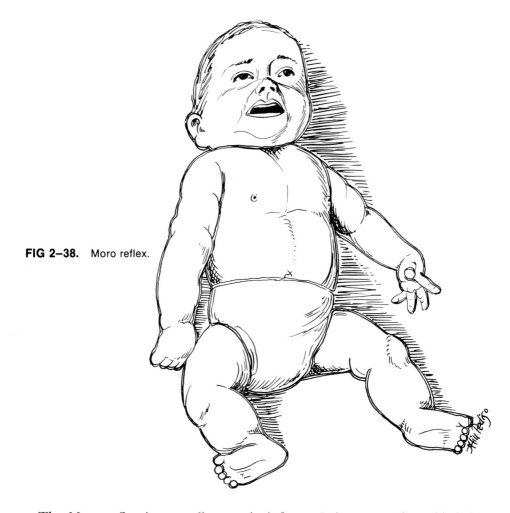

FIG 2–38. Moro reflex.

The Moro reflex is normally seen in infancy. It is present from birth but usually disappears between 16 and 20 weeks of age. It may not be elicited if the infant has a brachial plexus injury, hemiparesis, or fracture of the clavicle. It is obtained in the infant by supporting the infant in the supine position with the neck slightly flexed. The head is dropped briefly, gently, and rapidly through an arc of 30°. A positive response consists of symmetric abduction, extension, and circumduction of the upper extremities and flexion of the lower extremities (see Fig 2–38).

Deep Tendon Reflexes

Deep reflexes, or muscle stretch reflexes are produced by the percussion of the tendons at their insertions. The state of the deep reflexes in different disease states can be clinically important. In acute disease of the anterior horn cell, for example, the deep reflexes are lost rapidly, whereas they are more slowly lost with peripheral neuropathic lesions. The shoulder girdle reflexes and signs are defined as follows:

Scapulohumeral Reflex

The inferior angle of the scapula is tapped. This normally causes the scapula to move in a medial direction along toward the midline with slight adduction of the arm. Here, the rhomboids are especially active. If the test does not produce results on one side in a very muscular individual, it is not clinically significant.

Pectoral Reflex

With the subject's arm semiabducted, the examiner places his thumb over the pectoralis major tendon near its insertion on the humerus. A sharp blow is struck upward toward the armpit. The contraction of the muscle may be seen and palpated and causes the arm to internally rotate slightly and adduct at the same time.

Biceps Reflex

With the subject's arm semiflexed at the elbow, and the forearm moderately pronated, the examiner places his thumb over the biceps tendon at the elbow and strikes the tendon. This normally produces a contraction of the muscle and flexion of the forearm.

Triceps Reflex

The patient's elbow is approximately positioned the same as for the biceps reflex test, or it may be held at a right angle. With the subject's arm internally rotated, the triceps tendon is struck directly just above the olecranon. The triceps muscle contracts and the elbow extends.

Clavicular Reflex

It is elicited by tapping the lateral portion of the subject's clavicle, resulting in an extensive contraction of various muscles in the upper limb. It may be used for demonstrating differences in deep reflex irritability between the two upper limbs. The degree of contraction of the tested muscles may be graded 0, 1, 2, or 3, the higher numbers indicating a greater amount of contraction.

Superficial Reflexes

Superficial reflexes are elicited by stimulating the skin. Muscle responses are produced by way of the reflex arc in which the stimulus is achieved by stroking a sensory zone. Scapular and interscapular reflexes are obtained by scratching the patient's skin over the scapula or interscapular surface, which results in contraction of the scapular muscles. An important superficial reflex seen in infancy is the Moro reflex.

"Shoulder Pad" Sign

Striking fullness of the shoulder may exist because of an extensive amyloid infiltration of periarticular and synovial tissue. Patients with cervical syringomyelia who have advanced neuropathic joint disease may show a mass of soft tissue swelling of the shoulder (Fig 2–39).

Modified Adson's Test

Starting from the same position as that used for the Adson test, the patient's arm is abducted to 90° and externally rotated with the elbow flexed. The subject's

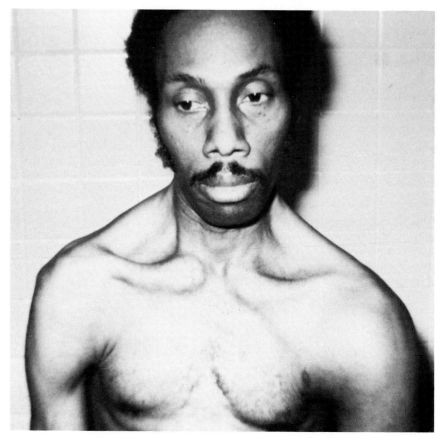

FIG 2–39. Patient with cervical syringomyelia is shown. Patient had a neuropathic joint and shows a "shoulder pad" sign as demonstrated.

head is turned as far as possible to the examined side. The pulse is palpated while the patient holds a deep breath and then coughs. Diminution or disappearance of the pulse represents a positive result of the test (see Fig 2–11).

Costoclavicular Maneuver

Examiner palpates the radial pulse with the patient sitting in a relaxed position. A stethoscope is placed over the mid aspect of the clavicle. The patient is asked to extend and depress the shoulders, with the examiner exerting pull on the arm in the same direction. Change in the pulse or production of a bruit is recorded.

An alternate method of this maneuver can be performed if the arm is placed backward with abduction of the shoulder and flexion of the elbow to 90°. Changes in the pulse or findings of venous obstruction are noted.

Hyperabduction Syndrome Test

With the patient sitting in a relaxed position, the examiner palpates the radial pulse and listens for a bruit beneath the clavicle or in the axilla. The patient's arm is then hyperabducted while changes in the pulse are noted. Obstruction in this syndrome is caused by compression of the artery at the level just beneath the insertion of the pectoralis minor tendon. In partial obstruction, a bruit is heard over the subclavian artery. When there is complete obstruction, no bruit is heard.

Modification of this maneuver can be performed with the patient sitting relaxed, arm abducted to 135° and externally rotated, and the head turned as far as possible from the examined side. When the patient holds a deep breath, the radial pulse is palpated and the changes in the pulse are noted.

Nerve entrapment and even compression of the median nerve at the wrist, and compression about the neck, thoracic outlet, and compression due to a supracondylar process in the lower humerus can cause shoulder pain. A thorough evaluation of these conditions must be included in any physical examination when other causes of pain are excluded.

References

1. Cave EF, Roberts SM: A method for measuring and recording joint function. *J Bone Joint Surg* 1936; 34:455.
2. Heuter C: Zur Diagnose der Verletzungen des M biceps Brachii. *Arch Klin Chir* 1864; 5:321–323.
3. Ludington NA: Rupture of long head of biceps cubiti muscle. *Am J Surg* 1923; 77:358.
4. Mayo Clinic and Mayo Foundation: *Clinical Examination in Neurology*, ed 3. Philadelphia, WB Saunders Co, 1971.
5. Monrad-Krohn GH: *The Clinical Examination of the Nervous System*, ed 8. New York, Paul B. Hoeber Inc, 1947.
6. Russe O, Gerhardt JJ, King PS: *An Atlas of Examination: Standard by Otto Russe*. Baltimore, Williams & Wilkins Co, 1972.
7. Steegmann AT: *Examination of the Nervous System*, ed 2. Chicago, Year Book Medical Publishers Inc, 1962.
8. Yergason RM: Supination sign. *J Bone Joint Surg* 1931; 13:160.

CHAPTER 3

Physical Examination of the Elbow

Bernard F. Morrey, M.D.

General Observations

The evaluation of any musculoskeletal process generally includes three distinct but closely related elements: (1) a careful history that is designed to localize and determine the level and implications of involvement; (2) a physical examination usually directed by the history; and (3) the radiographic assessment and any special diagnostic techniques that may better elucidate the pathology. With current trends to rely more heavily on sophisticated and revealing laboratory tests, it is appropriate to emphasize the extreme value of a carefully conducted physical examination. In this chapter we will also discuss the significance of some of the physical findings.

It is obvious that the physical examination should be directed and influenced by a careful history of the chief complaint. With elbow involvement, the patient may be initially seen with a primary complaint of loss of strength but in fact may be demonstrating reflex inhibition due to a chronic or subtle pain pattern. Similarly, the chief complaint of motion loss may actually be due to reflex inhibition from pain or, less commonly, weakness of the elbow flexors or extensors.

To properly appreciate the possible source of pathology, it is essential to recognize the major functions of the elbow, which may be summarized as follows: (1) serves to work in concert with the shoulder to place the hand in space; (2) functions as an essential linkage for the development of the stability necessary for fine work of the distal unit, the hand; and (3) supplies power to perform work.

With any joint, three inherent features uniquely defined by the anatomy determine both the normal as well as pathologic function. Simply stated these include motion, strength, and stability. Yet, as is also true with all articular link systems, to a greater or lesser extent, elbow dysfunction may be compensated for by other joints. For example, upper extremity dysfunction may be compensated for by the motion of the shoulder and of the wrist. To perform activities of daily living and personal care, some function may be compensated for by motion at the spine, hip, or knee.

A careful history involving elbow dysfunction is directed not just to the major complaint but its impact on activity, such as essential daily activities of personal hygiene, occupational activities, or recreational pursuits. The temporal features of the condition are also eminently important: Was the onset acute or insidious? Can the duration be measured in weeks, months, or years? In a recent discrete period of time, are symptoms getting better, worse, or staying the same? Localization of the symptoms is best determined by asking the patient to point if possible to the one area causing the most symptoms. In some classic conditions, this can almost be diagnostic, for example, tennis elbow. The character of pain: dull, aching, sharp, burning, a dead feeling, or an electrical-type sensation, helps to distinguish the possible soft tissue, articular cartilage, or neurovascular causation. Any possible secondary gain, litigation, workman's compensation, or other underlying distraction should be noted and considered.

Anatomy

A detailed and thorough knowledge of the specific anatomy of the elbow joint is essential to complement a careful history and to properly assess this joint. It is helpful in the course of the physical examination to consider various anatomical aspects of both the congruent articular surface, the unique arrangements of the collateral ligament structure, the role of the anterior capsule, and the flexor and extensor motors, as well as the intimate association of the nerves.

Articulation. This is a very highly congruent joint. The very close articular tolerance provides a great deal of inherent stability but also contributes to the frequent loss of elbow motion after trauma (Fig 3–1).

Capsule. The anterior capsule provides varus-valgus stability in extension but its sensitivity to trauma contributes to the well-recognized tendency for the elbow to develop flexion contracture after often trivial insults.

Surface Landmarks. Because the elbow is a subcutaneous joint, several bony landmarks are readily available to the examiner and aid in both the assessment and therapeutic measures, such as aspiration. The medial epicondyle is more prominent than the lateral and the two serve as a rough estimation of the axis of elbow rotation (Fig 3–2). Posteriorly, the tip of the olecranon forms a definite relationship with the epicondyles as the apex of an equilateral triangle when the elbow is flexed, and lies in a straight line when the elbow is extended. The lateral triangle is defined by the lateral epicondyle, olecranon, and radial head. A final landmark of significance with respect to considering a surgical approach is the avascular or safe interval of the lateral supracondylar bony column.

Muscle. Because of the tight constraints of the joint and near hinge motion, the major elbow flexors are discrete and include the biceps and brachialis muscles. The brachioradialis muscle serves as a secondary flexor while the remaining muscles participate very minimally in this activity. Similarly, extension is solely a function of the triceps mechanism. The remaining musculature crossing the joint originates medially and laterally, but serves as motors for the forearm, wrist, and fingers, with the exception of the stabilizing role of the anconeus and extensor carpi ulnaris.[16,6]

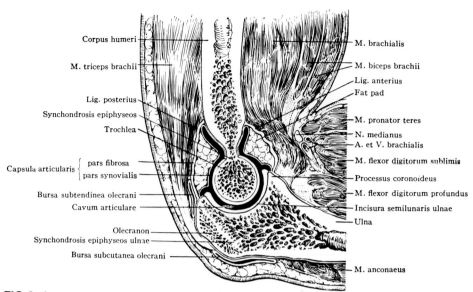

Corpus humeri — — M. brachialis

M. triceps brachii — — M. biceps brachii
— Lig. anterius
— Fat pad

Lig. posterius —

Synchondrosis epiphyseos —
— M. pronator teres
Trochlea — — N. medianus
— A. et V. brachialis
— M. flexor digitorum sublimis
Capsula articularis { pars fibrosa
{ pars synovialis — — Processus coronoideus
— M. flexor digitorum profundus
Bursa subtendinea olecrani — — Incisura semilunaris ulnae
Cavum articulare — — Ulna

Olecranon —
Synchondrosis epiphyseos ulnae —
Bursa subcutanea olecrani —
— M. anconaeus

FIG 3–1. Sagittal section demonstrating the close congruity of ulnohumeral joint as well as the muscular covering of joint both anteriorly and posteriorly. (From Anson BJ, McVay CB: *Surgical Anatomy,* ed 5. Philadelphia, WB Saunders Co, 1971, vol 2. Reproduced by permission.)

Nerves. Finally, this is the only joint in which a major nerve is in such intimate association with the joint itself (Fig 3–3). Thus, traumatic conditions,[22] as well as inflammatory arthritides may be associated with ulnar nerve dysfunction. Furthermore, on occasion, even the medial and radial nerve may be injured from elbow trauma.[16, 24] The ulnar nerve may be implicated in such clinical conditions as medial epicondylitis and be irritated by valgus axial deformity, and instability.

Inspection

The elbow and entire upper extremity should be assessed by simple visual inspection.

Axial Alignment. The normal valgus position of the forearm with respect to the humerus, the so-called carrying angle, is associated with a great deal of individual variation. This has been studied extensively by several investigators and has been found to average approximately 10° for males and 13° for females (Fig 3–4).[4, 7, 20, 21] The most common alteration of this angle is the relationship to the childhood supracondylar fracture producing the so-called gunstock or varus deformity. The valgus angular deformities are usually of cosmetic significance and do not significantly interfere with function. Rotary alignment abnormalities may occur but are not well recognized clinically because this particular deformity is so well compensated for by motion in the shoulder.

Form. The soft tissue contour of the elbow joint consists of the anterior biceps and posterior triceps expansion, with medial and lateral muscle masses originating from the region of the epicondyles. Gross joint destruction, for example, in advanced rheumatoid arthritis, and fracture deformity, obliterates these landmarks, as does fracture through the distal humerus or proximal radius and ulna (Fig 3–5).

Anterior. Anteriorly, the antecubital fossa is the most significant landmark. This is composed of the lateral mobile wad of muscles as well as the medial flexor pronator group (Fig 3–6). It is unusual to observe specific pathology in the region of the antecubital fossa, unless perhaps a large lipoma or soft-tissue mass is present.

Posterior. Posteriorly, a prominent bony protuberance may suggest ruptured triceps tendon forming an indentation above the tip of the olecranon. This

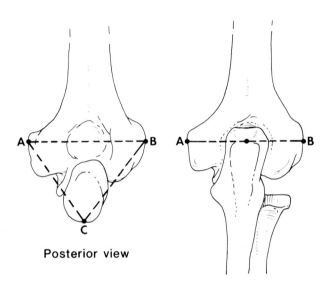

Posterior view

Lateral view

FIG 3–2. Palpable bony landmarks of elbow include the medial and lateral epicondyles (*A* and *B*), which serve as an estimation of the axis of rotation. With elbow extended, tip of the olecranon is in line with these two landmarks. With elbow flexed, equilateral triangle (*A-C*) is formed. On the lateral side, lateral epicondyle, head of the radius, and tip of olecranon form an important triad for assessment of synovitis, as well as a location for insertion of needle for aspiration or injection (*B-D*).

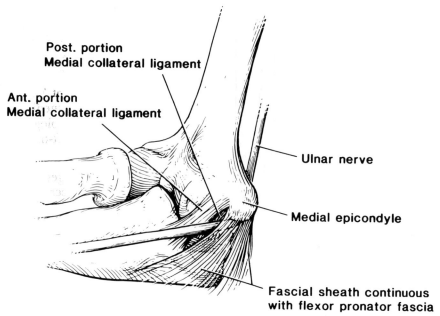

FIG 3–3. Ulnar nerve is tightly constrained under medial epicondyle by forearm fascia but is also intimately associated with posterior portion of ulnar collateral ligament, thus accounting for its vulnerability to injury. (Courtesy of Baylor College of Medicine.)

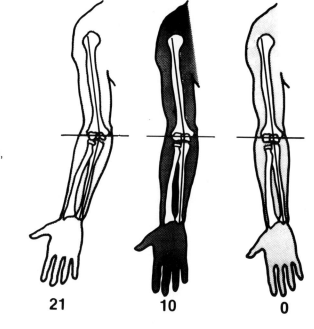

FIG 3–4. Significant normal variation in carrying angle exists, with normal being about 10°.

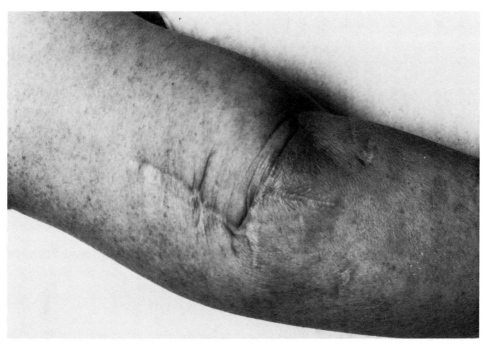

FIG 3–5. Gross destruction from rheumatoid arthritis or, as in this case, trauma, results in disturbance of the normal soft tissue contour.

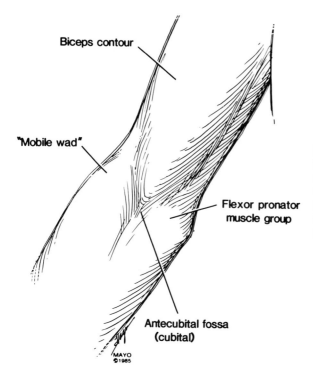

Biceps contour

"Mobile wad"

Flexor pronator
muscle group

Antecubital fossa
(cubital)

MAYO
©1985

FIG 3–6. The antecubital fossa is bounded by medial flexor pronator and lateral "mobile wad" muscle masses originating from epicondyles, as well as the biceps musculature and elbow crease, proximally.

should be easily diagnosed due to the loss of function. The posterior olecranon bursa is obvious if inflamed (Fig 3–7). A distinction between the infected and noninfected bursitis can usually be made by the associated redness, warmth, and tenderness that is associated with the infected bursa. A dislocated or subluxed joint presents with gross distortion of the contour, usually with a posterior prominence of the displaced ulna (Fig 3–8). This instability may be associated with articular erosions and spontaneous dislocation as in rheumatoid arthritis. Furthermore, rheumatoid nodules occur on the extensor surface of the elbow and may present as a discrete mass or prominence over the olecranon.

Medial. The medial aspect of the joint is not very characteristic with respect to its contour. Few visual clues are available. The medial epicondyle can be seen and occasionally a subluxing ulnar nerve can be identified with anterior subluxation during flexion and reduction of the nerve behind the epicondyle with extension. A malunited fracture of the medial epicondyle might also be evident as an increased osseous or bony prominence medially.

Lateral. Inspection of the lateral aspect of the joint is most rewarding to detect effusion and synovitis (Figs 3–9, A and B). Dermal atrophy may be ob-

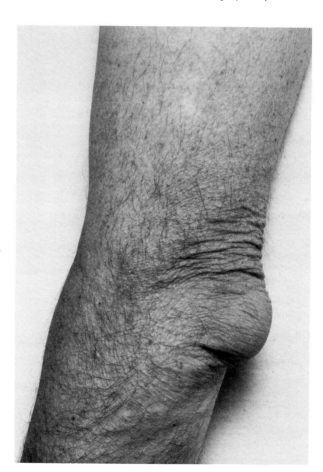

FIG 3–7. A distended olecranon bursa is readily diagnosed by inspection and palpation.

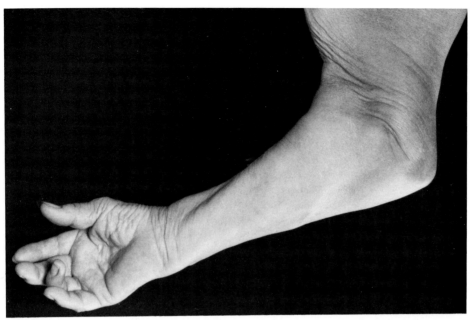

FIG 3–8. Posterior displacement and prominence of the olecranon in a patient with an ununited supracondylar fracture.

served in patients who have undergone repeated cortisone injections for chronic lateral tennis elbow syndrome.

Palpation

Because the elbow is a subcutaneous joint, as mentioned above, palpation is very rewarding. Several bony landmarks are available to the examiner, the medial lateral epicondyles as well as the tip of the olecranon, the radial head and the lateral supracondyle bony ridge (see Fig 3–2).

Anterior. A mass of the antecubital fossa may represent a lipoma or a ganglion. Synovitis is not appreciated because of the muscular covering of the joint anteriorly (see Fig 3–1). The anterior lateral muscle mass includes the origin of the brachioradialis muscle and extends quite far up the lateral aspect of the distal humerus. This muscle is readily palpated with resisted elbow flexion as the forearm is placed in neutral rotation. The biceps tendon and muscle are easily palpated. Medially, the lacertus fibrosis can be identified and the leading edge defined (Fig 3–10). The brachial artery may be identified under the biceps aponeurosis just medial to the biceps tendon. The median nerve is medial to the artery.

Posterior. The triceps tendinous attachment to the tip of the olecranon is rather discrete and can be palpated with resisted extension of the joint at 90°. The medial and lateral epicondyles and the tip of the olecranon are not only

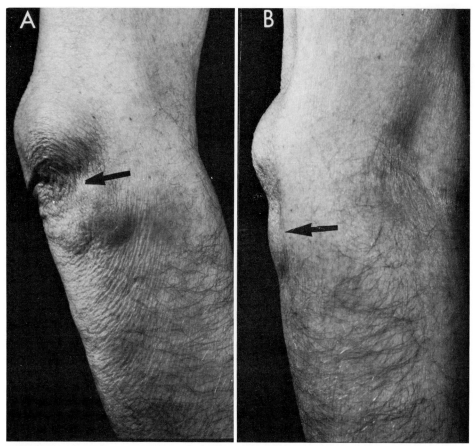

FIG 3–9. Synovitis or effusion is difficult to appreciate in the elbow and is most obvious at soft triangular space between lateral epicondyle, head of the radius, and tip of olecranon. **A,** normally, this area may be observed to be depressed (*arrow*), **B,** but fills out in the presence of effusion or synovitis (*arrow*).

observable but also palpable from the posterior aspect of the joint. Palpation of the distal humerus may reveal the altered relationship of these three bony landmarks, which indicates a structural pathologic process (Fig 3–11). When the elbow is flexed to 90°, the region of the olecranon fossa may also be palpable and the presence of osteophytes, ectopic callus, or spur formation determined (Fig 3–12).

Medial.   The medial epicondyle is the most prominent of the bony landmarks and serves as the superior border of the cubital tunnel. The ulnar nerve can be palpated behind the medial epicondyle (Fig 3–13). Mobility, tenderness, and a Tinel sign are readily tested. Sometimes this nerve can sublux either on a congenital or acquired basis.[10] Synovitis is rarely palpable since the medial capsule is quite strong owing to the reinforcement by the ulnar collateral complex. Palpation of the flexor-pronator group of muscles may be enhanced when this is performed while resisting these motions.

Lateral.   The lateral epicondyle and the lateral supracondylar bony column are readily palpated (Fig 3–14). Distally, the radial head is identified and when deformed, can be the source of significant symptoms. Pronation and supination with the elbow extended and flexed 90° helps to localize this articulation (Figs 3–15, A and B). The anconeus muscle is descernible at the lateral aspect of the olecranon inferior to the radial head and becomes prominent during resisted elbow extension. Effusion or synovitis is palpable in the lateral triangle defined above.

Motion

The elbow is a trochoginglymoid joint, meaning it provides 2 *df*, flexion-extension, and pronation-supination.[26] Each of these functions occurs independently through discrete articulations of the ulnohumeral and proximal radioulnar joints, respectively. This unique articular arrangement of the elbow joint allows for the hand to be placed in a great variety of positions in space.

The normal arc of flexion-extension with some variation is about 0° to 145° to

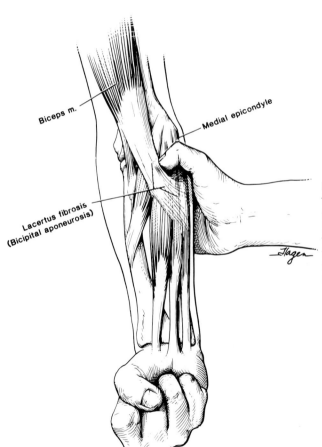

Biceps m.

Medial epicondyle

Lacertus fibrosis
(Bicipital aponeurosis)

FIG 3–10.   The lacertus fibrosis may be readily palpated by resisting elbow flexion at 90° and placing the thumb just medial to biceps tendon. Leading edge of lacertus fibrosis or bicipital aponeurosis is readily appreciated.

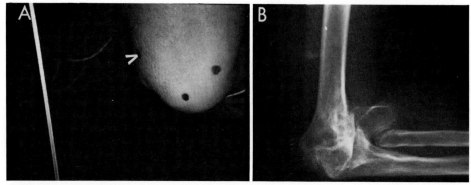

FIG 3–11. **A,** distortion of landmarks comprising epicondyles and tip of the olecranon demonstrates skeletal abnormality. **B,** in this instance, patient had a nonunion of an intercondylar fracture.

150° (Fig 3–16).[1,9] Even more normal variation occurs in the arc of pronation-supination. Generally, this motion can be considered to average 75° pronation and 85° supination (Fig 3–17).[31]

The reliability of the hand-held goniometer to measure elbow flexion and extension has been shown to be reliable to within about 5° of accuracy.[17] Pronation and supination are more difficult motions to consistently measure. Using the brachium as the reference, the angle made by a linear object held in the hand is the measurement technique most commonly used clinically. A more accurate

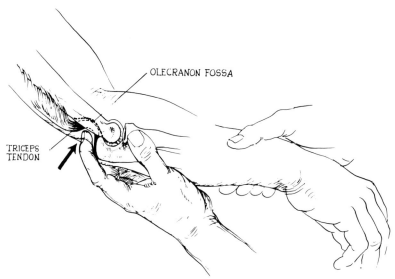

FIG 3–12. By flexing elbow to 60° and with patient relaxed, olecranon fossa can be palpated in some thin individuals. (From Hoppenfeld S: *Physical Examination of the Spine and Extremities.* New York, Appleton-Century-Crofts, 1976. Reproduced by permission.)

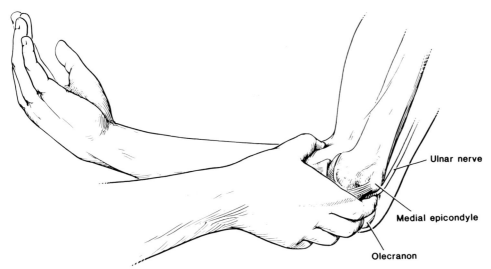

FIG 3–13. Ulnar nerve may be examined by rolling fingers under medial epicondyle with the elbow relaxed at 90°. If symptoms are present in this area, it is helpful to flex and extend elbow to assure that ulnar nerve does not sublux. This maneuver or taping the nerve may elicit Tinel's sign.

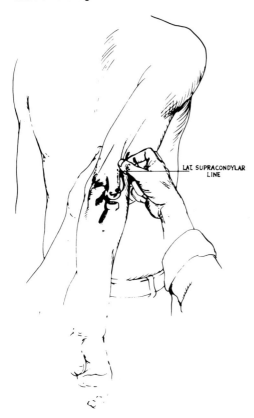

FIG 3–14. Supracondylar bony column is a valuable landmark for certain surgical exposures and is readily identifiable between flexor and extensor muscle masses, proximal to lateral epicondyle. (From Hoppenfeld S: *Physical Examination of the Spine and Extremities.* New York, Appleton-Century-Crofts, 1976. Reproduced by permission.)

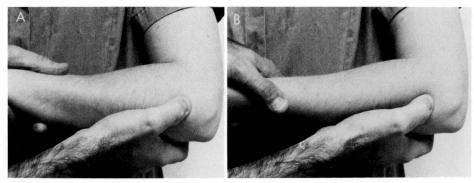

FIG 3–15. **A,** radial heat palpation should be done gently with the elbow flexed at 90° and forearm gently pronated. **B,** and supinated. Presence of crepitus with forearm rotation as well as flexion and extension should be noted.

method might use the plane of the wrist as the forearm reference, thus eliminating additional motion that occurs at the wrist and hand.

Unlike the shoulder, the rigid soft tissue constraints do not allow much additional elbow passive motion. When present, reflex inhibition due to pain is the most common cause of the disparity. The quality of the motion should also be enlisted by palpating the joint to discern if crepitus is present.

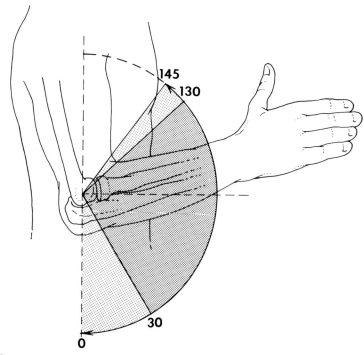

FIG 3–16. Normal range of elbow flexion is about 0° to 145°. However, functional arc of motion is somewhat less, and most activities can be performed with flexion of 30° to 130°.

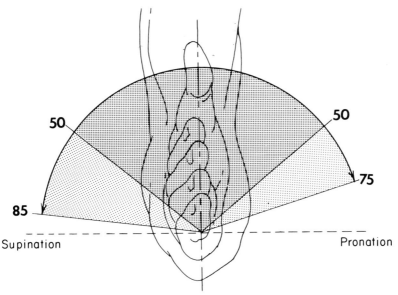

FIG 3–17. Pronation and supination motion averages 75° to 85°, respectively. Most activities of daily living, however, can be accomplished with 50° of each motion.

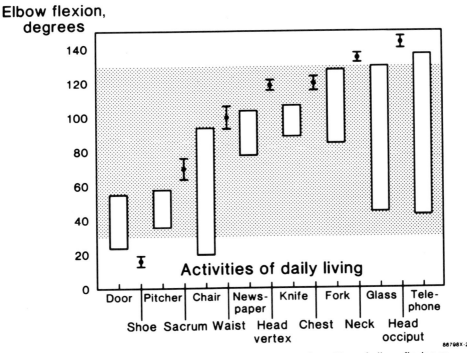

FIG 3–18. Fifteen daily activities demonstrating the arc and position of elbow flexion required. It is noted that most of these activities are accomplished within 30° to 130° flexion range.

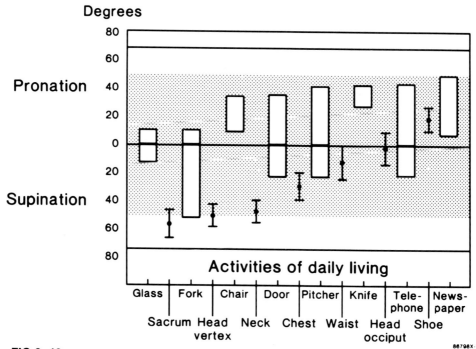

FIG 3–19. Fifteen activities of daily living are noted to be accomplished with pronation and supination of 50°, respectively.

As is true with other joints, most individuals do not use or require the full potential arcs of motion that exist at this joint. The so-called functional arc of motion has been studied in the laboratory.[26] Fifteen activities of daily living and personal hygiene were found to be generally accomplished with arcs of 30° to 130° of flexion and 50° of pronation and 50° of supination (Figs 3–18 and 3–19). Also, unlike other joints, there is no optimum position for a stiff elbow. The unique function of this joint, serving to link the hand to the shoulder, implies the

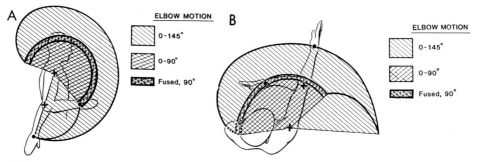

FIG 3–20. With normal elbow motion, hand may be placed in almost an infinite variety of positions in space (large surface). With motion of 0° to 90°, area of reach is dramatically reduced (smaller space). **A,** arthrodesis or ankylosis at 90° allows only a certain discrete distance from shoulder to be attainable (*arc*). **B,** sagittal plane, transverse plane.

ability to bring the hand closer to or further from the body for optimum function. The linkage with the shoulder may allow for compensated positioning of the hand in space but always at a discrete distance from the individual. Thus, elbow ankylosis is well tolerated for certain power activity but is quite disabling with respect to positioning of the hand in space. The significance of loss of elbow motion is demonstrated in Figure 3–20.

Associated Joint Involvement and Assessment

When the other joints of the upper extremity are involved with significant motion loss or pain, the normal function of the elbow is variously curtailed. Limitation of elbow flexion and extension is even more extreme if shoulder motion does not allow the extremity to be raised above the horizontal. Similarly, significant wrist involvement alters pronation and supination. When the elbow only is involved, the normal function of the other joints provides significant compensation for loss of elbow motion. Thus, these joints must be considered and assessed when the clinical circumstances warrant.

Strength

Assessment of strength is performed with the patient comfortable and the elbow at 90° of flexion.[11, 14] Clinically, most strength tests are of the isometric type in which extension and flexion are resisted by the examiner (Fig 3–21).[12, 18, 23] The elbow is supported and the wrist grasped by the opposite hand, thus avoiding wrist or hand pathology. Pronation and supination strength should also be determined. The position of the forearm also influences the maximum flexion and extension strength obtained.[19, 29] For example, muscle power is greatest during flexion with forearm supination and weakest in pronation. Extension, on the other hand, is most powerful with the forearm in pronation and is strongest at elbow positions of 90° to 120°.[14, 28, 32] The strongest supination effort is observed when the forearm is fully pronated and, conversely, when the forearm is fully supinated, the greatest pronation strength is enlisted. However, because the examination will frequently be conducted on patients with injury and a normal arc of forearm motion is not obtainable, most observers perform these strength studies with the forearm in the neutral rotation as a more reliable standard starting point (Fig 3–22). Once again, the elbow or distal humerus is supported and resistance exerted at the wrist.

Recent attempts are being made to objectively document elbow strength. Isometric strength may be measured clinically with a simple spring device or more sophisticated torque dynamometers. Assessment of fatigue and endurance may be documented with more complex devices that measure isokinetic muscle contracture.

Because of the rapid increase of interest in such devices, the orthopedic surgeon should have a reasonably clear understanding of the relationship between the various modalities of strength testing. Simply stated, isometric testing is performed when the elbow and the muscle are undergoing maximum contraction but no motion of the joint is occurring. Isotonic contracture and testing are performed with a constant load being applied to the joint but with the muscle either shortening (concentric) or lengthening (eccentric). Finally, the commonly

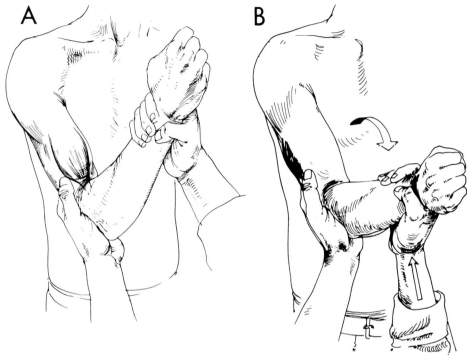

FIG 3–21. **A,** flexion and **B,** extension strength is best measured with the forearm in neutral rotation and elbow flexed at 90°. The elbow is supported and examiner resists each respective motion. (From Hoppenfeld S: *Physical Examination of the Spine and Extremities.* New York, Appleton-Century-Crofts, 1976. Reproduced by permission.)

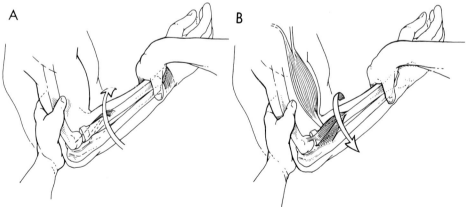

FIG 3–22. **A,** pronation and **B,** supination strength is most commonly measured with the elbow supported and flexed 90°. Forearm is in neutral position and each motion is resisted at the wrist by examiner. (From Morrey BF: *The Elbow and Its Disorders.* Philadelphia, WB Saunders Co, 1985. Reproduced by permission.)

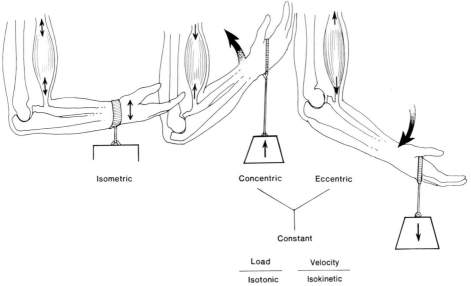

Isometric

Concentric   Eccentric

Constant

Load	Velocity
Isotonic	Isokinetic

FIG 3–23. Three types of muscle contracture might be measured during examination. Isometric contracture is the most commonly used and is the simplest method. Isokinetic and isometric contractures may be both concentric or eccentric and require more sophisticated equipment to accurately measure. (From Morrey BF: *The Elbow and Its Disorders.* Philadelphia, WB Sanders Co, 1985. Reproduced by permission.)

discussed isokinetic muscle contracture is one in which a constant velocity of contracture is maintained and the muscle is either shortening or lengthening. The distinction between these three types of muscle test is illustrated in Fig 3–23. The relationship of these various testing modalities has yet to be clearly defined. In general, it can be stated that isometric testing serves as a valid test of maximum muscle contracture but is inadequate to test endurance strength.[3, 5, 8, 13]

The opposite extremity serves as a basis to estimate the extent of strength loss. If both extremities are involved, some normal standard should be consulted. Moreover, to more fully appreciate the differences between the various muscle functions, some understanding of their relationship is worthwhile. In our experience involving more than 100 normal subjects, it was noted that males are approximately twice as strong as females in all functions, and extension strength is about 60% to 70% that of flexion strength.[2, 23] Supination is slightly stronger (about 15%) than pronation. Finally, the dominant extremity is stronger than the nondominant side by about 4% to 8% (Fig 3–24).

Reflexes

The evaluation of three cervical nerve roots may be examined by reflexes of muscle about the elbow. The biceps reflex is performed with the forearm resting comfortably over the examiner's arm and the elbow flexed about 90° and tests the competency of the C5 root (Fig 3–25). The triceps reflex is again elicited with the elbow flexed approximately 90° and the forearm resting over the examiner's

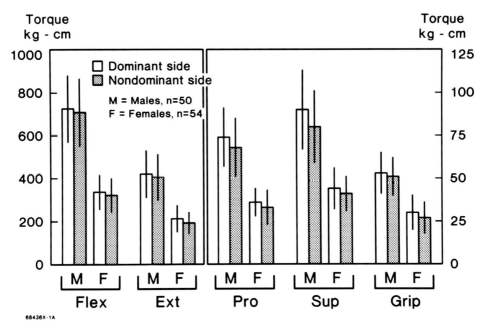

FIG 3–24. Relationship between dominant and nondominant extremities, as well as between males and females, of various functions of the elbow. (From Morrey BF: *The Elbow and Its Disorders.* Philadelphia, WB Saunders Co, 1985. Reproduced by permission.)

FIG 3–25. Biceps reflex is performed with the patient relaxed and the elbow in 90° of flexion, forearm being supported by examiner. This tests the C5 nerve root. (From Hoppenfeld S: *Physical Examination of the Spine and Extremities.* New York, Appleton-Century-Crofts, 1976. Reproduced by permission.)

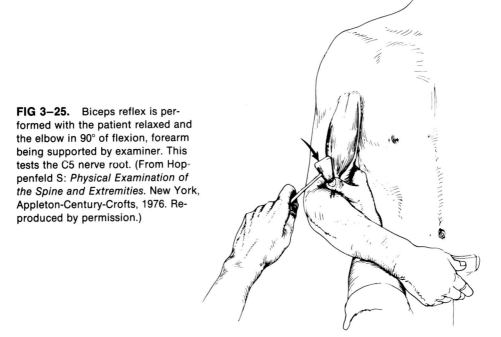

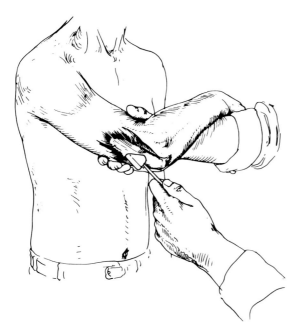

FIG 3–26. The C7 nerve root is tested with triceps reflex. Elbow is relaxed and supported by examiner at about 90° of flexion. (From Hoppenfeld S: *Physical Examination of the Spine and Extremities.* New York, Appleton-Century-Crofts, 1976. Reproduced by permission.)

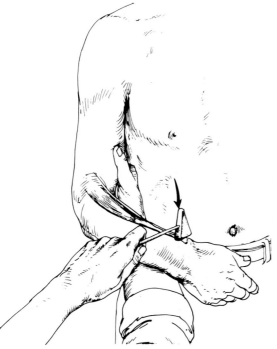

FIG 3–27. The C6 reflex is examined distally near the wrist, but tests the brachioradialis and is performed with elbow in neutral or the pronated position and flexed approximately 90°. (From Hoppenfeld S: *Physical Examination of the Spine and Extremities.* New York, Appleton-Century-Crofts, 1976. Reproduced by permission.)

arm, and tests the C7 cervical root (Fig 3–26). The triceps reflex is not as vigorous as is that of the biceps, so with this test the muscle should be observed for contracture. The brachioradialis reflex is elicited at the wrist again with the forearm flexed 90°, usually in a neutral rotation, and is an assessment of the competency of the C6 nerve root (Fig 3–27).

Stability

As discussed in the section on anatomy, elbow stability results from the relationship of the articular cartilage and the soft tissue constraints of this joint. As the most congruous joint in the body, significant stability may be observed even in the face of the lack of competent soft tissue constraints. On the other hand, removal of articular cartilage due to fracture of the radial head or of the olecranon is not generally associated with elbow instability if the anterior capsule and collateral ligament structures are intact. Studies have suggested that the radial collateral ligament is taut throughout the entire arc of motion.[25] The anterior portion of the medial collateral ligament is taut after the first 20° of flexion, and the posterior portion of the medial collateral ligament becomes taut only after 60° or more of flexion.

Thus, varus-valgus stress testing of this joint in approximately 10° to 15° of

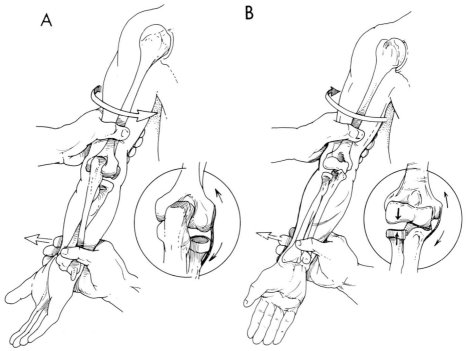

FIG 3–28. A, varus instability of elbow is measured with humerus in full internal rotation and an outward force applied to slightly flexed forearm. **B,** valgus instability is evaluated with elbow slightly flexed and humerus in full external rotation. (From Morrey BF: *The Elbow and Its Disorders.* Philadelphia, WB Saunders Co, 1985. Reproduced by permission.)

flexion does provide valuable information with respect to the integrity of the collateral ligaments. However, testing of these ligaments is difficult due to the axial motion that occurs at the shoulder joint. Thus, for varus instability, the humerus is fully internally rotated and an outward force is applied to the forearm (Fig 3–28). This tests the radial collateral ligament. Outward force on the forearm with the humerus fully externally rotated tests the medial collateral ligament complex (see Fig 3–28). Anterior and posterior instability is usually obvious. The magnitude can be readily assessed with the elbow in 90° of flexion while grasping the distal humerus and anteriorly and posteriorly displacing the forearm. Finally, superior and inferior instability of the joint is rarely in question, and usually would be demonstrated only after significant joint erosion from rheumatoid arthritis or from excision of the proximal ulna. This is examined in a manner similar to anterior posterior instability with the force being directed superiorly and inferiorly.

Localization of Pathology

To resolve questions that may arise as to whether the primary pathology is intra-articular or extra-articular is the use of a diagnostic injection of xylocaine hydrochloride. The joint is entered through the lateral triangle (Fig 3–29). Any fluid that is obtained is sent for the appropriate studies. This aspiration is particularly easy if effusion is present, since the bulging capsule allows ready access of the needle. After a small amount of xylocaine has been introduced into the joint,

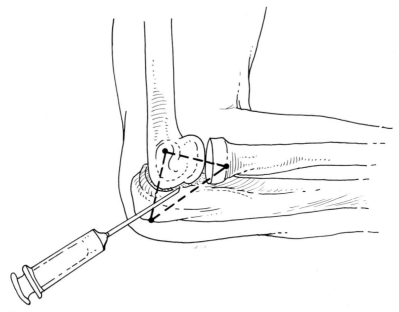

FIG 3–29. Palpation of three prominent landmarks on lateral aspect of elbow, lateral epicondyle, head of the radius, and tip of olecranon provides an accurate landmark for aspiration or injection of the joint. (From Morrey BF: *The Elbow and Its Disorders*. Philadelphia, WB Saunders Co, 1985. Reproduced by permission.)

improved motion due to relief of pain clearly documents reflex inhibition as a major cause of the patient's complaint. Additional functional improvement, for example, increased ability to lift weight without pain, may also be observed.

References

1. American Academy of Orthopaedic Surgeons: *Joint Motion: Method of Measuring and Recording*. Chicago, American Academy of Orthopaedic Surgeons, 1965.
2. Askew LJ, An KN, Morrey BF, et al: Functional evaluation of the elbow: Normal motion requirements and strength determination. *Orthop Trans* 1981; 5:304.
3. Asmussen E, Hansen O, Lammert O: The relation between isometric and dynamic muscle strength in man. *Comm Dan Nat Assoc Infant Paral* 1965; 20.
4. Atkinson WB, Elftman H: The carrying angle of the human arm as a secondary symptom character. *Anat Rec* 1945; 91:49.
5. Barnes WS: The relationship between maximum isokinetic strength and isometric endurance. *Res Q Exerc Sports* 1980; 51:714.
6. Basmajian JV, Griffin WR: Function of anconeus muscle. *J Bone Joint Surg* 1972; 54A:1712–1714.
7. Beals RK: The normal carrying angle of the elbow. *Clin Orthop* 1976; 119:194.
8. Berger RA: Comparison of static and dynamic strength increases. *Res Q* 1962; 33:329.
9. Boone DC, Azen SP: Normal range of motion of joints in male subjects. *J Bone Joint Surg* 1979; 61A:756.
10. Childress HM: Recurrent ulnar nerve dislocation at the elbow. *Clin Orthop* 1975; 108:168.
11. Clarke HH, Elkins EC, Martin GM, et al: Relationship between body position and the application of muscle power to movements of the joint. *Arch Phys Med* 1950; 31:81.
12. Daniels L, Williams M, Worthingham C: *Muscle Testing: Techniques of Manual Examination*, ed 2. Philadelphia, WB Saunders Co, 1946.
13. Doss WS, Karpovich PV: A comparison of concentric, eccentric, and isometric strength of the elbow flexion. *J Appl Physiol* 1965; 20:351.
14. Elkins EC, Ursula ML, Khalil GW: Objective recording of the strength of normal muscles. *Arch Phys Med* 1951; 33:639.
15. Field JH: Posterior interosseous nerve palsy secondary to synovial chondromatosis of the elbow joint. *J Hand Surg* 1981; 6:336–338.
16. Funk D: *EMG Investigation of Muscular Contractions About the Human Elbow*, thesis. Mayo Graduate School of Medicine, Rochester, Minn, 1984.
17. Hellebrandt FA, Duvall EN, Moore ML: The measurement of joint motion: Part 3. Reliability of goniometry. *Phys Ther Rev* 1949; 29:302.
18. Hoppenfeld S: *Physical Examination of the Spine and Extremities*. New York, Appleton-Century-Crofts, 1976.
19. Jorgensen K, Bankov S: Maximum strength of elbow flexors with pronated and supinated forearm. *Med Sports Biomechan* 1971; 6:174.
20. Keats TE, Teeslink R, Diamond AE, et al: Normal axial relationships of the major joints. *Radiology* 1966; 87:904.
21. Lanz T, Wachsmuth W: *Praktische Anatomie–Arm*. Berlin, Springer-Verlag, 1959.
22. Malkawi H: Recurrent dislocation of the elbow accompanied by ulnar neuropathy: A case report and review of the literature. *Clin Orthop* 1981; 161:170–174.
23. McGarvey S, Morrey BF, Askew LJ, et al: Reliability of isometric strength testing: Temporal factors and strength variation. *Rel Res Clin Orthop Rel Pres* 1984; 185:301.
24. Millender LH, Nalebuff EA, Holdsworth DE: Posterior interosseous nerve syndrome secondary to rheumatoid synovitis. *J Bone Joint Surg* 1973; 55A:753.
25. Morrey BF, An KN: Functional anatomy of the elbow ligaments. *Clin Orthop* 1985; 20:84–90.

26. Morrey BF, Askew LJ, An KN, et al: A biomechanical study of normal functional elbow motion. *J Bone Joint Surg* 1981; 63A:872.
27. Morrey BF, Chao EY: Passive motion of the elbow joint: A biomechanical study. *J Bone Joint Surg* 1979; 61A:63.
28. Provins KA, Salter N: Maximum torque exerted about the elbow joint. *J Appl Physiol* 1955; 7:393.
29. Rasch PJ: Effect of position of forearm on strength of elbow flexion. *Res Q* 1955; 27:333.
30. Simmons JW, Rath D, Merta R: Calculation of disability using the Cybex II system. *Orthopedics* 1982; 5:181.
31. Wagner C: Determination of the rotatory flexibility of the elbow joint. *Eur J Appl Physiol* 1977; 37:47.
32. Williams M, Stutzman L: Strength variation through the range of motion. *Phys Ther Rev* 1959; 39:145.

CHAPTER 4

Physical Examination of the Wrist

Ronald L. Linscheid, M.D.
James H. Dobyns, M.D.

The wrist lends itself well to physical examination. It may be easily positioned and compared with the opposite wrist. Almost all the structures that comprise or pass the wrist may be palpated or tested by various maneuvers. The wrist contains four joint systems: the distal radioulnar, which supports rotatory motion of the hand; the radiocarpal and midcarpal joints, which provide flexion-extension and radial-ulnar deviation; and the carpometacarpal joints, which provide rigid fixation for the second and third metacarpals and significant mobility for the first, fourth, and fifth metacarpals to aid in spatial adaptation of the palm during grasping. The wrist is the most complex joint in the human body. It acts as the final adjustable linkage for placing the hand in a functional position.

The nature of the patient's complaint and many other items of the history will alert one to the area of interest at the physical examination. An important fact to be obtained is the patient's finger-touching demonstration of the area or areas of pain and tenderness. It is desirable to have a standard approach to physical diagnosis for thoroughness's sake.

Inspection

The forearm should be uncovered to well above the elbow and all jewelry removed. The injured or "complaint wrist" should be compared with its opposite member. Deformity (engorgement, inflammation, color, fullness, swelling, or a different configuration) should be observed, as well as skin damage, nail changes, and crease alterations. Fractures, sprains, arthritides, congenital variations, and other diseases (infections, tumors, paralyses, and other nerve abnormalities) will all provoke such changes. In addition to appearance, inspection can reveal the range of motion. Rotation is checked with both elbows firmly adducted against the trunk. The hands are turned from a palm up to a palm down position. Pronation is considered normal from 0° to 60° through 90°, and supination from 0° to 45° through 80°, with the majority of people having a range of approximately 80° in either direction. With one limb of the goniometer laid across the flexion crease of the wrist and the other limb in line with the humerus, a reasonably accurate angular measurement can be obtained. Limitation of motion may occur anywhere in the forearm or wrist.

Wrist flexion is measured with the goniometer laid on the dorsal surface of the forearm and over the third metacarpal for palmar flexion. Placement on the palmar aspect of the forearm and contacting the third metacarpal area of the palm measures dorsiflexion. These positions give values slightly higher than those obtained from laying the goniometer along the side of the wrist, but are quite reproducible. Dorsiflexion from 60° to 80° is usual, with palmar flexion being slightly greater. Radial and ulnar deviation are measured with the hand flat and the goniometer parallel to the third metacarpal and longitudinal axis of the forearm. Radial deviation from neutral to 15° through 25° and ulnar deviation from 0° to 30° through 45° are usual. Limitation of motion follows a host of conditions. Repeated measurements of wrist motions provide one way of recording improvement.

Strength tests, both for grip and for wrist motions, are quite helpful in following the progress of a wrist problem. One of the standard grip meters is used for three trials of the affected hand, which are interposed between three trials for the normal hand. The patient should be instructed to grip as firmly as possible, then release. The grip size is adjusted according to the size of the hand. The nondominant hand is usually 10% to 15% weaker. Inconsistent efforts and tremulousness are suggestive of anxiety, depression, inattention, or other reaction to injury. Weakness, inconsistent with the appearance and muscle bulk, suggests conscious motivational problems (malingering). Isometric testing of wrist extension, flexion, and deviation power is also useful.

Palpation

The structures of the wrist are readily palpated. One's own wrist is a convenient place to begin learning the amount of pressure necessary and the characteristic features of each anatomical point during palpation. Starting with the skeletal prominences and beginning on the radial aspect of the wrist in ulnar deviation, the radial styloid is identified (Fig 4–1, A). One centimeter proximally, the sharp ridge dividing the first dorsal compartment for the abductor pollicis longus and the extensor pollicis brevis may be felt running at a 30° oblique course from proximal and lateral to palmar and distal. Running a finger dorsally reveals another prominent bony ridge, Lister's tubercle, which serves as a fulcrum for the angulation of the extensor pollicis longus. It is felt just radial to the midline of the wrist. Moving ulnarly, a flat firm area representing the dorsoulnar angle of the radius is present. The ulnar head is next palpable as a smooth, rounded prominence, much more evident in pronation. The ulnar styloid process extends distally, but its position appears to change from full pronation to full supination as the radius rotates around the ulnar head. It lies dorsally in supination and ulnopalmarly in pronation. The palmar aspect of the radius is largely covered by the flexor tendons except for the palmar aspect of the styloid processus radial to the flexor carpi radialis and below the radial artery (Fig 4–1, B). The palmar aspect of the ulnar head, though covered with soft tissue structures, is palpable in the supination position.

The body of the scaphoid is felt in the anatomical "snuff box," the hollow just

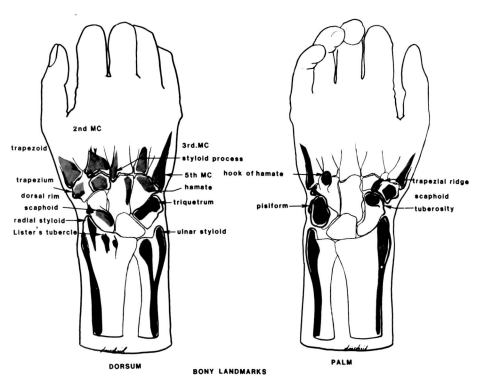

FIG 4–1. Dorsum of the wrist, identifiable bony prominences stippled (*left*); palmar identifiable bony prominences stippled (*right*).

distal to the radial styloid lying between the abductor pollicis longus and extensor pollicis longus, and near the surface in ulnar deviation. The scaphoid tuberosity is a hard, rounded prominence approximately 0.5 cm in diameter, lying distal and palmar to the radial styloid. It is readily identified during extension. Just distal and in seemingly continuity is the trapezial ridge, which overlies the flexor carpi radialis at the beginning of the thenar eminence. The dorsal rim and proximal pole of the scaphoid become obvious on wrist flexion, lying just distal to Lister's tubercle dorsoradially (see Fig 4–1, A).

The scapholunate interval may be felt between the scaphoid and lunate during ulnar deviation. The lunate is largely covered by the finger extensors and is less palpable. Over the distal scaphoid is a sulcus that admits the pulp of the index finger. Beyond this is the trapezoid in the index finger axis and the trapezium in the thumb axis. The base of the index metacarpal and the chevron-shaped interval representing the second carpometacarpal joint lie next in line for the index ray and the thumb carpometacarpal joint and its margins for the thumb ray. The dorsal surface of the distal capitate is felt by deflecting the extensor tendons with direct pressure downwards in the center of the wrist. The styloid process of the third metacarpal is felt between the capitate and trapezoid. Directly proximal to the third carpometacarpal area is a central wrist sulcus overlying the proximal capitate.

Returning proximally and ulnarly, the triquetrum is palpable just distal to the ulnar head, with the lunate and lunotriquetral interval becoming apparent on radial deviation. Distal to the triquetral ridge is the hamate. The motion between the two is readily discernible on radial-ulnar deviation motions. Next distal, the fourth and fifth metacarpal bases are palpable; both active and passive motion in the carpometacarpal joints are readily appreciated.

On the ulnar aspect of the wrist there is a sulcus between the ulnar head and the triquetrum, followed distally by another sulcus for the triquetrohamate interval, then the base of the fifth metacarpal.

On the palmar aspect of the wrist, beginning ulnarly, one notes the pisiform bone just distal to the distal wrist crease in the emerging hypothenar eminence (see Fig 4–1, B). This is distractible from its triquetral articular partner by exerting to-and-fro motions. One centimeter distoradially, one can feel the sharp prominence of the hook of the hamate through the thickened overlying palmar tissues. The palm is thickened from these bony landmarks across to the trapezial ridge and scaphoid tuberosity over the transverse carpal ligament that connects them.

Using these bony landmarks for identification, it is possible to identify most of the soft tissue structures of the wrist (Fig 4–2). Over the radial styloid, the cephalic vein is recognizable, especially if the hand is dependent or the venous drainage temporarily occluded. In this same area, one or more branches of the dorsal sensory radial nerve can be rolled between the fingertip and bone. The tendons of the abductor pollicis longus and extensor pollicis brevis are palpable

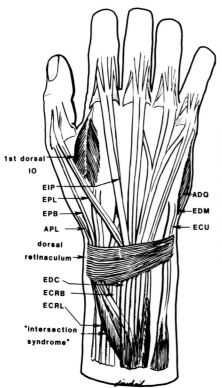

1st dorsal
IO

EIP
EPL
EPB
APL

dorsal
retinaculum

EDC
ECRB
ECRL

"intersection
syndrome"

ADQ
EDM
ECU

FIG 4–2. Dorsal soft tissue structure, usually identifiable by palpation. *EIP* indicates extensor indicis proprius; *EPL*, extensor pollicus longus; *EPB*, extensor pollicus brevis; *APL*, abductor pollicus longus; *EDC*, extensor digitorum communis; *ECRB*, extensor carpi radialis brevis; *ECRL*, extensor carpi radialis longus; *ADQ*, abductor digiti quinti; *EDM*, extensor digiti minimi; and *ECU*, extensor carpi ulnaris.

proximal and distal to the radial styloid where they are covered by the dorsal retinaculum as the first dorsal compartment. Their muscle bellies cross the radial wrist extensors where the muscle prominence is seen proximally. Tendon excursion and tension are easily palpated.

The extensor pollicis longus stands out on extension and abduction of the thumb, delineating the dorsal and ulnar boundary of the snuff box. The extensor carpi radialis brevis and longus are palpated best just distal and ulnar to the extensor pollicis longus when wrist extension is being resisted. By comparing the relative tension in the tendons as first resisted wrist extension with radial deviation and then neutral wrist extension are tested, the extensor carpi radialis brevis and extensor carpi radialis longus can usually be differentiated. The finger extensors are easily visualized and palpated in the mid-wrist area. They are most prominent when active extension of all fingers is being carried out against some resistance. The extensor digiti minimi and extensor indicis proprius are noted in the same way, with active extension of both index and little fingers without the other digits or of either alone. At the wrist level, the extensor indicis proprius is palpated just distal and a finger's breadth ulnar to Lister's tubercle; the extensor digiti minimi is palpated at the dorsoulnar angle of the radius. The extensor carpi ulnaris lies dorsal to the ulnar styloid and thus is ulnarly placed in pronation and dorsally placed in supination. Its course to the base of the fifth metacarpal is accentuated during forced ulnar deviation. The dorsal sensory branch of the ulnar nerve, although small, may be identified in thin individuals by rolling it between a finger and the triquetrum as it courses obliquely dorsally (Fig 4–3).

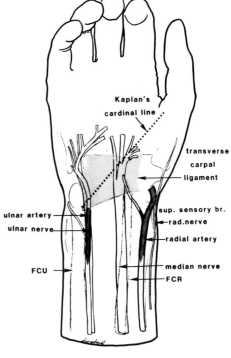

FIG 4–3. Identifiable soft tissue structures on the palmar aspect of the wrist and their relationships. Finger flexor tendons occupying central aspect of distal forearm and palmaris longus, which often overlies the median nerve, are deleted. *FCU* indicates flexor carpi ulnaris; and *FCR,* flexor carpi radialis.

VESSELS & NERVES

The flexor carpi ulnaris produces a prominence on the ulnovolar aspect of the wrist as it courses to the pisiform. The ulnar artery pulse is identifiable just radial to this and occasionally, the cordlike ulnar nerve may be rolled between a finger and the ulnar head. The palmaris longus, present in approximately 80% of individuals, strongly marks the center of the palmar aspect of the wrist with resisted "cupping" of the palm. The median nerve usually lies under the radial aspect of this tendon or in its absence a finger's breadth ulnar to the flexor carpi radialis. A positive Tinel sign may be elicited by tapping or rolling the nerve beneath a finger in many individuals. The flexor tendons to the fingers are palpable proximal to the wrist crease, especially with resisted finger flexion.

The flexor carpi radialis provides the landmark tendon radiopalmarly, which also is most prominent on resisted flexion. The radial artery is palpable radial to this over the radial styloid palmar surface (see Fig 4–3).

Diagnosis by Testing

With reasonable adeptness in localizing the various anatomical structures, a systematic approach to diagnosis is more easily accomplished. Most patients will be initially seen with pain; therefore, the elicitation of tenderness or reproduction of their pain by maneuver is helpful. Other patients will present with deformity, limitation of motion, or tumoral prominences. Localization is equally important to identify the system involved.

To avoid missing clues to a systemic or more extensive process, it is useful to survey the entire upper extremity before localizing one's examination to a specific locale on the wrist. Following a systematic examination procedure will minimize overlooking relevant findings. Inspection and palpation circumferentially around the wrist, range of motion determination, and estimates of strength-endurance will obviate most errors of omission in examination. Palpation should be light (searching for alterations in contour, configuration, and structure) and heavy with discrete localization (searching for and assigning priority to the areas of tenderness). Localization of the diagnosis may be categorized by systems as skeletal, articular, ligamentous, tendinous, nervous, vascular, and epidermal.

Skeletal Conditions

Some of the more important areas are as follows:

Scaphoid. Classic scaphoid fractures are diagnosed by tenderness in the anatomical snuff box. Simultaneous pressure over the dorsal pole and tuberosity may elicit pain from a waist fracture and is more likely to find a tuberosital fracture or dorsal pole fracture.

Trapezium. A palmar ridge fracture has point tenderness at the insertion of the transverse carpal ligament, while a body fracture presents with generalized trapezial tenderness and is most easily demonstrated radiodorsally.

Lunate. A fracture or Kienböck's disease presents with central tenderness aggravated by clamping the lunate between the forefinger and thumb and moving the carpus. Direct compression through the central carpus is also provocative.

Triquetrum. A dorsal ridge fracture produces tenderness directly dorsally over the triquetrum when grasped between the forefinger and thumb. Triquetral body fractures are demonstrated either dorsally or laterally (ulnarly) by direct pressure or provocation stress (compression or tension).

Hamate. Other than the scaphoid, the fracture most often missed in the carpus is a fracture of the hook of the hamate. Pain on direct palmar pressure over the hook is highly suggestive. Pain is also produced by stressing the fracture site either by resisted abduction of the little finger or resisted flexion of the profundi with the wrist ulnarly deviated. The direct and indirect stress provocation described for carpometacarpal and triquetrohamate joints will also identify hamate body fractures.

Capitate. Fractures of the waist and proximal articular surface result in pain and tenderness of the central dorsal wrist sulcus, just distal to the lunate. Damage to the expanded distal portion is diagnosable by the usual local changes of swelling, bruising, inflammation, and tenderness; stress provocation is as described for the carpometacarpal area.

Marked deformity such as seen with perilunate fracture-dislocations is marked by gross alterations of carpal contour and requires roentgenologic examination for differentiation.

Radius and Ulna. Undisplaced fractures of the radius usually present with well-localized tenderness, as does the ulna. Styloid fractures of both are usually palpable.

Articular and Ligamentous Conditions

Clinical diagnosis of the large variety of sprains of the wrist has been significantly improved in the last two decades both by improved recognition and by appreciation of the persistently disabling character of these entities.

Scaphotrapezial. Trapezoidal tenderness may be generalized or fairly discrete at palmar, radial, or dorsal margins. Crepitus on forced motion or tuberosital displacement is suggestive of isolated degenerative joint disease or traumatic chondromalacia. Involvement of this joint may severely limit wrist motion.

Scapholunate Joint. This area is one of the most frequent pain-tenderness foci in the wrist as a result of its susceptibility to injury. Point tenderness suggests an occult ganglion arising from the scapholunate ligament, scaphoid or lunate impaction syndrome, or scapholunate tear. Even minor degrees of the latter may result in painful motion; when more severe, the result is rotatory subluxation of the scaphoid. The dorsal pole is prominent and often ballotable, as it has escaped from its ligamentous attachment to the lunate. In this situation, the wrist may also have a dorsal prominence as the capitate is displaced dorsally on the unstable dorsiflexed lunate (dorsal intercalated segment instability). Distraction of the wrist or palmar translocation of the distal carpus will correct the deformity.

Lunotriquetral. Lunotriquetral tenderness implies similar problems: a tear, partial or complete, of the lunotriquetral interosseous membrane. Local tenderness, crepitus, and a jump or click with radial-ulnar deviation are suggestive of instability at this level. A positive ballottement test is further confirmation and is performed by grasping the triquetrum between the thumb and forefinger of one hand and the lunate similarly with the other hand (Fig 4–4). Displacement of the triquetrum up and down on the lunate demonstrates laxity, crepitus, and pain.

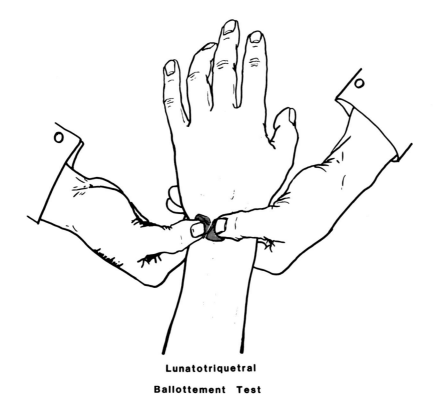

Lunatotriquetral

Ballottement Test

FIG 4-4. Lunatotriquetral ballottement test for lunatotriquetral interosseous membrane dissociations.

With complete lunotriquetral dissociation, the midcarpal joint collapses, with the lunate palmar flexing, giving the wrist a fork-shaped deformity known as a volar flexed intercalated segment instability.

Triquetrohamate. Pain elicited by passive, forced extension-ulnar deviation with tenderness at the triquetrohamate interval is suggestive of a triquetrohamate impingement syndrome. There may be a suggestion of dorsal subluxation of the hamate with excessive mobility.

Pisotriquetral. Pisotriquetral joint pain, crepitus, and tenderness are suggestive of a fractured pisiform, degenerative joint disease, or osteochondromatosis and are easily provoked by manipulation.

Carpometacarpal Joints. Second, third, fourth, and fifth carpometacarpal joint localized tenderness may be seen individually or in combination. Chronic sprains of these joints are uncommonly recognized. Testing is performed by firmly holding the proximal bone: e.g., capitate, flexing and extending the distal bone, e.g., third metacarpal. Complaints of pain with this motion, localized tenderness, or crepitus are suggestive of injury to the carpometacarpal joint(s). A more forceful injury results usually in dorsal subluxation of the metacarpal bases with palmar angulation of the metacarpals. The acute injury is associated with soft tissue swelling directly over the carpometacarpal joints.

Distal Radioulnar Joint. The distal radioulnar joint is often the site of pain after injury, which is usually brought on by rotatory motions of the forearm. Prominence of the ulnar head on pronation greater than the opposite wrist suggests dorsal subluxation. This infers attenuation of the triangular fibrocartilage, dorsal radioulnar ligament, or fracture of the base of the ulnar styloid. Ballottement of the ulnar head is usually positive and painful crepitus suggests chondromalacia of the convex surface within the sigmoid notch of the radius.

Reduction of the ulnar head with simultaneous realignment of the ulnar carpus by support beneath the pisiform often relieves the patient's discomfort. Rotating the wrist to full supination also leads to relief in most instances. The site of chondromalacia on the articular head may sometimes be determined by ballotting it as the wrist is rotated through several positions.

Occasionally the ulnar head will sublux palmarly on supination, providing a protrusion proximal to the pisiform. Reduction occurs with pronation.

Crepitus and pain at the distal radioulnar joint may also occur from triangular fibrocartilage tears or lunate-ulnar impingement usually associated with an ulnar-positive variant. This is usually due to degenerative changes occurring on the lunate and ulnar head through a defect in the triangular fibrocartilage. The latter is a roentgenologic diagnosis. The pain is accentuated by ulnar deviation and manipulation of the ulnotriquetral area. Catching or clicking may accompany these maneuvers and are meaningful if different from the other side or painful or both.

Rheumatoid arthritis affects all of the above articulations often simultaneously, and may result in similar instabilities. There is usually generalized swelling of the wrist and frequently tendinous involvement as well.

Tendon Conditions

All of the tendons that cross the wrist with the exception of the palmaris longus and flexor carpi ulnaris are enveloped by a tendon sheath mechanism that enhances their frictionless excursion. Interference with this excursion by damage, deformity, or swelling of the tendons or their sheaths is a common problem.

Tendons on the dorsum of the wrist are constrained into six dorsal compartments by the dorsal retinaculum (see Fig 4–2). The digit flexors are held within the carpal tunnel by the transverse carpal ligament and the flexor carpi radialis within an adjacent but separate compartment. The tenosynovium within these compartments may react with inflammation or hypertrophy under certain conditions. Catching, triggering, painful motion—even rupture—may occur.

Stenosing Tenosynovitis. Stenosing tenosynovitis is often associated with hypertrophy of the overlying ligament as well as thickening of the tenosynovium. An inflammatory response is more common in rheumatoid arthritis though the distinction between the extremes of these two conditions is often ill defined. Stenosing tenosynovitis at the wrist is seen in each tendon compartment though with different symptomatic manifestations. Women are affected four times as commonly as men.

Stenosing tenosynovitis of the first dorsal compartment associated with pain on thumb motion and/or wrist ulnar deviation is also known as de Quervain's disease. There is tenderness directly over the radial styloid. The underlying retinacular hypertrophy may be obvious and occasionally a small ganglion protrudes from the area. A proximal effusion along the abductor pollicis longus and extensor pollicis brevis may be present. A positive Finkelstein test is suggestive confirmation (Fig 4–5). This test is classically performed by having the patient clench the thumb under the grasping fingers, with pain produced on acute wrist ulnar deviation of the wrist. Sharp pain experienced at the radial styloid represents a positive test. When performed forcefully, this test may also be positive in normal patients and is often positive in those with basilar thumb joint arthrosis unless the stress is modified to avoid first metacarpal depression. Rarely "triggering" of the extensor pollicis longus is seen and a nodule may be palpated slipping past Lister's tubercle.

Stenosing tenosynovitis of the flexor carpi radialis is seen in patients who repetitively flex and extend the wrist. Tenderness proximal to the trapezial ridge, aggravated by resisted flexion, is present. Motion may be limited and painful.

Tenosynovial hypertrophy within the carpal tunnel usually results in median nerve symptoms. Though age is a factor, repetitive overuse at any age may result in this condition with its other findings of local tenderness, stretch pain, and swelling.

Tenosynovitis in the second, third, fourth, fifth, and sixth dorsal compartments is more apt to have an associated effusion or inflammatory tenosynovitis. Involvement of the fourth compartment is associated with an effusion confined over the metacarpal bases but moving to-and-fro with finger motion. Less commonly, a dumbbell swelling to either side of the dorsal retinaculum is seen. The

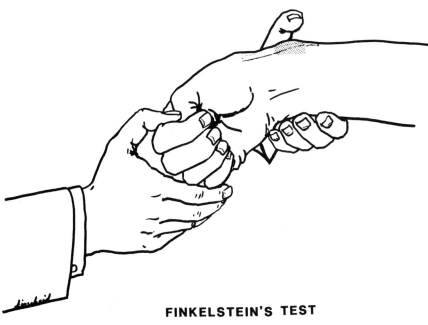

FINKELSTEIN'S TEST

FIG 4–5. Finkelstein's test for de Quervain's disease.

sixth compartment involvement often manifests as a nodular, ropy appearance with a fluctuant cystic consistency. Similar but less obvious involvement is noted in the other compartments.

The extension-intersection syndrome is a unique problem that occurs between and around the more superficial abductor pollicis longus-extensor pollicis brevis and the deeper extensor carpi radialis longus and brevis tendons where they intersect three finger breadths proximal to Lister's tubercle (see Fig 4–2). Symptoms usually develop after a period of intense wrist activity and are accompanied by swelling of the abductor pollicis longus-extensor pollicis brevis muscular compartment, with tenderness to direct pressure and pain on thumb or wrist motion. At the peak of reaction most cases display a uniquely palpable and audible crepitus on wrist flexion-extension that has been compared to two pieces of wet leather gliding on each other. Distinction from de Quervain's disease is necessary.

Dysfunction Associated With Musculotendinous Anomalies

Linburg's syndrome is associated with vague discomfort in the palm and wrist often associated with a persistent pinch position (Fig 4–6). Carpal tunnel symptoms may be present. The condition is caused by an interconnection between the flexor pollicis longus and index profundus, which is an anomalous tendinous

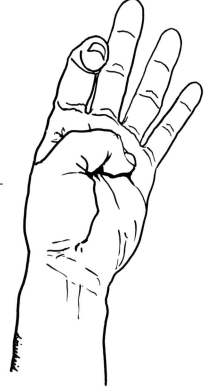

FIG 4–6. Linburg's test for symptomatic interconnection between flexor pollicis longus and flexor index profundus.

Linburg's test

condition seen in 10% to 15% of hands. Linburg's sign is elicited by flexing the thumb maximally onto the hypothenar eminence and actively stretching the index finger into extension. Limitation of extension and pain denote a positive sign.

Nerve Conditions

Two major compound nerves, the median and ulnar, cross the palmar aspect of the wrist. Several sensory nerves may also be symptomatic. The latter are usually painful as a result of injury or compression and often develop a traumatic neuroma. Only syndromes (contusion, stretch, and compression) of the major nerves will be addressed here. For any of these nerves, prolonged localized (thumb-tip) pressure directly over the site of nerve damage will often recapitulate the bothersome symptom complex.

Radial Sensory Nerve. The radial sensory nerve divides into several branches over the radial styloid and is most susceptible to injury in that location. Wartenberg's cheiralgia is due to nerve irritation in this location, usually secondary to compression from cast, splint, or watch band. The condition may be neuropraxic, improving with time, or present a chronic problem due to an intraneural neuroma. Occasionally, the paresthetic pain is quite disabling. A positive Tinel sign or local tenderness related to a palpable nerve is diagnostic.

Similar findings are seen with the dorsal sensory branch of the ulnar nerve, usually where it is in close proximity to the triquetrum, as well as the palmar cutaneous branch of the median nerve between the palmaris longus and flexor carpi radialis; and the terminal thenar branch of the lateral antebrachial cutaneous nerve at the base of the thenar eminence.

A traumatic neuroma of the posterior interosseous nerve as it runs beneath the finger extensors may elicit pain, particularly from wrist flexion. An enlargement (ganglion of nerve) may occur in this location. Tenderness in the scapholunate area is often hard to differentiate and requires further testing.

Median Nerve. The median nerve is susceptible to compression within the carpal canal as a result of a disparity between the cross-sectional area of the canal and its contents. The name "carpal tunnel syndrome" has thus stuck as the descriptive term. Numbness and tingling in the median distribution with nocturnal and use exacerbation are characteristic. Hypohidrosis of the thumb and index finger are common and thenar atrophy is usually seen late. Onset of symptoms within 60 seconds of full wrist flexion was described by Dr. George Phalen as a useful test for establishing the diagnosis and has since borne his name. Reverse Phalen's test in extension, sustained grip test, and 60 seconds of direct pressure at the wrist crease will also frequently elicit the symptoms. A positive Tinel sign is helpful but not diagnostic. Differentiation from other common injury sites, such as cervical root, brachial plexus, and pronator teres causes should be excluded.

Ulnar Nerve. The ulnar nerve is much less frequently involved at the wrist but may be irritated by ganglion, lipoma, or a vascular mass in Guyon's canal. There may also be mechanical aggravation by direct pressure or by the indirect irritation of distal ulnar instability or carpal instability. Ulnar nerve symptoms may be affected by direct pressure between the pisiform and hammulus, or by compressing the nerve against the ulnar head. Weakness of one or more intrinsic muscles requires careful evaluation.

Tumoral and Other Conditions

"Carpe bossu" or carpal bossing is a dorsal protrusion occurring at the second or third carpometacarpal joint. It is usually asymptomatic except for susceptibility to being bumped. It is hard because of an underlying bony protrusion at either side of the joint.

Ganglia occur frequently at the wrist. Dorsoradial ganglia occur commonly from early adolescence to middle age, and are seen more frequently in women but may also be seen in children or the aged (most intratendinous ganglia are in this group). The usual appearance consists of an irregular smooth prominence with a rubbery consistency. Palmar flexion increases the prominence usually at the scapholunate ridge, but occasionally the ganglion presents distal to the scaphotriquetral ligament and may present anywhere over the dorsum of wrist or hand. Pain, if present, occurs at the extremes of flexion and extension, or from direct compression.

Radiopalmar ganglia occur proximal to the scaphoid tuberosity, usually following the tenosynovial sheath of the flexor carpi radialis. Some penetrate the weak capsular area overlying the palmar projecting distal scaphoid; for the rest, the stalk usually proceeds to the ulnar aspect of the scaphotrapeziotrapezoidal joint. Ganglia in this area are irregular, often multilobulated, and in close proximity to the radial artery. They have a feel similar to other ganglia and will transilluminate like most ganglia—except when ruptured, bloody, or subcapsular.

Occasionally, ganglia present at the distal radioulnar joint; within tendons, vascular walls, nerves, or fascia such as the dorsal retinaculum. They may also occur within the various compartments or within the carpal tunnel. These are difficult to detect on physical examination.

Other lumps and bumps include lipomas, xanthomas, rheumatoid nodules, fibromas, keratoacanthomas, inclusion cysts, and osteochondromas. There are rare malignant tumors in the wrist region. These include squamous cell carcinomas, synoviomas, rhabdomyosarcomas, fibrosarcomas, malignant histiocytomas, epithelioid sarcomas, clear-cell sarcomas, and very infrequent bone or joint malignancies. These are usually very firm, fixed, nontender, slowly growing tumors that are difficult to differentiate from some benign tumors and require excisional biopsy, with immediate provision for definitive surgical care.

Vascular Conditions

The radial pulse is readily detected at the palmar aspect of the radial styloid. It may be followed dorsodistally into the snuff box area and the interval between the bases of the first and second metacarpals. In thin individuals, the thenar branch may be detected between the palmar wrist creases running alongside the flexor carpi radialis tendon. On the ulnar side of the wrist, the ulnar artery is often detectable alongside the ulnar aspect of the flexor carpi ulnaris and into Guyon's canal. The deep and superficial arches of the hand are parallel to Kaplan's cardinal line by 1 cm proximally and distally, respectively (see Fig 4–3). On the dorsal aspect of the wrist, the dorsal arch or one of the dorsal metacarpal arteries may be detected along the bases of the second or third metacarpals.

Allen's test, named for Dr. Edgar Allen, assesses the relative contribution to the circulation of the hand from the radial and ulnar arteries. The hand is exsanguinated by having the patient make a firm fist in rapid sequence three times while the examiner has his fingers over the respective arteries at the wrist (Fig 4–7). These are compressed firmly with the last fist formation, and the patient is allowed to open the hand, but in relaxed fashion rather than tautly extended. The latter position interferes with circulatory return in many individuals. The ulnar artery is then released and the flow of arterial blood into the hand is inferred by the pink color return to the palm. If the hand remains blanched longer than 30 seconds, interference of the ulnar circulation may be inferred. The test is repeatable for the radial artery by releasing the radial artery after exsanguination and compression. The use of the hand-held Doppler testing apparatus allows a more thorough evaluation of the superficial arch and its branches with and without testing.

Loss of ulnar arterial filling of the hand suggests occlusions that may occur from thrombosis, previous traumatic interruption, or external compression. A firm, ropelike, tender mass in Guyon's canal may signal thrombosis or a thrombosed aneurysm. The latter is usually larger and the artery convoluted; characteristic sounds are noted on auscultation. A history of using the palm to strike objects, "hypothenar hammer," or the use of vibrating implements is often elicited. Heavy smoking is also often implicated in patients with this problem.

There is occasionally a strong urge to rely on roentgenograms for definitive diagnosis at the wrist. Most of the conditions described above would be overlooked with this stratagem. Conversely, a careful, thorough physical examination may suggest specific roentgenologic views or techniques that will help to

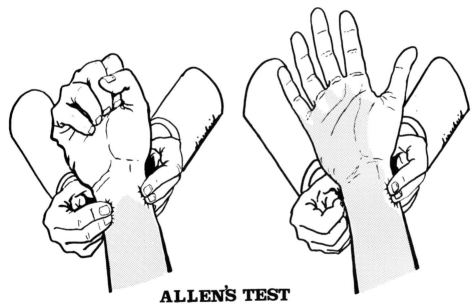

ALLEN'S TEST

FIG 4–7. Allen's test is to assess relative blood flow into hand between the radial and ulnar artery, and to assess patency of the arteries.

establish diagnoses. Occasionally injections of local anesthetic such as lidocaine into a specific area, with prompt pain relief, will also aid diagnosis. This must be done with anatomical certainty to be of real value. Nothing suffices for improved performance in physical diagnosis more than repetition.

Bibliography

1. Allen EV: Thromboangiitis obliterans: Methods of diagnosis of chronic occlusive arterial leisons distal to the wrist with illustrative cases. *Am J Med Sci* 1929; 178:237–244.
2. de Quervain F: *Clinical Surgical Diagnosis for Students and Practitioners,* ed 4, Snowman J (trans). New York, William Wood and Company, 1913.
3. Finkelstein H: Stenosing tenovaginitis at the radial styloid process. *J Bone Joint Surg* 1930; 12:509–540.
4. Fiolle J: Le 'Carpe Bossu.' *Bull Mem Soc Nat Chir* 1931; 57:1687–1690.
5. Kaplan EB: *Functional and Surgical Anatomy of the Hand,* ed 2. Philadelphia, JB Lippincott Co, 1965.
6. Linburg RM, Comstock BE: Anomalous tendon slips from the flexor pollicis longus to the flexor digitorum profundus. *J Hand Surg* 1979; 4:79–83.
7. Phalen GS: The carpal tunnel syndrome: 17 years experience in diagnosis and treatment of 654 hands. *J Bone Joint Surg* 1966; 48-A:211–228.
8. Tinel J: *Nerve wounds: Symptomatology of peripheral nerve lesions caused by war wounds,* Joll CA (ed), Rothwell F (trans). New York, William Wood and Co, 1918.

CHAPTER 5

Functional and Physical Examination of the Hand

Michael Jablon, M.D.
Harold E. Kleinert, M.D.

The hand may reflect a disease process that exists elsewhere in the body. Because the hand is the distal functional end of the upper extremity, a basic knowledge of the neuromusculoskeletal system of the entire upper extremity is necessary in order to perform a meaningful physical examination. A complete examination of the hand must integrate the local anatomy with its normal function.

History

The setting in which the history is taken may determine its completeness. An interested and sincere expression of concern for the patient is necessary to establish a good rapport with the patient, which is essential to the physical examination. The details of the history may vary according to the complexity of the injury. A brief history is sufficient for a simple laceration whereas a more exacting one will be necessary for more complicated injuries and diseases. Important recorded data should include the age of the patient, dominant hand, sex, and occupation, as well as any important avocations. Any previous hand injuries or surgical procedures should be noted.

Always and especially when dealing with work-related injuries, it is necessary to record the time of injury, the time that has elapsed since the injury, and if any previous treatment has been administered. Knowing the precise mechanism of injury is important to accurately evaluate the amount of crushing and blood loss, while information on the position of the hand at the time of injury can supply the physician with information useful in determining the level of injury to the gliding parts of the hand. The nature of the injury; whether burning occurred, either electrical, thermal, or chemical; and if the wound was contaminated in an industrial setting or in a dirty environment, such as with soil in a farm accident, should be determined.

In nontraumatic cases, it is necessary to establish when the patient first noted the pain, sensory change, swelling, or contractures. Ask the patient if the hand problem impairs occupational performance or limits any activities of daily living, and if there are any specific activities that accentuate the problem. Establishing the time of day or night when the patient experiences more pain is helpful in determining if specific activities are aggravating the patient's problem. If joints or tendons in other extremities are similarly affected a more generalized disease process is probable.

When thoracic outlet syndrome and brachial plexus injuries are being evaluated, one should record the impaired dermatome distribution in the upper extremity, as this will help pinpoint lesions, such as those of a cervical disk, brachial plexus, or thoracic outlet compression.

A general assessment of the medical condition of the patient is necessary since common problems such as myocardial disease may lead to hand and arm pain, or diabetes may lead to peripheral neuropathy. A brief social and family history should be taken. The family history is especially important in congenital abnormalities.

Physical Examination

The examination of a patient in the emergency room differs markedly, in scope and detail, from one done in the office. Information obtained in the emergency room will determine if the patient will require immediate surgical intervention or not. It is essential to record both those hand functions that are present as well as those that are absent to accurately determine a plan for treatment. Proper timing of the examination is essential for accurate information. For example, sensation must be mapped in the case of a finger laceration before local anesthesia is applied. However, all physical examinations must include a thorough assessment of the skin, vascular system, neurologic system, bones, joints, tendons and ligaments, motor function, and other common clinical conditions as applicable.

In order to perform a complete physical examination, the entire upper extremity of the involved hand and the cervical spine should be evaluated. The opposite hand and upper extremity are used for comparison. Therefore, the patient should be undressed to the waist at the time of the examination.

The chief goal of the hand surgeon is to restore normal form and function to the hand, which includes the basic postural functions such as pinch, hook, and grasp. It is important to remember that the hand, like the face, is exposed, and therefore, cosmetic and psychological results should be considered.

In order to confirm a suspected diagnosis, electromyography and nerve-conduction velocity studies may be necessary to verify nerve function. During the first interview, observation of the hand provides important information about the postural integrity of the hand, as well as about the condition of the skin. Because form and function are interrelated, any disruption of either will lead to dysfunction.

The Skin

Inspection and Palpation

The skin is examined for color and consistency (Fig 5–1). Comparison with the other extremity is useful. Normal circulation is indicated by normal warmth and color. Trophic changes such as tight shiny skin often accompany vascular

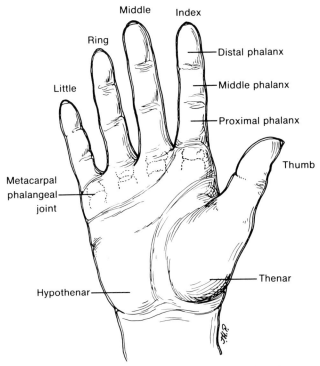

FIG 5–1. Volar surface anatomy of the hand.

and neurologic disorders. Loss of hair suggests that circulation is inadequate, while increase in hair growth is associated with sympathetic dystrophy. The lack of nerve supply will alter the normal pattern of perspiration. The skin is a good monitor of the degree of hydration.

There is no "extra" skin found on the palmar aspect of the hand. Any significant skin loss will lead to contractures and loss of function with a corresponding decrease in the range of motion at the joint closest to the loss of skin. Skin on the dorsal aspect of the hand may be pinched and elevated when the fingers are extended. Normally, this skin will immediately resume its original shape. In conditions of illness, dehydration, or senility, the skin remains wrinkled. The glabrous palmar skin is thickened and fixed by the longitudinal bands of the palmar fascia. It may be reasoned that the thick palmar fascia enables man to firmly grasp tools and other objects because it prevents the skin from moving or slipping. Contractures in the palmar skin may be due to palmar fibromatosis from scars or Dupuytren's disease. Thus, when examining the range of motion, it is important to note the presence of any underlying cords or dimples in the palmar skin.

All scars should be noted as to their healing characteristics (i.e., keloid), orientation, length, and any associated restriction of motion. Scars appropriately oriented along the lines of tension, or Langer's lines will not interfere with the normal pattern of motion. Knowledge of the lines of tension is essential in planning elective surgical skin incisions.

Skin lesions and their size and consistency should be recorded. Characteristics such as whether the lesion is raised or recessed, pigmented or hair bearing, or tender or painful to palpation need to be recorded during the examination. Determining if the lesion is limited to the skin or if there is a mass beneath the skin; whether it is firm, soft, or fluctuant; and if the lesion moves with motion of the hand or fingers, helps to establish a working diagnosis. For example, a ganglion on the dorsum of the wrist may be confused with a dorsal tenosynovitis; however, evaluation of size, location, diffuseness, and motion can differentiate the two diagnoses. The ganglion will not move with the flexion and extension of the fingers; however, the tenosynovitic tissue will.

Skin Injuries

Lacerations are often classified as "tidy" and "untidy" wounds. The care of a tidy wound that has minimal or no devitalized tissue differs from the care of untidy, devitalized, contaminated tissue. Burns are classified by their depth and degree of involved tissue. A first-degree burn involves the superficial skin layer and is characterized by erythema. A second-degree burn blisters the skin. Third-degree burns involve full-thickness skin and are usually less painful since nerve endings are destroyed. Fourth-degree burns extend beyond the skin, damaging the deeper tissues.

Vascular Examination

The ulnar and radial arteries provide an excellent blood supply to the hand through the palmar arches. The superficial palmar arch is supplied by the ulnar artery. It contributes the major part of the circulation to the ulnar digits. The deep arch through the radial artery is the principal supply of blood to the thumb. Patency may be interrupted by thromboembolic disease, vascular occlusive disease or vessel injury of the palmar arches.

The Allen test (Fig 5–2) is used to assess vascular competence. First the patient is told to "make a fist," which exsanguinates the hand, causing blanching of the skin. Then the physician occludes both the radial and ulnar arterial pulses with digital pressure applied at the wrist. The patient then opens his hand and allows it to relax. Thereafter, one artery is released and the digits are observed for return of the normal vascular blush. The return of normal color will be abnormally slow or absent in all or some of the digits if there is an incomplete arch or vascular system. The test is then repeated releasing the other artery. The uninjured hand should also be checked for comparison.

A digital Allen test is used to assess vascular competence in the fingers. It is performed by "milking" the blood out of the involved digit, which is held outstretched by the examiner. The test is conducted by simultaneously kneading the finger in a distal to proximal direction along both neurovascular bundles. While pressure is maintained on the ulnar digital artery, it is released from the radial digital artery. The vascular refill of the digit is observed. The test is repeated, maintaining pressure on the radial digital artery while releasing pressure on the ulnar digital artery. Often, with lacerations of the volar aspect of a digit, injury to one of the digital arteries may go unrecognized if not specifically tested for. All patients with lacerations on the volar surface of a finger should be carefully tested for injuries of the digital nerves and arteries.

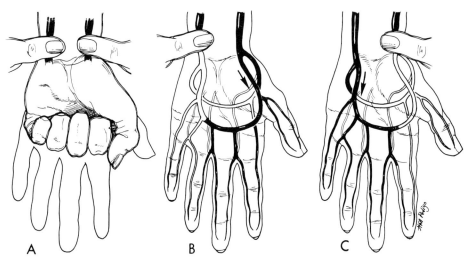

FIG 5–2. Allen test to assess vascular competence.

Vascular disease is manifested by cold intolerance, trophic change, or loss of normal hair growth. If the Allen test reveals an intact, functioning palmar arch, when findings consistent with vascular disease are present, then a proximal lesion should be considered. For example, vascular compromise may be associated with compression of the axillary artery in thoracic outlet syndrome.

The hypothenar hammer syndrome is thrombosis of the ulnar artery, which can be diagnosed by the Allen test. Occlusion of the ulnar artery will be apparent as no blood flow into the hand will occur through the thrombosed ulnar artery. Symptoms may be noted especially in the little finger. The possibility of more proximal vascular disease should be remembered. Venous obstruction, especially proximal, may lead to generalized edema in the upper extremity and hand. Thrills may be palpable and bruits may be ausculted. An additional tool that can be used in the diagnosis of venous obstruction is the Doppler flow instrument, which assesses and localizes vessel blood flow.

Neurologic Examination

The general sensory examination is probably the most subjective and least quantifiable aspect of the physical examination. The two-point discrimination (Fig 5–3) is widely used in determining the presence and extent of nerve dysfunction in the hand and digits. A bent paper clip or a caliper is used for this test. The patient is asked not to watch as the physician tests the pulp of each digit on both the ulnar and radial aspects, by lightly touching the area with both of the points of the paper clip or caliper. The patient is asked to report whether he feels one or two points of pressure. The ability to feel two points spaced approximately 4 mm apart is considered normal at the fingertips.

A "moving" two-point discrimination test is performed by slightly moving the points when touching the skin. This test is more sensitive and most patients will be able to discriminate two points that are 4 mm apart.

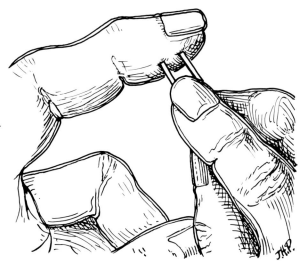

FIG 5–3. Two-point discrimination tested with a paper clip.

Tinel's sign is the shocklike sensation elicited when the examiner taps the extremity over a sensitive nerve. Striking the "funny bone" at the medial side of the elbow is actually a Tinel's sign that occurs when the ulnar nerve is struck at the level of the proximal medial epicondyle of the humerus. The Tinel sign is used to assess neurologic dysfunction. Peripheral nerves involved in compression neuropathies are sensitive when struck over the joint of compression. For example, tapping over the volar part of the wrist (Fig 5–4) in a patient with a carpal tunnel syndrome will lead to an electric shocklike sensation at the distribution of that nerve. After a laceration of a nerve, or nerve repair, the Tinel test may be used as one of the signs indicating healing. Healing progresses at the rate of approximately 1 mm per day after the completion of wallerian degeneration. Tinel's sign is a sensitive guide in that it advances along with the leading edge of the healing nerve. If regrowth is not occurring, the Tinel sign will remain at the same level, whereas advancement of the Tinel sign corresponds to nerve regeneration. Therefore, accurate measurements and recordings of the Tinel sign are essential to proper evaluation of nerve regeneration.

Electromyographic and nerve-conduction velocity tests are also useful in the analysis of nerve function. These tests are adjuncts to the physical examination and are helpful in differentiating nerve lesions and their locations.

Three peripheral nerves (Fig 5–5) innervate the hand; the ulnar nerve, the median nerve, and the radial nerve. Entrapment or compression of these nerves may occur at various points in their course through the arm to the hand.

The ulnar nerve is responsible for the innervation of the muscles and skin on the ulnar side of the forearm and hand. It enters the forearm through the cubital tunnel, around the medial epicondyle of the humerus. This is a common site of nerve compression. The nerve then enters the hand through Guyon's canal at the wrist. On entering the hand, the ulnar nerve divides into sensory digital branches that innervate the little finger and the ulnar half of the ring finger, and the motor branch. The dorsal cutaneous branch of this nerve supplies sensibility to the dorsal aspect of the hand over the little and ring metacarpals, the dorsum of the little finger, and the dorsoulnar half of the ring finger.

Ulnar nerve sensory function is tested by examining the cutaneous sensory area on the pad over the little fingertip, since this area is totally supplied by this nerve.

The following muscles are innervated by the ulnar nerve: the palmaris brevis, the hypothenar muscles, the seven interosseous muscles, the two ulnar lumbrical muscles, and the adductor pollicis. The flexor pollicis brevis may also be partially or totally innervated by this nerve.

Compression of the ulnar nerve leads to paresthesias and motor abnormalities in the hand. The finely balanced motor function of the hand depends on ulnar nerve innervation of the intrinsic muscles that stabilize the metacarpophalangeal joints, providing the balance against the pull of the extrinsic flexors and extensors, preventing an ulnar claw posture. The intrinsic muscles abduct the fingers from the "fixed" long finger, and act as metacarpophalangeal joint flexors and interphalangeal joint extensors. Motor function is evaluated by the patient's ability to abduct, and then adduct the fingers, especially the little finger. A quick examination to determine ulnar nerve injury at the level of the wrist involves testing of the flexor digiti minimi. The patient is asked to raise the small finger vertically, flexing the metacarpophalangeal joint to 90° while maintaining the hand flat, with the palm up and the interphalangeal joints straightened. The patient will be unable to perform this task if there is a lesion to the ulnar nerve.

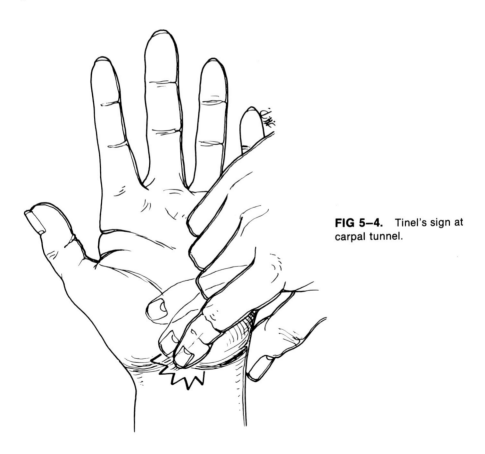

FIG 5–4. Tinel's sign at carpal tunnel.

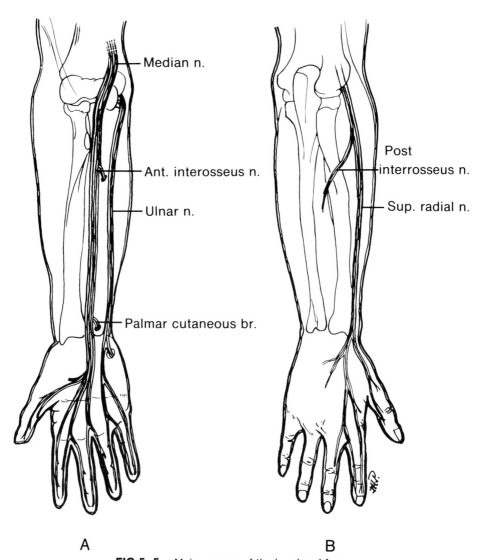

FIG 5–5. Major nerves of the hand and forearm.

Froment's paper sign tests the motor function of the branch of the ulnar nerve that innervates the thumb adductors. The patient is told to secure a piece of paper, which is placed between the thumb and the radial side of the index finger, while the examiner pulls on it. If the patient flexes the interphalangeal joint of the thumb and fails to hold the paper, the test is considered positive for an ulnar lesion. In this event, the flexor pollicis longus overpowers the interphalangeal extensors, which have been weakened by the absence of the adductor pollicis.

The median nerve innervates the radial side of the flexor portion of the forearm and hand. It enters the forearm, piercing the two heads of the pronator muscle. It then enters the hand through the carpal tunnel, after which it branches several times, innervating the volar surface of the thumb, the dorsal and volar surfaces of the index and middle fingers, and the radial side of the ring finger.

The following muscles are innervated by the median nerve: the abductor pollicis brevis, the opponens pollicis, the two radial lumbricals, and the superficial head of the flexor pollicis brevis.

Compression of the median nerve at the wrist is called carpal tunnel syndrome. Phalen's test, which is performed by allowing the wrist to fall into complete volar flexion for one minute, aids in the diagnosis of a carpal tunnel syndrome by accentuating the compression symptoms of the median nerve. In carpal tunnel syndrome the thenar muscles may atrophy and diminish abductor pollicis brevis function (loss of palmar abduction).

The pronator teres syndrome represents a compression neuropathy of the median nerve in the proximal forearm. This condition resembles the carpal tunnel syndrome; however, numbness occurs in the palm because of involvement of the palmar cutaneous nerve. The pronator test may elicit these symptoms if it is conducted by holding the patient's hand and resisting an effort to pronate the forearm, with the elbow extended.

Knowledge of the sensory distribution of the palmar cutaneous nerve, a branch of the median nerve, will aid in establishing the site of median nerve entrapment. The palmar cutaneous nerve innervates the central portion of the palm and does not pass through the carpal tunnel. Loss of sensation in the distribution of this nerve indicates a lesion of the medial nerve at a site more proximal than the carpal tunnel.

Median nerve integrity can be determined by asking the patient to flex the distal phalanx of the index finger. The patient's inability to perform this movement indicates injury to the median nerve above the level of innervation of the flexor digitorum profundus.

The motor nerves, such as the anterior interosseous nerve, branches from the median nerve at the level of the pronator teres in the proximal forearm. This nerve innervates the flexor digitorum profundus to the index and long fingers, the flexor pollicis longus, and the pronator quadratus. Compression of the anterior interosseous nerve will result in a weakened pinch since active flexion is lost at the thumb interphalangeal joint and the index and long-finger interphalangeal joints. Tenderness may or may not be present in the proximal volar forearm. When the recurrent motor branch of the median nerve is affected in the carpal tunnel syndrome, the thenar muscles may be atrophied. With advanced compression, there may be an absence of abductor (rheumatoid arthritis).

The radial nerve enters the forearm by passing directly over the anterior ligament at the articulation between the capitulum of the humerus and the head of the radius. It then enters the hand and the thumb dorsally.

The radial nerve does not innervate any intrinsic muscles of the hand. Its important motor function is to innervate the muscles of the forearm necessary for extension of the wrist and metacarpophalangeal joints.

The posterior interosseous nerve is the motor branch of the radial nerve that arises at the level of the supinator muscle at the arcade of Froshe. It innervates all the dorsal forearm muscles except the brachio radialis, extensor carpi radialis longus, and occasionally, the extensor carpi radialis brevis. Neurologic dysfunction must be distinguished from other causes of loss of digital extension. If a Tinel sign is present at the level of the arcade of Froshe, the diagnosis of compression at that site can be made. Another cause for loss of finger extension includes attrition ruptures of the extensor tendons.

When weakness or a loss of extension is due to neurologic compression, the supinator test may be positive. This test is conducted as the patient with the elbow extended attempts to supinate the forearm against resistance by the examiner. This test is positive if pain is produced over the radial nerve distribution of the hand. Weakness in the extensors may be produced at the level of the arcade of Froshe. This condition is frequently confused with and accompanied by signs of tennis elbow. With radial epicondylitis, or tennis elbow, maximum tenderness occurs over the epicondyle, whereas with posterior interosseous nerve compression, maximum tenderness is between the fixed and mobile muscle wads (short forearm muscles and long, i.e., brachio radialis, and radial wrist extensor muscles).

Bones

The hand is composed of 27 bones which are divided into three groups: the carpus, the metacarpus, and the phalanges (Fig 5–6).

The bony structure of the wrist is based on the eight carpal bones that lie in two rows, called the proximal and distal carpal rows. The bones of the proximal carpal row, starting from the radial side, are called the scaphoid, lunate, triquetrum, and pisiform bones. The bones of the distal carpal row, from radial to ulnar side, are the trapezium, trapezoid, capitate, and hamate bones.

The first metacarpal and trapezium are uniquely articulated to form what is sometimes referred to as a "saddle joint." The architecture of this joint allows for the wide range of thumb motion.

The second and third metacarpals, which make up the bases of the index and middle fingers, are firmly attached to the distal carpal row rendering them immobile. This fixation provides the stability needed for the pinch mechanism and other fine movements of the hand.

The fourth and fifth metacarpals, which make up the bases of the ring and little fingers, are mobile. This mobility provides the necessary range of motion, allowing the ulnar side of the palm to adapt and close around various shaped objects supplying the grasp mechanism of the hand.

There are 14 phalanges in each hand, two in each thumb and three in each finger. The interarticulations of these phalanges, called the proximal and distal interphalangeal joints, are mobile.

Clinical examination of the skeletal system with regards to pain when pressure is applied, crepitation, or swelling, can aid in the evaluation of the hand; however, roentgenograms are essential in supplying more complete information.

Lateral films of the hand should be taken with the fingers separated to avoid superimposition of fingers on the roentgenogram. Special views of the carpal tunnel help evaluate the carpal tunnel and the hook of the hamate. Scaphoid views with radial and ulnar deviation of the hand aid in the evaluation of this commonly injured carpal bone. Brewerton views are used to evaluate the metacarpophalangeal joint, especially in the rheumatoid arthritic hand. These views are taken by positioning the hand at an angle to the anteroposterior plane. Before

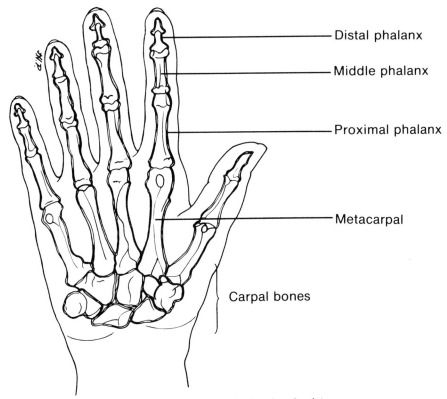

Distal phalanx

Middle phalanx

Proximal phalanx

Metacarpal

Carpal bones

FIG 5–6. Bones of the hand and wrist.

reducing a dislocation or fracture, roentgenograms should be studied to completely evaluate the pathology.

Bone deformity may represent an acute injury, malunion from a previous injury, the presence of a bone lesion, or the result of a growth disturbance. Common bone lesions in the hand include enchondroma bone cysts, osteochondromas, osteoid osteomas, and giant cell tumors. Malignant tumors are rare, but may show up as metastatic bone tumors.

Joints

Examination of the joints of the hand includes the measurement and recording of the ranges of motion of each joint. A chart is drawn to record extension and flexion at each joint. By convention, neutral or 0° describes full extension of the hand. Lack of extension is recorded in negative degrees. When passive motions exceed active motions, the range of passive motion is recorded in parentheses. The long finger is a reference point, and motion of the other fingers away from this finger either on its radial or ulnar side represents abduction, while motion towards the long finger is considered adduction.

Normal joint function is essential for a normal range of motion. It must be kept in mind that normal joint motion from a functional standpoint is dependent on many factors, including: intact and supple skin, normal joint architecture, ligaments and underlying bone structures, and intact gliding tendons with normally innervated functioning muscles. An abnormality in any one of these structures can result in restricted motion.

Movements to be examined in order to determine limitation in wrist function are flexion and extension, radial and ulnar deviation, and supination and pronation of the forearm. Flexion to about 80°, and extension to about 70° from the neutral or straight position is considered normal.

To test ulnar and radial deviation, the patient is asked to extend his hand in the neutral position and move it from side to side. Since the ulna does not extend distally as far as the radius, and it is not articulated to the carpal bones, the range of ulnar deviation is greater. Normal ulnar deviation ranges to approximately 30°, while radial deviation ranges to approximately 20°.

Supination and pronation of the forearm are limited by the amount of rotation of the radius around the ulnar. Problems occurring at the elbow or in the radioulnar articulation of the wrist can limit such rotation. To test the range of supination and pronation, the patient is told to flex his elbow to 90°, securing his elbow at the waist. This prevents him from using shoulder adduction and flexion during this test. For supination, the patient starts with his palm facing downward. He is asked to secure a pencil and rotate his hand until his palm is facing upward. The pencil should be parallel to the floor at the start and finish of the test. To test pronation, the patient starts with his palm upward and grasping the pencil, rotates his hand until the palm is facing downward. The normal range of motion for supination and pronation is 180°, and any limitation of this range suggests pathology at the elbow, in the forearm, or at the radioulnar joint in the wrist.

The ranges of motion to be tested in the fingers are: flexion and extension of the metacarpophalangeal and interphalangeal joints of the fingers; finger adduction and abduction at the metacarpophalangeal joints; flexion and extension of the thumb at the metacarpophalangeal and interphalangeal joints; thumb adduction and abduction; and opposition.

The test for finger flexion and extension is performed by having the patient make a fist and then having him slowly extend his fingers. In flexion, the fingers should move uniformly into a fist, resting near the distal palmar crease in the palm. In normal extension, the fingers should move uniformly into or past the neutral or straight position. Observations should be made as to whether or not the patient has difficulty performing these movements with any of his fingers.

Abduction and adduction of the fingers are tested by asking the patient to spread his fingers apart and then to bring them back together again. In normal abduction, the distance between each finger should measure about 20°. In normal adduction, the fingers should close until touching.

Thumb flexion at the metacarpophalangeal and interphalangeal joint, or transpalmar abduction, is tested by having the patient open his hand, palm up, and touch the base of his little finger with his thumb. In the test for thumb extension, or radial abduction, the patient starts with his palm up, fingers together, and then moves his thumb horizontally away from his fingers. The extension is measured by the angle between his thumb and index finger, normal being approximately 50°.

Palmar abduction is the measurement of the angle between the index finger and the thumb when the thumb is moved vertically away from the index finger while the hand is opened and extended with the palm up. A normal angle for this test is approximately 70°. Bringing the thumb back in approximation with the index finger demonstrates palmar adduction. Opposition is performed by asking the patient to touch his thumb to the tips of each of his fingers, especially the little finger.

The ligamentous integrity of each joint should be tested. The radial and ulnar collateral ligaments maintain joint stability. The ligaments should be tested with the interphalangeal joints both in extension and flexion (Fig 5–7).

The ligamentous stability at the metacarpophalangeal joints should be tested in flexion when the collateral ligaments are normally taut. Instability in hyperextension usually indicates an injury to the volar plate, which restrains the joint. If the history suggests a dislocation, then roentgenograms should be obtained to evaluate the possibility of any intra-articular or small avulsion fractures.

Painful joint motion may be indicative of other abnormal conditions. Flexor tendon injuries, fractures, and ligamentous injuries must be investigated. If painful joint motion is associated with swelling and inflammation, then an infectious process must be distinguished from an arthritic condition. Joint swelling accompanied by exquisite tenderness with any motion favors the diagnosis of pyarthrosis. Suppurative tenosynovitis is associated with Knavel's cardinal physical findings, which are joint flexion and fusiform swelling of the digit, tenderness on passive extension and to palpation over the flexor sheath (Fig 5–8), and warmth and erythema in the finger.

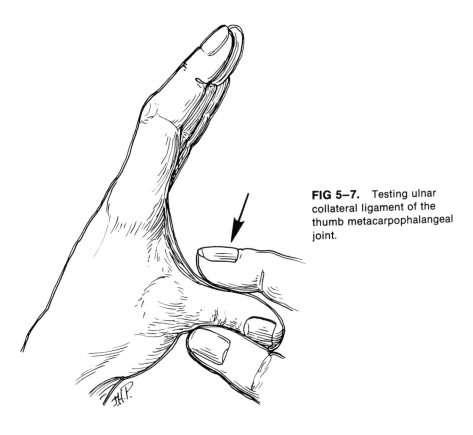

FIG 5–7. Testing ulnar collateral ligament of the thumb metacarpophalangeal joint.

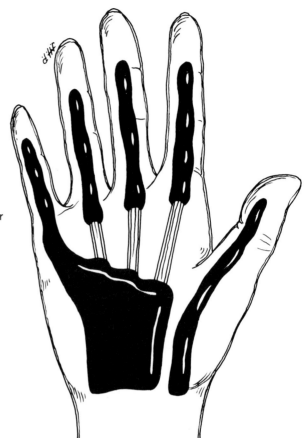

FIG 5–8. Location of flexor tendon sheaths.

Arthritides

Degenerative osteoarthritis may cause deformity and limited painful joint motion. Osteoarthritis is commonly associated with joint swelling at the distal interphalangeal joints (Heberden's nodes) or at the proximal interphalangeal joints (Bouchard's nodes). Roentgenograms show a characteristic loss of the joint space, which is due to the loss of articular cartilage. In rheumatoid arthritis, demineralized bone is associated with subchondral cysts and bone erosion. Swelling in the arthritic joints is caused by synovitis, and boggy synovium may be fluctuant to palpation.

Pain at the carpometacarpal joint may denote osteoarthritis, which must be distinguished from de Quervain's tenosynovitis. The torque or grind test, which is performed by compressing the carpometacarpal joint and gently rotating the proximal phalanx, will elicit pain in osteoarthritic joints. In de Quervain's tenosynovitis, pain radiates along the dorsal and radial aspect of the thumb, across the radial aspect of the wrist, and sometimes into the forearm when the thumb is clasped in the palm and the hand is ulnarly deviated (Finkelstein's test, Fig 5–9).

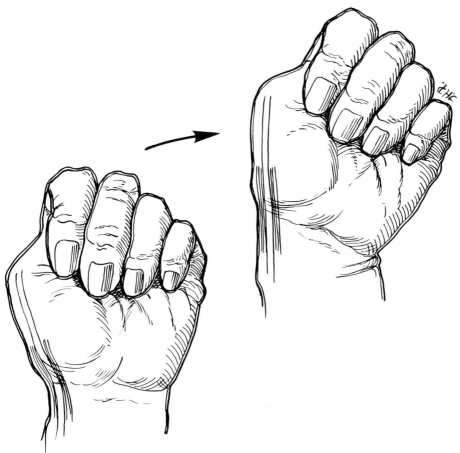

FIG 5–9. Finkelstein's test, ulnar deviation causing pain—for de Quervain's tenosynovitis.

Calcific Tendinitis

A less common cause of painful joint motion may be associated with erythema and swelling, which can be diagnosed by the presence of an amorphous calcified density near a joint on the roentgenogram.

Muscles and Tendons

A careful examination of the muscles and tendons of the hand depends on a thorough knowledge of the anatomy. The muscles of the hand are customarily divided into extrinsic muscles or intrinsic, depending on their origins and insertions. Extrinsic muscles have their origins in the forearm and their insertions in the hand, while intrinsic muscles have their origins and insertions in the hand.

The extrinsic muscles can be further divided into extensors or flexors. The extension tendons run along the dorsum of the forearm entering the hand along

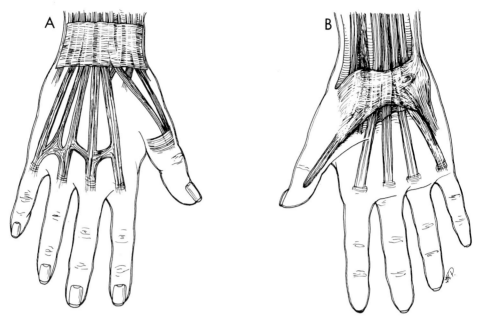

FIG 5–10. Flexor and extensor tendons at the wrist.

the back and lateral side of the wrist (Fig 5–10). They are held in place within the bony grooves by transverse fibrous bands called the extensor retinaculum. Fibrous partitions divide this retinaculum into six compartments that house the nine extensor tendons.

The first dorsal compartment of the wrist contains the tendons of the abductor pollicis longus and the extensor pollicis brevis. The abductor pollicis longus inserts at the base of the first metacarpal, on its radial side. It is responsible for the abduction of the thumb. Continued action causes the abduction of the wrist. The extensor pollicis brevis inserts at the base of the first phalanx of the thumb and is required for extension of the phalanx. Continued action also contributes to abduction of the wrist. Evaluation of these two tendons is done by asking the patient to extend his thumb. The taut tendons can be palpated on the radial side of the wrist.

The second dorsal compartment of the wrist contains the extensor carpi radialis longus, which inserts at the base of the index metacarpal, and the extensor carpi radialis brevis, which inserts at the base of the third metacarpal. Radial wrist extensor tendons (extensor carpi radialis longus and extensor carpi radialis brevis) are responsible for extension and abduction of the hand. These tendons can be palpated when the patient makes a fist, simultaneously bringing his hand into extreme flexion or extension.

The extensor digitorum communis tendons and the extensor indicis proprious tendon pass through the fourth compartment of the extensor retinaculum. The extensor digitorum inserts at the level of the metacarpophalangeal joint to the extensor hood of the fingers. The extensor indicis inserts on the ulnar side of the extensor digitorum of the index finger. These tendons are solely responsible for extension of the metacarpophalangeal joints of the fingers. These muscles are tested by having the patient extend his fingers.

The fifth compartment of the extensor retinaculum contains the extensor digiti minimi. Beyond the wrist, this tendon branches in two and joins the expansion of the extensor digitorum on the dorsum of the proximal phalanx of the little finger. It is responsible for little finger extension and can be tested by asking the patient to straighten his little finger alone.

The sixth dorsal compartment houses the extensor carpi ulnaris. The point of insertion of this tendon is at the base of the fifth metacarpal. Its action is necessary for extension and adduction of the hand and can be palpated when the hand is held in adduction.

The extensor muscles of the forearm are innervated by the radial nerve. The four most superficial flexor tendons are the pronator teres, the flexor carpi radialis, the palmaris longus, and the flexor carpi ulnaris.

The pronator teres lies on the flexor surface of the forearm, originating at two heads, the humeral and the ulnar. Insertion is on the lateral surface of the body of the radius. Contraction of this muscle results in pronation of the hand. It is innervated by the branch of the median nerve.

The flexor carpi radialis inserts at the base of the second metacarpal bone, sending a slip to the base of the third metacarpal. The palmaris longus inserts onto the central part of the flexor retinaculum and the palmar aponeurosis, or palmar fascia. The flexor carpi ulnaris inserts at the pisiform bone. These tendons are all inserted on the relatively fixed wrist bones, not the mobile ones and are responsible for the flexion of the wrist, while the flexor carpi ulnaris plays an important role in wrist adduction, acting in conjunction with the extensor carpi ulnaris. The flexor carpi radialis and the palmaris longus are innervated by a branch of the median nerve, while the flexor carpi ulnaris is innervated by a branch of the ulnar nerve. These tendons can be palpated when the patient flexes his wrist.

Just below these muscles, in a middle layer, lies the flexor digitorum superficialis. It is the largest of these superficial flexors, dividing in its course through the hand, finally supplying two slips that insert on the sides of the middle phalanx of each finger. Flexion of the fingers at the proximal interphalangeal joint is controlled by this tendon. The examiner can test for each tendon by holding adjacent fingers in extension (Fig 5–11), and asking the patient to bend his middle joint. This tendon is innervated by a branch of the median nerve.

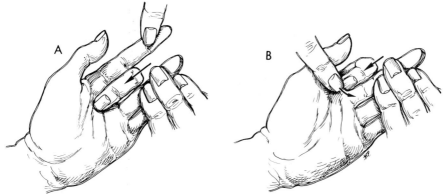

FIG 5–11. Testing for function of the superficialis tendons. Note that distal interphalangeal joint of index finger must be lax to test for superficialis tendon function of index.

In the deep layers of the forearm lie the flexor digitorum profundus and the flexor pollicis longus muscles. The flexor digitorum profundus tendons insert into the bases of the distal phalanges of the fingers, while the flexor pollicis longus inserts into the base of the distal phalanx of the thumb. These tendons are responsible for the flexion of the distal phalanges of the fingers and thumb and can be tested by securing the fingers in extension at the proximal interphalangeal joint and asking the patient to bend the tip of his fingers or thumb (Fig 5–12). These tendons (for thumb, index, and middle fingers) are innervated by the anterior interosseous nerve, which is a branch of the median nerve.

The intrinsic muscles of the hand can be divided into the thenar muscles, the adductor pollicis, the hypothenar muscles, the lumbricals, and the interossei muscles.

The thenar muscle group is made up of the abductor pollicis brevis, opponens pollicis, and the flexor pollicis brevis. These muscles act on the thumb at the metacarpal and proximal phalanges and are responsible for abducting and flexing, or opposition of, the thumb. They can be tested by asking the patient to touch the tip of his little finger with his thumb. They can also be tested by having the patient perform palmar abduction and palpating the muscle group. This muscle group is usually innervated by the motor branch of the median nerve; however, in some patients it is possible that the ulnar nerve is also involved in its

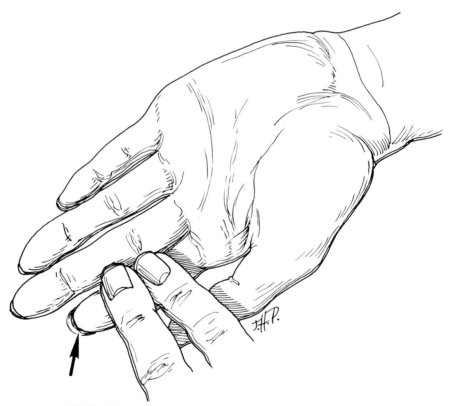

FIG 5–12. Testing flexor digitorum profundus tendon function.

innervation. It is important to test the uninvolved hand for any deviations in these muscles.

The adductor pollicis divides into two slips that insert at the proximal phalanx of the thumb. Because this muscle is innervated by the ulnar nerve, it can be evaluated using the Froment paper test, previously described.

The hypothenar muscle group is composed of the abductor digiti minimi, flexor digiti minimi, and the opponens digiti minimi. These muscles are necessary for abduction and flexion of the little finger. They act together, allowing the patient to move his little finger away from his hand. A branch of the ulnar nerve is responsible for innervation of these muscles.

Four intrinsic muscles associated with the tendons of the flexor digitorum profundus are called the lumbricals. They insert into the extensor digitorum, by way of the radial lateral bands of each finger, and are responsible for flexing the metacarpophalangeal joints and extending the interphalangeal joints. The lumbricals of the index and middle fingers are innervated by branches of the median nerve in the palm, while the lumbricals of the ring and little fingers are innervated by branches of the ulnar nerve in the palm.

A set of muscles that occupy the intervals between the metacarpals make up the interosseous muscle group. Adduction and abduction of the fingers is the result of the action of these muscles. If contraction occurs when the first dorsal interosseous muscle is palpated with the fingers spread, this group is intact. Another test can be performed by asking the patient to lift his middle finger and move it from side to side while keeping his hand, palm down, flat on a table. These muscles are innervated by motor branches of the ulnar nerve.

Intrinsic tightness of the finger may cause the proximal interphalangeal joint to be limited in extension. The severity of radial and ulnar intrinsic tightness can be differentiated by deviating the examined digit radial and ulnarward.

The fibrous tendon sheaths, which are strong ligamentous tunnels surrounding the tendons, maintain the gliding mechanism of the fingers. If a finger triggers, or clicks, wherein the patient may actively flex, but is unable to actively extend his finger, he may be afflicted with a stenosing tenosynovitis, or trigger finger. This condition is related to a localized constriction of the lumen of the tendon sheath, and swelling about the tendon.

A volar laceration that results in a straight finger that is not in line with the normally flexed posture of adjacent fingers when the extremity is relaxed, is indicative of flexor tendon injury. Partial laceration may be determined by decreased muscle tone when gentle pressure is applied against the involved fingertips. The presence of pain on attempted flexion is a result of blood in the sheath.

The forces of extension should be balanced by the forces of flexion at each joint. When the imbalance occurs secondary to tendon laceration, or any other reason, the posture of the hand or fingers changes. The normal tone and balance of the extensor and flexors allows for passive flexion and extension of the fingers with motion only at the wrist. This is called the "tenodesis effect." When the wrist is extended, the tension in the resting flexors increases, and the digits flex down to the palm. Conversely, with wrist flexion, the flexors are relaxed and the relative tension in the extensors increases, extending the digits. This principle is essential in tendon transfers and other reconstructive procedures to restore function for nerve paralysis. For example, the tenodesis effect can be augmented to maximize grasp and release in the quadriplegic patient by using available motors to power the wrist extensor while tethering the flexor tendons.

Keeping this concept of the tenodesis effect in mind when examining the hand, it is useful to observe finger position relative to wrist position.

Postural Deformities

Loss of balance combined with loss of motion leads to joint contractures in the hand. Motion is crucial for the hand because it is necessary to maintain suppleness. Any immobilization of the hand must be as brief as possible, while motion and function are maintained in the unaffected portions of the hand. Joint contractures can be minimized if the hand is maintained in a functional or "safe position" when immobilized. The wrist should be extended 15°, the metacarpophalangeal joints flexed 65° to 70°, and the interphalangeal joints maintained in relative extension.

Common postural deformities, all of which center on an imbalance at one or more joints, include claw hand, boutonnière deformity, swan neck deformity, and mallet finger deformity.

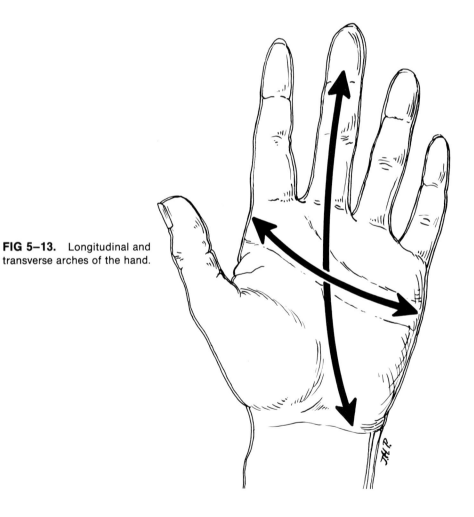

FIG 5–13. Longitudinal and transverse arches of the hand.

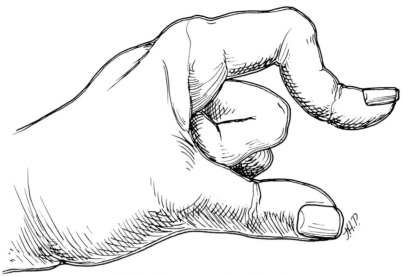

FIG 5–14. Boutonnière deformity.

A claw hand is the result of an imbalance of the intrinsic and extrinsic muscles. Since the intrinsic muscles are weakened, either by injury or disease, the extrinsic muscles cause a flattening of the metacarpal arch (Fig 5–13), hyperextension of the metacarpophalangeal joint, and flexion of the proximal interphalangeal and distal interphalangeal joints. This deformity can occur with lesions to the ulnar nerve alone, or combined with the median nerve, brachial plexus injuries, spinal cord injuries, and in some generalized disease processes.

A boutonnière deformity (Fig 5–14) is recognized as flexion at the proximal phalangeal joint and extension of the distal interphalangeal joint. Any injury or disease that disrupts the insertion of the extensor tendon at the base of the middle phalanx can cause this deformity. The remaining lateral bands sublux and slip volar to the axis of the proximal interphalangeal joint. Often, this deformity does not appear immediately after injury, but develops later, as the lateral bands tear, stretch and eventually sublux and become flexors of the proximal interphalangeal finger joints.

The swan neck deformity (Fig 5–15) is maintained by a hyperextension of the proximal phalangeal joint and flexion at the distal interphalangeal joint. This muscle imbalance may be the result of volar plate injury, flexor digitorum superficialis weakness, or synovitis in the rheumatoid hand. A terminal extensor tendon injury that causes relative overpull of the extensors at the proximal interphalangeal joint may have the same result.

A mallet finger deformity (Fig 5–16), or baseball finger, occurs from injury at the insertion of the extensor tendon, which causes avulsion of the tendon or an avulsion fracture of the distal phalanx in which a piece of the bone remains attached to the extensor tendon. Loss of extension at the distal interphalangeal joint occurs. A laceration at the distal joint that severs the extensor tendon also results in this deformity.

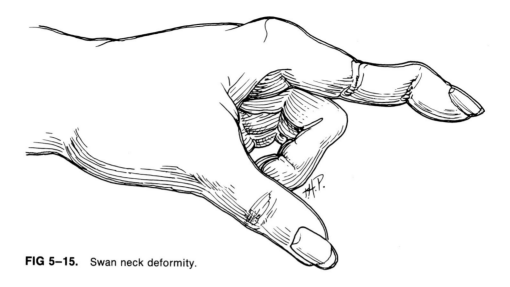

FIG 5–15. Swan neck deformity.

Structural abnormalities leading to abnormal posture include Dupuytren's contracture, camptodactyly, and clinodactyly.

A Dupuytren's contracture occurs when there is an abnormal proliferation of tissue in the palm of the hand. It may cause a postural deformity when volar cords in the skin tether the involved digits in flexion. This more commonly involves the little and ring fingers. If the condition is not alleviated, associated joint contracture may develop at the proximal and metacarpophalangeal joints.

Camptodactyly is a congenital flexion contracture, usually of the little finger, seen in children. This contracture develops into a postural deformity by abnormally shortening the flexor tendon unit of the involved digit.

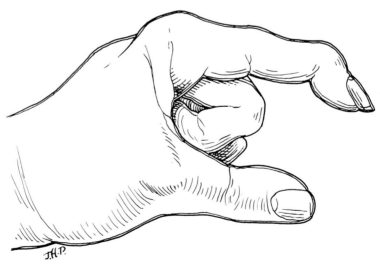

FIG 5–16. Mallet finger deformity.

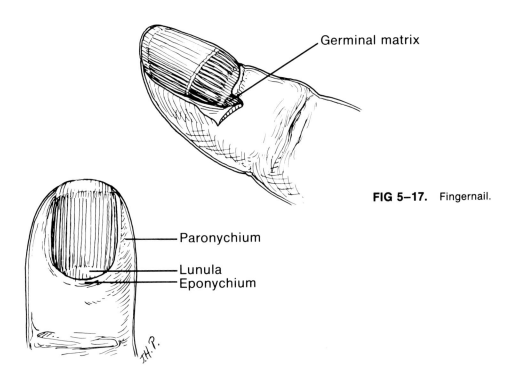

Germinal matrix

FIG 5–17. Fingernail.

Paronychium

Lunula
Eponychium

Clinodactyly refers to the abnormal angulation of bony origin of a finger. It is a structural abnormality of the middle phalanx of the involved digit, usually the little finger, which leads to joint angulation in the coronal plane.

Nail Examination

The nail plate (Fig 5–17) is formed by the cells of the germinal matrix. Growth disturbances of the nail result from injuries and diseases of the germinal matrix or from metabolic disturbances.

A common cause of disruption of nail growth is the "mucous cyst," which is actually a ganglion that arises from the distal interphalangeal joint, producing pressure on the nail plate and causing subsequent deformity. Nail plate infections, particularly those involving fungi, produce severe deformities. The resulting rigid and split nails catch on clothes and other objects further aggravating the injury. Proper repair of nail-bed lacerations is necessary to minimize these disturbances.

Traumatic subungual hematoma produces acute and increasing pain and may be recognized by the presence of dark blood beneath the nail plate.

Further Readings

1. American Society for Surgery of the Hand: *The Hand: Examination & Diagnosis.* Edinburgh, Churchill Livingstone, 1983.

2. Flatt AE: *The Care of Congenital Hand Anomalies.* St Louis, CV Mosby Co, 1977.
3. Green DP: *Operative Hand Surgery.* New York, Churchill Livingstone, 1982.
4. Lamb DW, Kuczynski K: *The Practice of Hand Surgery.* Oxford, Blackwell Scientific Publications, 1981.
5. Lister GD: *The Hand: Diagnosis and Indications.* Edinburgh, Churchill Livingstone, 1977.
6. Spinner M: *Injuries to the Major Branches of Peripheral Nerves of the Forearm.* Philadelphia, WB Saunders Co, 1978.

CHAPTER 6

Physical Examination of the Cervical Spine

Melvin Post, M.D.

The spine is the central part of the axial skeleton. The cervical spine portion supports the head and protects the spinal cord as it emerges from the base of the neck. The spinal cord and the nerves that originate from it are especially vulnerable in the cervical region because of the forces it often receives in serious accidents and because of the wide ranges of motion of which it is capable. It is axiomatic that a thorough knowledge of the anatomy and physiology of this region is crucial, especially in the neck region, if the medical examiner is to correctly assess the complaints of a patient and integrate the physical findings in order to establish a correct diagnosis. Specifically, it is essential to understand from what levels the nerves emerge from the spinal cord and the corresponding foramina of the cervical spinal, and to whence they are distributed. A knowledge of the distribution of the motor nerves and sensory dermatomes is essential if the examiner is to fully comprehend his own findings.

Inspection

The patient is asked to undress to the waist. Shorts are worn. Females should be appropriately dressed and the whole torso and all four extremities observed as the patient ambulates. Gait patterns are recorded (see Chapter 8). Posture and positioning of the torso and extremities are observed. Contractures of the extremities are noted. Evidence of cerebellar ataxia is recorded. Does the patient compensate by standing on a broad base, or sway? Is the gait pattern based on organic disease (hemiplegia, spastic or ataxic, parkinsonian, or waddling) or is it hysterical in nature?

Facial expressions and movements of the extremities should be recorded. Fast, jerking, purposeless, unsustained involuntary movements usually suggest choreatic motions that may relate to one group of muscles and then another. The face may assume a grotesque expression and become contorted. Athetosis may become apparent when involuntary movements are slower and almost continuous, with the facial expression appearing more sustained, and may subside during periods of sleep. Wild flailing of the extremities, either unilateral or bilateral, may be related to a hemiballismus. Localized muscle spasms and tics should be differentiated from movements of a psychogenic origin.

Following completion of the general inspection portion of the examination, the position of the head is noted. Obvious protruding masses, scars, and skin changes are recorded. For example, a scar on the lower half of the lateral neck may be related to a lymph node biopsy that may have injured the spinal accessory nerve and caused a paralysis of the trapezius and winging of the scapula (see Chapter 2). Is a surgical scar on the anterior part of the neck related to a previous anterior cervical disk fusion?

Range of Motion

Normal passive and active motions of the cervical spine should be recorded (Fig 6–1). Pure motions consist of flexion, extension, rotation, and lateral tilt (see Fig 6–1). Normally, there are 80° of flexion, 40° of extension, 65° of rotation to the right and left, and 45° of lateral tilt to the right and left. These motions are used in combination and allow a wide range of combined motions of the cervical spine. About half of rotation motion occurs between C-1 and C-2 while half of flexion motion occurs between the occiput and C-1. The other half of flexion-extension motion occurs between the remaining cervical vertebrae. Anything that interferes with normal facet articulation will limit motion. This may include surgical, congenital, or acquired fusion, dislocations, or subluxations of the facets, and fractures or congenital anomalies such as Klippel-Feil deformity. These conditions represent mechanical incongruities or constraints between the normal articular relationship of the vertebral bodies. Muscle spasm in the neck may also severely limit normal neck motions and restrict head movements.

Normally, a patient should be capable of touching the chin to the chest during flexion, and look directly above in extension (see Fig 6–1). The head should rotate to each side in a smooth, synchronous manner unless there is muscle spasm or a mechanical bony block such as arthritis or subluxation of the facet

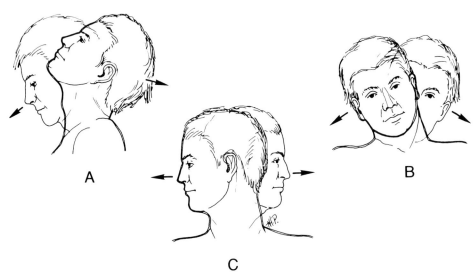

FIG 6–1. Motion of cervical spine. Flexion-extension (*A*), lateral tilt (*B*), and rotation (*C*).

joints. The head ordinarily can laterally tilt 45° to either side. The active and passive ranges of motions should be tested except where instability or fracture is suspected. In this case, roentgenograms should be taken first to rule out this possibility for fear of causing nerve or spinal cord injury.

Palpation

The neck should be palpated both in the erect and supine positions. Abnormal muscle spasm of the muscles of the neck may be more easily detected in the erect position when the muscle is required to act against gravity. In the supine position with the muscles relaxed, many of the deeper neck structures may be palpated, especially anteriorly.

The anterior structures include the hyoid bone above the thyroid cartilage opposite the level of the vertebral body of C-3. It is most easily palpated between the thumb and index digits. When the patient swallows the movement of the bone is felt. The thyroid cartilage lies inferiorly to the hyoid bone. Its superior notch lies in the midline. The top part of the cartilage rests opposite the level of the vertebral body of C-4. The lower part lies opposite C-5. Inferior to the sharp lower edge of the thyroid cartilage lies the first cricoid ring resting opposite C-6. It will move when the patient swallows. The examiner may palpate the anterior carotid tubercle, that is the anterior tubercle of C-6 transverse process. The tubercle is deep, but may be felt with the fingertips while pressing posteriorly with the patient supine. It is the point used to identify the level between C5-6 either for a planned disk fusion at this level or as the site of injection of the stellate ganglion.

The lateral and posterior portion of the neck should be examined in the supine and erect positions (Fig 6–2). The sternocleidomastoid muscle originates from the mastoid process and inserts at the region of the sternoclavicular joint (Fig 6–3). This structure serves as a landmark in separating the anterior triangle of neck from the posterior structures. Palpation of both sternocleidomastoid muscles should be performed with the neck in the neutral position and with the head turned to one side and then to the other side. In injuries of the neck this muscle may be tender or in spasm. When the head is turned to the opposite side and the chin tilted up slightly, the muscle away from which the head is turned is taut and easily palpated. If it is in spasm (as in torticollis), rotation motion of the neck will be painful and limited.

Lymph nodes can be palpated at the anterior border of the sternocleidomastoid muscle if they are enlarged (Fig 6–3). The thyroid gland straddles the thyroid cartilage. It ordinarily feels smooth, but may contain nodules. It may be enlarged on one or both sides. It should also be palpated while the patient swallows small sips of water or saliva.

The parotid gland lies opposite the angle of the mandible and may be felt if it is enlarged. In this case the gland may be tender if it is infected.

The carotid artery pulse can be palpated next to the carotid tubercle when the examiner presses posteriorly with the fingertips. The examiner should avoid palpating both carotid pulses simultaneously for fear of evoking a carotid reflex. Both pulses are palpated separately and compared.

The supraclavicular fossa is normally a depressed area above the clavicle. It may be lost when a fracture of the clavicle has occurred due to the deformity of a

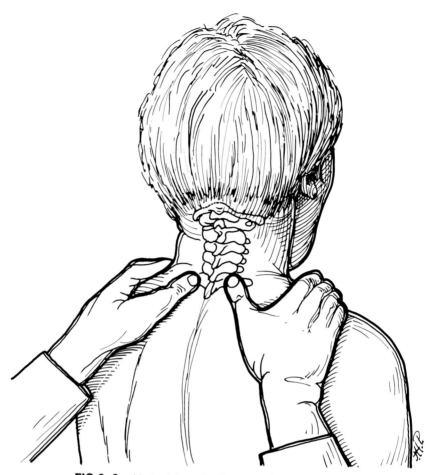

FIG 6–2. Method for palpating posterior element of neck.

displaced fracture and hemorrhage within the soft tissues. If a significant cervical rib is present, it also may be palpated in this fossa. The cupola of the lung resides in the base of the fossa and can easily be injured by infection or trauma.

Much of the posterior portion of the neck lies in the subcutaneous plane and is more easily palpated. Again, the neck should be palpated both in the erect and supine positions. In the erect position, the lateral fingers are placed over the top of the shoulders while the thumbs are used to feel the underlying bony parts (see Fig 6–2). The muscles are less tense with the neck in the supine position. In this case, each side of the head is cupped by the hands while the examiner is positioned above the head facing distally. The fingertips may then palpate the deeper parts. These include the occiput superiorly, the mastoid process, the spinous process of C-2 and the rest of the spinous processes of C-2 through T-1. During this part of the examination the normal lordosis of the cervical spine is felt. The spinous processes of C-7 and T-1 are larger than the others. All the spinous processes should be aligned. The muscles on either side of the posterior midline of the cervical spine are raised posteriorly and thus create a midline valley overlying the spinous processes. The facet joints lie about 2.5 cm lateral to the midline and can sometimes be palpated in very thin patients. They can be tender in patients with osteoarthritis.

Individual muscles, including the trapezius and sternocleidomastoid, should be palpated (see Chapter 2). They may be tender, and a paralysis of the spinal accessory nerve will affect both muscles. Other structures such as the greater occipital nerve lying high in the posterior cervical region can be palpated, especially if they are inflamed. Moreover, when this nerve is so affected, it may be exceptionally tender and even cause headaches.

Neurologic Examination

Nowhere in the body is a thorough neurologic examination as important as in the cervical region in diagnosing disease relating to local and referred conditions. Precise levels of disease process may be inferred if the examiner has a

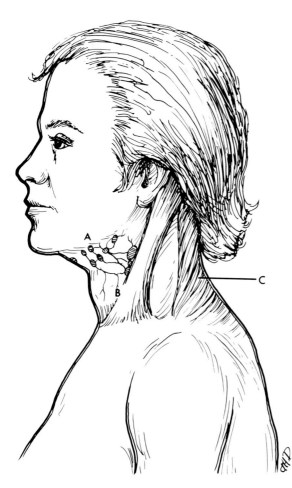

FIG 6–3. Lateral structures of the neck: neck glands (*A*), carotid pulse (*B*), and trapezius muscles (*C*).

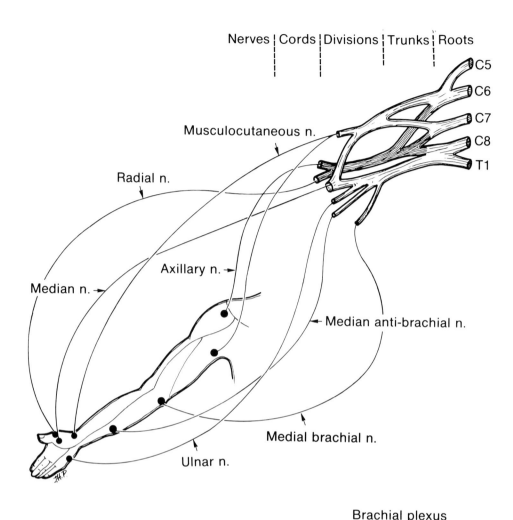

| Nerves | Cords | Divisions | Trunks | Roots |

Musculocutaneous n.

C5
C6
C7
C8
T1

Radial n.

Axillary n. →

Median n. →

← Median anti-brachial n.

Medial brachial n.

Ulnar n.

Brachial plexus

FIG 6–4. Constitution of brachial plexus and its peripheral nerve distribution.

thorough knowledge of the anatomy and physiology of the levels of the nerve roots, the brachial plexus, and the distribution of the corresponding peripheral nerves (Fig 6–4), and sensory dermatomes (see Fig 1–1).

Eight nerves emerge from the cervical spine, although there are only seven cervical vertebrae. The first seven cervical nerves exit superior to the corresponding cervical vertebra. The eighth cervical nerve emerges between the seventh cervical and first thoracic vertebra. It follows then that the T1 nerve exits below the first thoracic vertebra.

The brachial plexus is constituted of nerves that originate from the level of C-5 of the spinal cord through T-1 (see Fig 6–4). They are termed roots. The roots form from the anterior primary rami of C5 through C8 and a greater part of T1. The roots of C5 and C6 coalesce and form the upper trunk, while the nerve roots of C8 and T1 coalesce to form the lower trunk. The seventh cervical root alone constitutes the middle trunk. Each trunk splits into anterior and posterior divisions a short distance above the clavicle. The upper two anterior divisions unite to form the lateral cord. The lower anterior division forms the medial cord. All three posterior divisions form the posterior cord. From the lateral cord, the lateral pectoral nerve (C5, C6, C7) arises, as well as the musculocutaneous nerve (C5, C6, C7) and the lateral root of the median nerve (C5, C6, C7). From the medial cord arises the medial pectoral nerve (C8, T1), the medial cutaneous of the forearm (C8, T1), the medial cutaneous of the arm (T1, T2), the medial root of the median (C8, T1), and the ulnar (C7, C8, T1). Finally, from the posterior cord, the upper and lateral subscapular nerve (C5, C6) arises, as well as the nerve to the latissimus dorsi (C5, C6, C7), the circumflex (C5, C6), and the radial nerve (C5, C6, C7, C8, T1). The medial, lateral, and posterior cords reside at the level of the second portion of the axillary artery. The peripheral nerves originate from the cords. Tables 6–1, 6–2, and 6–3 show the muscles that control the neck, the upper extremity, and the shoulder girdle. Usually, the muscles of the neck can be grouped when examining the patient (Table 6–1).

Table 6–3 shows the principal nerves that arise from the cords of the brachial plexus. Figure 6–1 shows the sensory distribution and dermatomes of the upper extremity.

Neurologic Testing

When the examiner has mastered the pattern of the sensory dermatomes and the anatomical distribution of the peripheral nerves, the physical examination of the upper extremity will be performed with ease.

From the C-5 level originates the musculocutaneous nerve (Fig 6–5). It innervates the biceps and brachialis muscles that are flexors of the elbow. The biceps supinates the forearm. The biceps reflex is a function of the C-5 level of the spinal cord but also receives nerve fibers from C6. The fifth cervical root and its corresponding spinal cord level provide sensation to the lateral arm. Loss of sensation in the upper lateral arm indicates an injury to the axillary nerve.

The C6 nerve root and its corresponding level in the spinal cord innervate the wrist extensors (Fig 6–6). This group of muscles also receives nerve fibers from C7. The wrist extensor muscles include the extensor carpi radialis longus (C6), the extensor carpi radialis brevis (C6), and the extensor carpi ulnaris (C7). The biceps is innervated in part by nerve fibers from C6. The brachioradialis reflex is performed by percussion of the brachioradialis tendon above the wrist. The brachioradialis is innervated by the radial nerve (C5 and C6). However, the reflex is primarily related to the C-6 level (see Fig. 6–6). Since C-6 also is partly responsible for the biceps reflex, it too should be tested as a function of this level. Thus, neither the muscle action nor reflexes are purely C-6 in origin. The sixth cervical root provides nerve branches for sensation of the lateral forearm, the thumb, index, and half the middle finger (see Fig. 6–6).

The seventh cervical nerve root level provides nerve branches to the radial nerve, and to the triceps muscle. The wrist flexor group of muscles as well as the finger extensors are similarly supplied by nerve branches from C-7 (Fig 6–7).

The wrist flexor muscles include the flexor carpi radialis (median nerve C7) and the flexor carpi ulnaris (ulnar nerve C8) (Fig 6–8). The finger extensors include the extensor digitorum communis, the extensor indicis proprius, and the extensor digiti minimi that are primarily innervated by C7 and to a lesser extent

TABLE 6–1.
Muscles of Upper Extremity Controlling Forearm and Hand Motion*

MUSCLE	NERVE(S)	NORMAL FUNCTION(S)	PARALYSIS	TEST(S)
Biceps brachii	Musculocutaneous C5-C6	Flexes and supinates forearm	Elbow flexion and supination weakened	Flexion of supinated forearm against resistance
Brachialis	Musculocutaneous C5-C6	Flexes elbow	Weakened elbow flexion	Resist flexion at elbow
Extensor carpi radialis longus	Radial C5-C6	Extends hand, abducts wrist	Markedly weakened radial deviation of wrist	Resist wrist extension
Extensor carpi radialis brevis	Radial C5-C7	Extends hand, abducts wrist	Markedly weakened radial deviation of wrist	Resist wrist extension
Extensor carpi ulnaris	Radial C6-C8	Extends hand, adducts wrist	Weakened ulnar deviation of wrist	Resist wrist extension
Extensor digitorum communis	Radial C6-C8	Extends hand	Loss of extension of finger MP joints with weakened IP extension	Resist finger extension
Extensor indicis	Radial C6-C8	Extends hand, second finger	Finger extension weakened	Resist second finger extension
Extensor indicis minimi	Radial C6-C8	Extends fifth finger	Fifth finger extension weakened	Resist extension little finger
Brachioradialis	Radial C5-C6	Flexes forearm, aids forearm supination	Weakens supination of prone hand	With forearm in neutral rotation and the elbow flexed 90° against resistance the contracting muscle is seen and palpated
Triceps	Radial C5-C6	Extends elbow	Elbow extension lost	Resistance against extended elbow
Pronator teres	Median C6-C7	Pronates forearm and hand	Weakened pronation	On pronation of forearm against resistance, contraction of pronator teres palpated
Flexor carpi radialis	Median C7-C8	Extends hand, abducts wrist, aids pronation of hand	Wrist flexion, abduction weakened	Resist wrist flexion, abduction against closed hand

Muscle	Nerve and Root	Action	Effect of Weakness	Test
Flexor carpi ulnaris	Ulnar C7-C8	Flexes hand, adducts wrist, aids pronation of hand	Hand flexion, wrist adduction weakened	Resist wrist flexion, adduction against closed hand
Flexor digitorum superficialis	Median C7-T1	Flexes proximal interphalangeal joints	Weakened flexion proximal interphalangeal joints	Stabilize fingers in flexion while resisting attempt to straighten fingers
Flexor digitorum profundus	Median C7-T1 radial half; Ulnar C7-T1 ulnar half	Flexes distal, and proximal interphalangeal joints	Loss of flexion distal interphalangeal joints	(Same test as noted above)
Dorsal interossei	Ulnar C8-T1	Abducts fingers	Weakened finger abduction	Resist finger abduction
Palmar interossei	Ulnar C8-T1	Adducts fingers (excludes thumb)	Weakened finger abduction	Resist finger adduction
Abductor digiti quinti	Ulnar C8-T1	Abducts MP and CM little finger	Weakened fifth finger abduction	Resist fifth finger abduction
Lumbricales (digits 1, 2)	Median C7-T1	Flexes metacarpophalangeal joints, extends interphalangeal joints	Weakened metacarpophalangeal joints, extension and extension phalangeal joints	Resist MP and IP joint extension
Abductor pollicis brevis	Median C8-T1	Abducts thumb in plane of 90° to hand	Weakened thumb abduction	Resist thumb abduction
Opponens pollicis	Median C8-T1	Flexes and adducts thumb toward little finger; medial rotation and flexion of CM	Weakened thumb opposition	Resist opposition of thumb
Opponens digiti quinti	Ulnar C8-T1	Flexes and adducts little finger toward thumb	Weakened adduction little finger	(Same test as noted above)

* MP = metacarpophalangeal; IP = interphalangeal; CM = carpometacarpal.

TABLE 6–2.
Muscles Controlling Neck Motions

MUSCLE	NERVE(S)	NORMAL FUNCTION(S)	PARALYSIS	TEST(S)
Rectus capitus anterior	Suboccipital C1-C3	Flexes head	Head flexion weakened	Resist head flexion
Rectus capitus lateralis	Suboccipital C1-C4	Bends head to same side	—	—
Rectus capitus posterior	Suboccipital C1	Both muscles acting bilaterally extend head; one acting alone turns face to same side	Weakens bend of head to side muscle	Resist bend of head to side of muscle
Obliquus capitus inferior	Suboccipital C1	Turns face to same side	—	—
Obliquus capitus superior	Suboccipital C1	Extends head and to same side	Weakens head extension	Resist head extension and bend to same side
Splenius capitus	C2-C4	Extends head	Head extension weakened	Resist head extension
Splenius cervicis	C2-C4	Extends head	Head extension weakened	Resist head extension
Semispinalis capitus	C1-C4	Extends head	Head extension weakened	Resist head extension
Semispinalis cervicis	C3-C6	Extends head	Head extension weakened	Resist head extension
Longissimus capitus	C1-C8	Both muscles acting bilaterally extend head; acting alone head flexes toward same side	Head extension weakened	Resist head extension
Longissimus cervicis	C1-C8	(Same as noted above)	Head extension weakened	Resist head extension
Scalenus anterior	Anterior primary division lower cervical nerves C4-C7	Bends neck to same side	Weakens bending of head to side of muscle	Sitting or supine flexion of neck with chin on chest against resistance applied to forehead
Scalenus medius	C4-C8	Bends neck to same side	—	—
Scalenus posterior	C6-C8	Bends neck to same side	—	—

128

TABLE 6–3.
Origin of Peripheral Nerves From Cords of Brachial
Plexus

	CORD	PERIPHERAL NERVE
C-5–C-6	Lateral cord	Musculocutaneous, lateral branch to the median
C-7	Median cord	Ulnar, medial branch to median
C-8–T-1	Posterior cord	Axillary, radial

by fibers from C8. The triceps reflex is tested by percussing the distal triceps tendon at the elbow (see Fig 6–7). The sensory distribution is illustrated in Fig 6–7.

The eighth cervical nerve root and its corresponding cervical spinal cord innervate the flexor digitorum superficialis and the flexor digitorum profundis. Branches from the median nerve innervate the flexor digitorum superficialis while the branches of the ulnar nerve innervate half the flexor digitorum profundus on its ulnar side, while branches from the median nerve innervate the radial half of the same muscle. Branches of the ulnar nerve are also supplied to the interossei (see Fig 6–8). Sensation is supplied to the ring and little fingers and to the distal forearm (see Fig 6–8). There is no reflex at the C8 nerve root level.

The first thoracic nerve root and its corresponding cord level innervate the finger abductors, which include the dorsal interossei and the abductor digiti quinti. Sensation is supplied to the medial arm by the medial brachial cutaneous nerve (Fig 6–9). There is no reflex at this level.

Miscellaneous Tests

Compression-Extension of the Cervical Spine

When the cervical neural foramina are narrowed, as in osteoarthritis of the facet joints associated with cervical disk degeneration, compression of the cervical spine may reproduce or exacerbate pain in the upper extremity (Fig 6–10). This referred pain is probably caused by an impingement on the nerve roots as they traverse the foramina. Similarly, the foramina may be narrowed, causing referred pain into the upper extremity when the head is extended.

Distraction-Flexion

The diameters of the cervical spine foramina may be increased by distracting the cervical spine as in using traction. Distraction can be accomplished by cupping the patient's chin and occiput with each hand of the examiner. This maneuver may relieve muscle spasm in the neck and diminish referred pain in the upper extremity. Gentle flexion of the cervical spine may also increase the diameter of the cervical foramina.

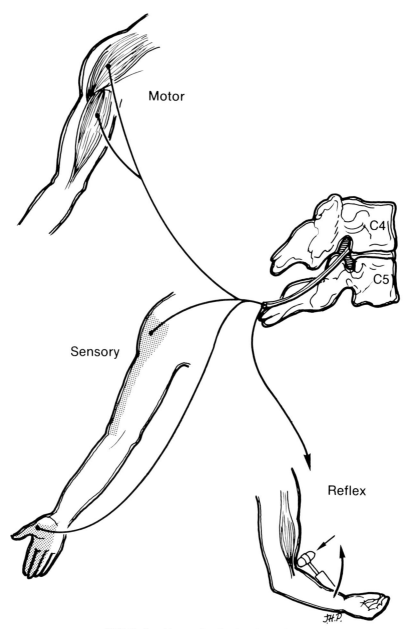

Motor

Sensory

C4

C5

Reflex

FIG 6–5. Nerve distribution from C-5.

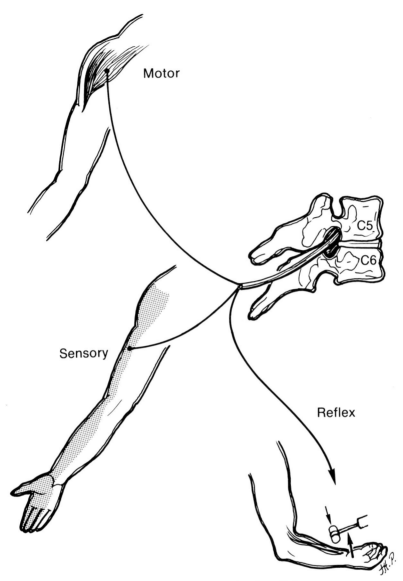

Motor

Sensory

Reflex

FIG 6–6. Nerve distribution from C-6.

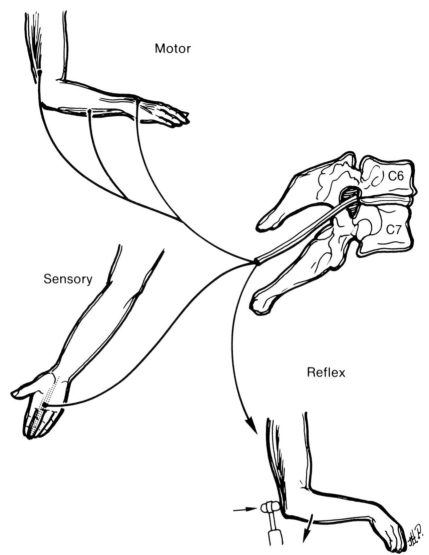

FIG 6–7. Nerve distribution from C-7.

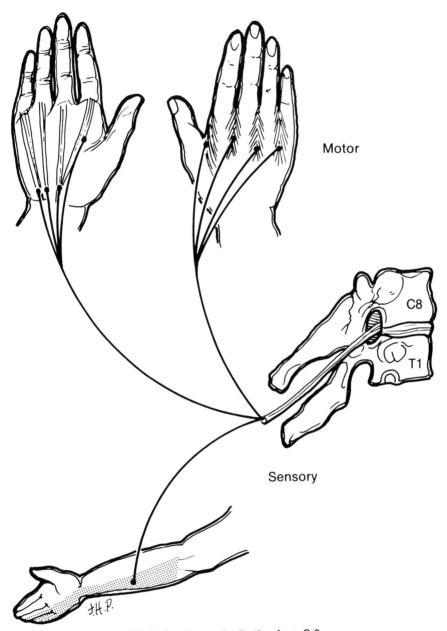

Motor

C8

T1

Sensory

FIG 6–8. Nerve distribution from C-8.

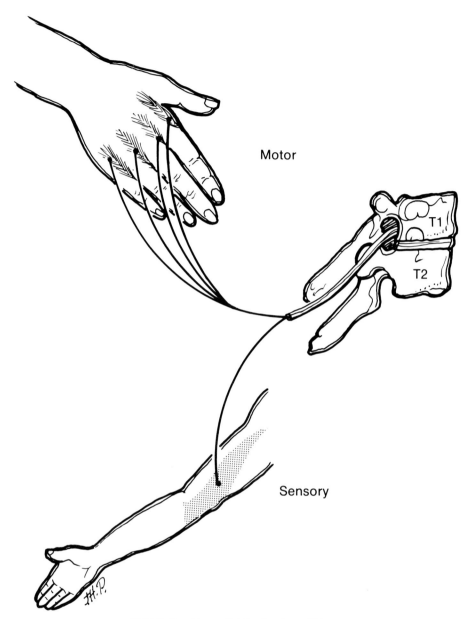

Motor

T1

T2

Sensory

FIG 6–9. Nerve distribution from T-1.

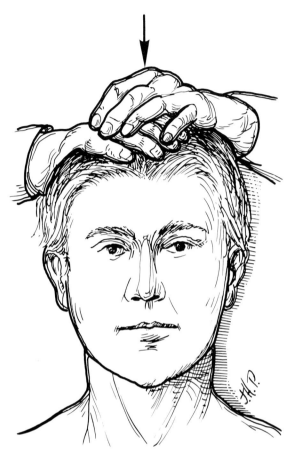

FIG 6–10. Compression test of the cervical spine.

Valsalva Maneuver

If a space-occupying lesion is present in the cervical canal, pain may be present. The pain can be referred to the corresponding dermatome in the upper extremity. In performing this test, the patient holds his breath and forces down against a closed glottis, as in moving the bowels. In a positive test pain is reproduced. Similar increased pain may be reproduced when there is an increase in the intraspinal pressure when radicular pain is exaggerated with space-occupying lesions. The pressure may be increased temporarily by sneezing or coughing or by digital compression of the jugular veins. Compression of the jugular veins is maintained until the patient complains of a fullness in the head, and should not be considered negative until venous return is blocked for at least two minutes. This last test is termed the Naffziger test.

References

1. Aird RB, Naffziger HC: Prolonged jugular compression: A new diagnostic test of neurologic value. *Trans Am Neural Assoc* 1940; 66:45–48.
2. DeJong RN: *The Neurologic Examination: Incorporating the Fundamentals of Neuroanatomy and Neurophysiology,* ed. 4. Hagerstown, Md, Harper & Row Publishers Inc., 1979.

CHAPTER 7

Examination of the Thoracic and Lumbar Spine

Melvin Post, M.D.

Back pain has been known to exist from time immemorial. However, it was only in the past several decades that various disease entities causing back pain have been differentiated. Like other regions of the body, it is still the history and physical examination on which the physician must rely to diagnose a disease state. The manifestations of disease that arise in the spine are protean and relate to pain and loss of function. Thus, as in the cervical spine, it is important to understand the physiology and anatomy of this region.

Inspection

Observation of the surface of the back, especially the skin, can provide useful information. Pigmented spots (cafe au lait), pedunculated polyps, rash, localized blisters (herpes zoster), hairy patches, and birthmarks may each be significant. Varying sizes of lipomas, which may be well circumscribed, diffuse over the back, or exist as an enlargement of the buttock, may indicate deeper involvement of the neural elements.

Before initiating a more detailed inspection of the back the examiner should know if the extremities are equal in length. Any discrepancy should be equalized by placing appropriate size blocks beneath the shortened extremity if the shortening is actual and not relative in nature (see Chapter 8). At this point the general posture should be noted from the front, sides, and back of the patient (Fig 7–1). Are the shoulders level and is the pelvis horizontal? When lumbar muscle spasm is present the patient may demonstrate an obvious list to one side, while the normal contours of the lumbar spine may be lost. A lumbar lordosis should be differentiated from the normal contour (Figs 7–2, A and B). Lateral bend or scoliosis may coexist with a lumbar lordosis (Fig 7–3). Is this finding structural or functional? The latter may be related to a shortened extremity or muscle spasm of the back muscles. When the spinal curve (scoliosis) is structural, the direction of the cavity and convexity should be recorded. The degree of compensation or decompensation should be recorded by dropping a plumb line

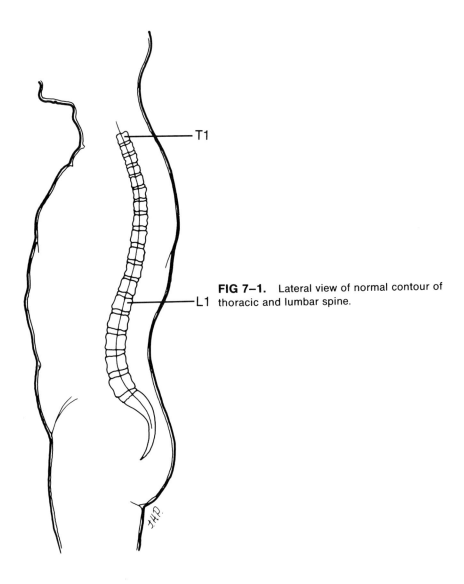

FIG 7–1. Lateral view of normal contour of thoracic and lumbar spine.

from the spinous process of C7. With compensation, the cord should fall in the midline of the natis. Similarly, it is important to know that in certain disease states, such as true disk herniation, when the disk herniation is lateral to the nerve root, the patient tilts away from the lesion. When the disk protrusion lies medial to the nerve root the patient will lean toward the side of the lesion. Other abnormalities of the alignment of the spine should be noted. Is there a gibbus observed in the dorsal region (Fig 7–4)? If so, it may be related to infection (tuberculosis), fracture, or a congenital bony anomaly of the spine. In an elderly female patient with back pain, a kyphotic deformity of the thoracic spine may indicate compression fracture(s) relating to idiopathic osteoporosis. In a young patient, excessive rounding may be related to an ankylosing spondylitis, or de-

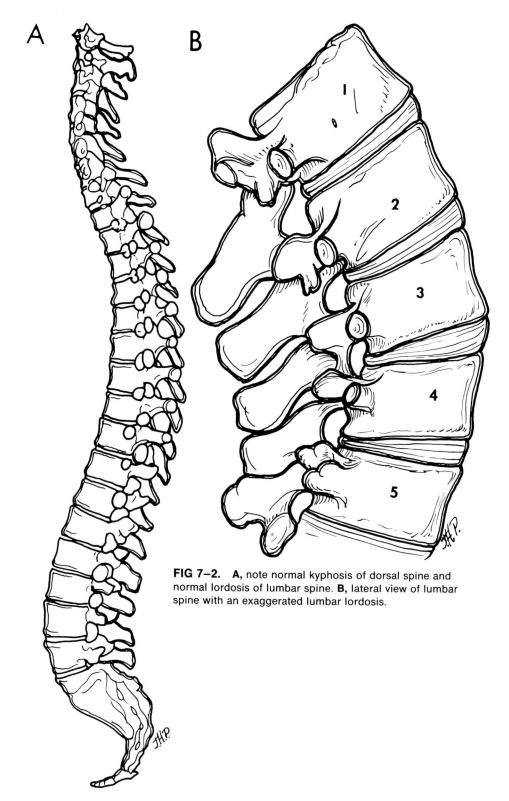

FIG 7–2. **A,** note normal kyphosis of dorsal spine and normal lordosis of lumbar spine. **B,** lateral view of lumbar spine with an exaggerated lumbar lordosis.

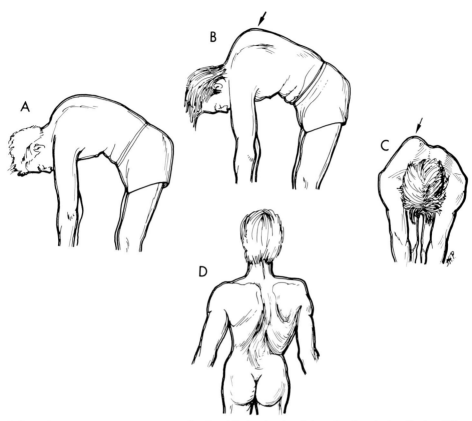

FIG 7–3. Normal flexion posture of spine (*A*); kyphosis of dorsal spine during flexion (*B*); humpback noted in scoliosis of spine (*C*); dorsolumbar scoliosis of spine (*D*).

crease of growth of the spine in Scheuermann's disease seen in the adolescent years.

It is equally important to observe the movement of the chest cage during respiration. There is relatively little motion between the thoracic vertebral bodies. However, disease in this region may limit excursion of the chest cage when rotated, and malaligned thoracic vertebral bodies and their attached ribs do not move synchronously. This is especially prevalent in ankylosing spondylitis.

Range of Motion

The spine is more flexible in youth and moves less with advancing age because of the greater elasticity of the soft tissues that connect the vertebral bodies in the young individual. In any event it should be noted if motion testing causes pain.

As in the cervical region, the ranges of motion occur in flexion-extension (Fig 7–5), right and left tilt (Fig 7–6), and rotation to the right and left (Fig 7–7). Normally, there is 80° of flexion, 25° of extension, 25° of rotation to the right and left, and 25° of lateral tilt to the right and left. Combinations of these motions

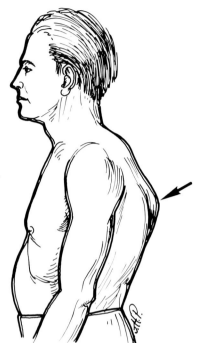

FIG 7–4. Gibbus of dorsal spine.

allow the patient to move into numerous positions. In general, motions of the lumbar spine occur in combinations.

As degenerative arthritic changes progress in the disks and facets, so too is there a corresponding decrease in normal motion. It is important to recall that normal lumbar flexion involves motion in the hips.

Gait

The gait pattern can be important in determining whether or not disease originates in the spine or the lower extremities. This has been discussed (see Chapter 8). In any event, observation of the gait can reveal obvious weakness and even atrophy of muscles that can affect normal gait.

Palpation

The examiner should palpate for muscle spasm while the patient is seated, standing, and during testing of motions. If the patient is malingering and will not flex the lumbar spine while erect, he should be asked to kneel on the padded seat of a chair facing the back rest. The muscles may relax and soften dramatically. In this case the lumbar spine may round out with ease. Are the paravertebral muscles extraordinarily firm and tender? Do they bulge as muscle spasm increases? Are they more prominent on one side of the midline of the spine? Can localized masses be palpated?

The spinous processes are not covered by muscle and are easily palpated. A tender spinous process can indicate disease including fracture, infection, or tumor. The iliac crests and sacrum should be palpated. Landmarks can be identified easily. For example, the tops of the iliac crests normally are aligned with the level of the fourth vertebral body (Fig 7–8). Similarly, the ischial tuberosity may be felt when the hip is flexed 90°.

Soft tissue palpation is important. The sciatic nerve emerges from beneath the pyriformis. The pyriformis tendon inserts into the posterior aspect of the greater trochanter. Beyond this point, the area of the sciatic nerve may be felt. Any tenderness should be recorded. The abdomen should be gently palpated while the hips are flexed and while the patient is supine in order to differentiate intra-abdominal disease from localized musculoskeletal conditions. The abdominal muscles as well as intra-abdominal organs, such as the liver and spleen, can be palpated. The inguinal region should be palpated for evidence of hernia.

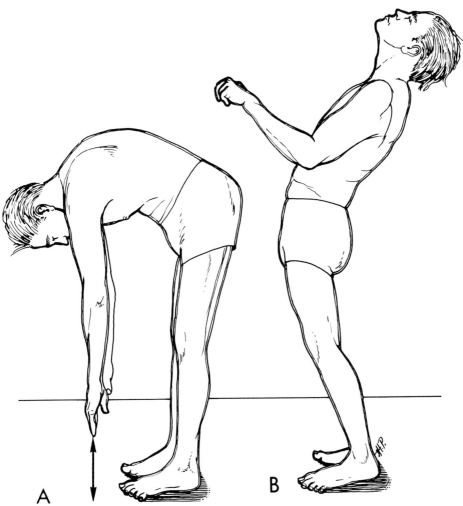

FIG 7–5. Normal flexion (*A*); extension motion of spine (*B*).

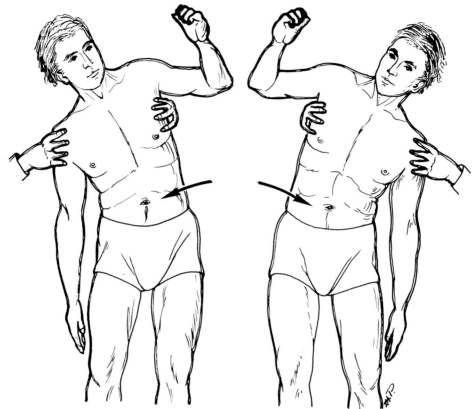

FIG 7–6. Normal right and left tilt of spine.

Neurologic Examination

The lumbar as well as the sacral and coccygeal plexus originate in the lower spinal cord (Figs 7–9 and 7–10). Their peripheral nerves emerge from specific sites and levels and travel into the lower extremity. Disease states that adversely affect these nerves in the spine can be detected by having a thorough knowledge of the sensory dermatomes and motor distribution in the lower extremity. Since the peripheral nerves contain fibers from different levels of the spinal cord, the examiner should keep this in mind.

Figures 7–9 and 7–10 show the composition of the lumbar and sacrococcygeal plexus. Figure 1–1 illustrates the sensory dermatomes of the lower extremity. Table 7–1 shows the nerve innervation of important muscles in the lower extremity.

The anterior abdominal muscles contract normally when the upper muscle fibers (T6-T9) and the lower muscle fibers (T10-L1) have normal innervation. If the abdominal muscles are weak in the presence of strong hip flexors, hyperextension of the lumbar spine will result when the patient tries to elevate the lower extremities or sit from a supine position.

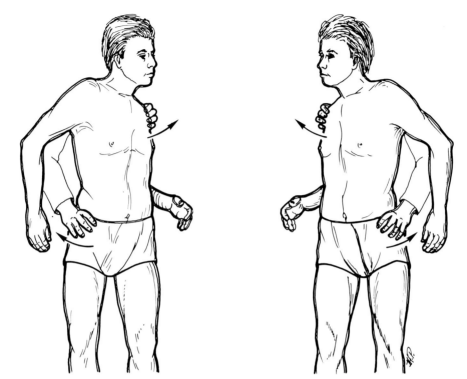

FIG 7–7. Rotation motion of spine.

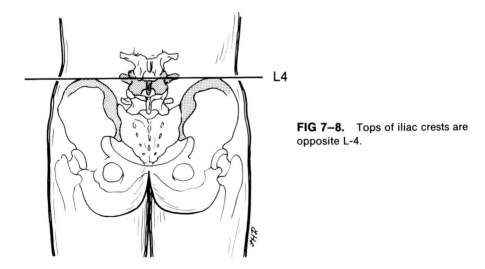

L4

FIG 7–8. Tops of iliac crests are opposite L-4.

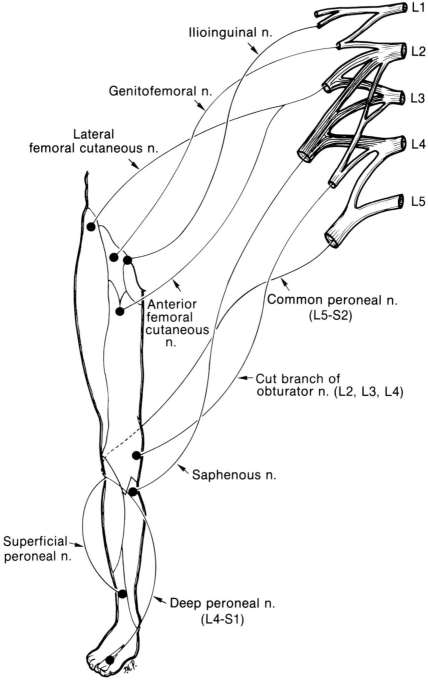

L1
L2
L3
L4
L5

Ilioinguinal n.

Genitofemoral n.

Lateral
femoral cutaneous n.

Anterior
femoral
cutaneous
n.

Common peroneal n.
(L5-S2)

Cut branch of
obturator n. (L2, L3, L4)

Saphenous n.

Superficial
peroneal n.

Deep peroneal n.
(L4-S1)

FIG 7–9. Lumbar plexus.

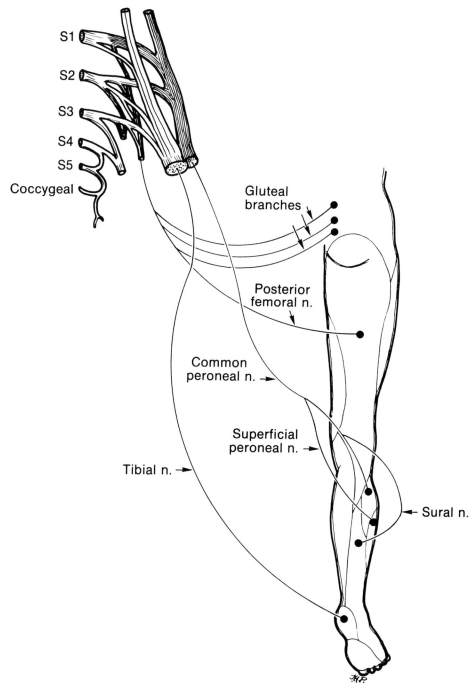

FIG 7–10. Sacral and coccygeal plexus.

TABLE 7–1.
Muscles of the Lower Extremity Controlling Motion

MUSCLE	NERVE(S)	FUNCTION(S)	PARALYSIS	TEST(S)
Psoas major	Lumbar plexus L1-L4	Flexion of hip	Weakened hip flexion	With thigh flexed, raise knee against resistance; with patient supine, raise extended extremity against downward resistance upon thigh
Ilicus	Femoral L2-L4	Flexion of hip	Weakened hip flexion	
Quadriceps femoris	Femoral L2-L4	Extends knee	Loss of active knee extension	Sitting or supine, extend leg against downward resistance against leg
Sartorius	Femoral L2-L4	Participates in hip flexion, lateral rotation	Weakened flexion and lateral rotation of hip	With knee extended, resist hip flexion*
Rectus femoris	Femoral L2-L4	Participates in hip flexion	Weakened knee extension	Resist extended leg
Gluteus maximus	Inferior gluteal L5-S1	Extension and lateral rotation of thigh	Hip extension weakened	Resist hip extension with patient prone
Gluteus medius	Superior gluteal L4-S1	Abducts hip	Abduction hip weakened	Resist hip abduction: sitting or supine separate knees against resistance
Gluteus minimus	Superior gluteal L4-S1	Abducts hip	Abduction hip weakened	Resist hip abduction
Tensor fascia latae	Superior gluteal L4-S1	Tensor assists flexion hip	Abduction of hip weakened	Resist hip abduction
Piriformis	To piriformis S1-S2	Abduction lateral rotation hip	Weakened lateral rotation abduction of hip	Resist lateral rotation, abduction of hip
Adductor longus	Obturator L2-L4	Adduction of thigh	Active adduction of thigh lost	Sitting or supine with knees together, patient resists separation of knee
Adductor brevis	Obturator L2-L4	Adduction of thigh	Same as above	(Same test as noted above)
Adductor magnus	Obturator L2-L4 Sciatic L4-L5 Supplies part of adductor magnus	Adduction and extension of thigh; also functions with hamstrings (medial rotation)	Adduction and extension thigh weakened	Resist adduction and extension of hip
Gracilis	Obturator L2-L4	Participates in adduction of thigh; flexion medial rotation of thigh	Adduction of thigh weakened	Resist thigh adduction
Gastrocnemius	Tibial L5-S2	Plantar flexion of foot also flexes knee but can't act with foot plantar flexes	Loss of plantar flexion of foot	Patient extends knee while plantar flexing foot against resistance; palpate muscle while testing

Muscle	Nerve & Root	Action	Loss	Test
Soleus	Tibial L5-S2	Plantar flexion of foot	Loss of plantar flexion of foot	Resist plantar foot flexion (same as above)
Biceps femoris	Tibial L5-S1	Flexion of knee	Active knee flexion weakened	While sitting flex knee against resistance or while prone with knee partly flexed, further flex against resistance
Semitendinosus	Tibial L5-S1	Flexion of knee; assists in hip extension	Active knee flexion, hip extension weakened; medial rotation of leg	With hip extended, resist knee flexion and medial rotation
Semimembranosus	Tibial L5-S1	Flexion of knee; assists in hip extension and medial rotation of leg	Active knee flexion, hip extension weakened; medial rotation of leg	(Same as noted above)
Tibialis anterior	Deep peroneal L4-S1	Dorsiflexes and inverts foot	Foot dorsiflexion and inversion lost	Dorsiflex and invert foot against resistance
Peroneus tertius	Deep peroneal L4-S1	Ankle dorsiflexion, tarsal eversion	Weakened ankle dorsiflexion, tarsal eversion	With foot dorsiflexed, resist eversion
Extensor digitorum longus	Deep peroneal L4-S1	Extension lateral four toes and dorsiflexes foot	Loss of toe extension eversion and ankle dorsiflexion	Resist toe extension
Extensor hallucis longus	Deep peroneal L4-S1	Extends big toe and dorsiflexes foot	Loss of big toe	Resist big toe extension
Extensor digitorum brevis	Deep peroneal L4-S1	Assists extension of toes except little toe	Loss of toe extension except little toe	Resist toe extension
Extensor hallucis brevis	Deep peroneal L4-S1	Extends big toe	Loss of big toe extension	Resist big toe extension
Peroneus longus	Superficial peroneal L4-S1	Eversion of foot and assists plantar flexion of foot	Loss of eversion of foot; weakened plantar flexion	With foot in plantar flexion resist eversion
Peroneus brevis	Superficial peroneal L4-S1	Eversion of foot and assists plantar flexion of foot	Loss of eversion of foot; weakened plantar flexion	With foot in plantar flexion resist eversion
Tibialis posterior	Posterior tibial L5-S1	Inversion and plantar flexion of foot	Inversion plantar flexion of foot weakened	While foot is plantar flexed, resist inversion
Flexor digitorum longus	Posterior tibial L5-S1	Plantar toe flexion especially at distal interphalangeal joints; assists plantar flexion of toes	Loss of toe flexion	Resist plantar flexion of toes
Flexor hallucis longus	Posterior tibial L5-S2	Plantar flexion of big toe and inversion	Loss of big toe flexion	Resist plantar flexion of big toe

* Muscles act in groups and often may be tested in groups.

In the presence of normal extensors of the back, if the examiner holds down the lower extremities with the patient in a prone position, the head and shoulders can be raised from the table.

The iliopsoas muscle is innervated chiefly by branches from (L1 to L4). It is the chief flexor of the hip. If it is weakened the patient will have difficulty in bring-

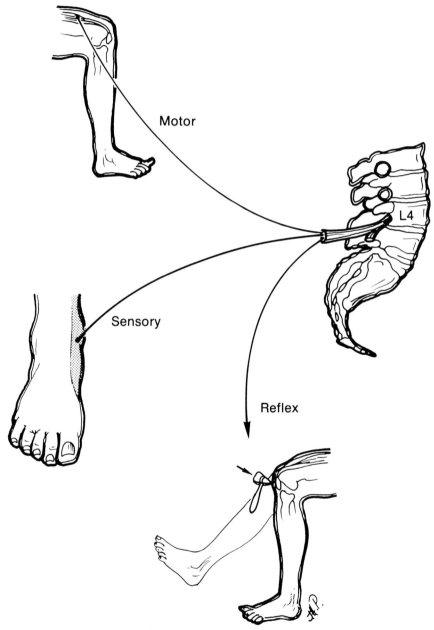

FIG 7–11. L-4 innervation.

ing the involved extremity forward. The examiner should also be certain the muscle is not contracted (see Hip, Chapter 8). The sensory dermatome pattern for these nerves is shown in Figure 1–1.

The adductors of the hip are innervated by nerve branches from the obturator nerve (L2-L4). They can be tested as a group. Similarly, the quadriceps muscles can be tested as a group. It keeps the knee actively extended when there is weight on the affected side. They are also innervated by the femoral nerve (L2-L4). The patellar reflex is possible primarily because of a corresponding intact spinal cord level at L-4.

The tibialis anterior is innervated by the deep peroneal nerve (L4-S1) (Fig 7–11). A weakened anterior tibial muscle can affect gait. The examiner should recall that the important patellar reflex arises from the L-4 level. If the nerve branch from the L-4 level is transected, the reflex can still be elicited since multiple nerve levels contribute to this reflex. Again, the sensory dermatome level is shown in Figure 1–1.

The neurologic level of L-5 can be tested by examining the strength of the extensor hallucis longus (Fig 7–12). It is innervated by the deep peroneal nerve

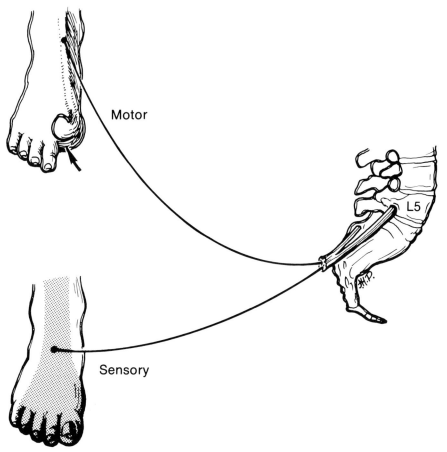

FIG 7–12. L-5 innervation.

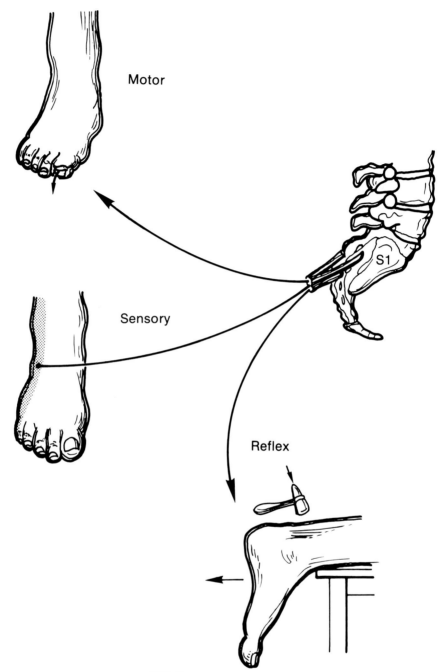

Motor

Sensory

Reflex

FIG 7–13. S-1 innervation.

(L4-S1). There is no reflex at this level. A compression of the L5 nerve root by a herniated disk at L4-5 will cause a weakness of this muscle.

The abductors of the hip (chiefly the gluteus medius and gluteus minimus) are innervated by the superior gluteal nerve (L4-S1). When these muscles are weakened the opposite side of the pelvis sags with a shift of body weight to the affected side (Trendelenburg's test).

To test the S-1 neurologic level, the muscle strengths of the peroneus longus and peroneus brevis should be examined (Fig 7–13). Similarly, the muscle strengths of the gastrocnemius-soleus group should be examined. A weakened gastrocnemius-soleus muscle group leads to difficulty in raising the heel during ambulation. This is commonly seen in a herniation of the L-5 disk. The achilles tendon reflex is present if the S-1 level is intact.

The nerves arising from S-2 to S-4 innervate the intrinsic muscles of the foot, and supply the muscle of the bladder.

Intermittent leg pain due to neural disease should be differentiated from intermittent claudication. Lumbar spinal stenosis may cause intermittent leg pain on one or both sides that can arise with activity and be relieved with rest. This should not be mistaken for vascular occlusive disease that causes leg pain with walking. A common cause of low back and leg pain is a herniated disk. Table 7–2 differentiates herniations at the fourth lumbar and fifth lumbar levels. Table 7–3 shows the principal muscles that control maneuvers of the lower extremity.

During any part of the neurologic examination the physician should keep in mind whether or not a patient is malingering and think of the whole person. Are the symptoms and findings localized or systemic? Are specific changes in the sensory pattern present that do not correspond to the anatomical nerve distribution? It is important to differentiate hysteria from malingering. The former may be related to a psychoneurosis. The patient has no control over his acts. With malingering the patient will willfully imitate disease. It may be difficult to differentiate these two conditions. Moreover, true spasticity of the muscle stretch reflex may be present and should be differentiated from disease not of organic nature. For example, disease associated with spastic paralysis is often characterized by a sustained contraction of specific muscle groups.

TABLE 7–2.
Neurologic Changes Associated With Common Lumbar Disc Herniations

LESION	L4 HERNIATION BETWEEN L4-5	L5 HERNIATION BETWEEN L5-S1
Affected nerve root	Fifth lumbar	First sacral
Pain pattern	Lateral thigh, anterolateral leg, dorsal aspect foot	Posterior thigh, posterolateral leg, lateral aspect foot, including heel and fourth and fifth toes
Sensory changes	Hypesthesia-anesthesia in areas where pain felt	Hypesthesia-anesthesia in areas where pain felt
Common muscle weakness	Extensor hallucis longus extensor digitorum brevis, and tibialis anterior	Plantar flexors of foot (triceps) and atrophy of posterior calf muscles
Reflex change	Tibialis posterior may be absent	Decreased or absent Achilles reflex

TABLE 7–3.

Principal Muscles Controlling Maneuvers of Lower Extremities

ACTION	MUSCLE(S)
Raise leg to step	Iliopsoas
Raising one side of body to step	Gluteus maximus and quadriceps
Shifting torso to side opposite raised leg during gait	Gluteus medius
Squatting and rising	Quadriceps
Walking on heels	Tibialis anterior and extensors of toes
Walking on toes	Gastrocnemius and soleus

Muscle Stretch Reflexes of the Trunk

Deep Abdominal Reflex.   The examiner may elicit this reflex by pressing on the abdominal muscles with a finger and tapping on the finger. If the deep abdominal reflex is exceptionally brisk, a pyramidal tract lesion should be suspect.

Back Reflexes.   With the patient prone, the examiner taps the lumbar and sacral areas of the spine. The erector spinal muscles contract.

Muscle Stretch Reflexes of the Lower Extremity

Patellar (quadriceps) Reflex.   This reflex is commonly termed the knee jerk. It is elicited when the patellar tendon is firmly tapped. In response the quadriceps femoris contracts. A similar response can be obtained by tapping the suprapatellar region when the patellar reflex is brisk.

Achilles (triceps surae) Reflex.   It is commonly termed the ankle jerk and is elicited by firmly tapping the achilles tendon above its insertion. During the testing of the reflex, the tendon is held taut by slightly dorsiflexing the foot. It is followed by a contraction of the gastrocnemius-soleus and plantaris muscles.

Adductor Reflex.   This reflex can be elicited by abducting the thigh slightly in order to stretch the adductor tendons, and then tapping in the area of the adductor tubercle. A response is obtained when the adductor muscles contract.

Internal-External Hamstring Reflex.   This reflex is elicited by tapping on the tendons of the semimembranosus and the biceps femoris muscles, respectively. A response is obtained when these muscles contract. The biceps femoris inserts into the fibula head and tapping the head of the fibula will cause a contraction of the muscle (fibular reflex).

Tensor Fasciae Latae Reflex.   This is elicited by tapping over the tensor fascia latae near its origin at the anterior superior iliac spine. The thigh will abduct in response.

Extensor Hallucis Longus Reflex.   This is obtained by tapping the examiner's finger while the finger exerts pressure over the terminal phalanx of the big toe.

Tibialis Posterior Reflex.   When this tendon is tapped behind the medial malleolus, a response is obtained when the foot inverts.

Brisk or diminished reflexes should not be interpreted as abnormal when isolated findings are discovered. If a reflex is diminished it may be reinforced by the Jendrassik maneuver. For example, on testing the patellar reflex the patient is asked to hook the cupped fingers together, placing the palm surfaces of the fingers of one hand into the others. While the patient pulls the fingers apart the tendon is tapped.

Superficial (Cutaneous) Reflexes

Superficial Abdominal Reflexes (Fig 7–14)

Epigastric Reflex.   Gently stroke from the tip of the sternum toward the umbilicus. A positive response follows with a contraction of the upper abdominal muscles.

Upper, Middle, Lower Abdominal Reflex.   The skin of each segment of the abdomen is stimulated in a diagonal manner. In response, the abdominal muscles of each segment should contract.

Bekhterev's Hypogastric Reflex.   The lower abdominal muscles contract when the inner aspect of the ipsilateral thigh is stimulated.

Cremasteric Reflex (Fig 7–15).   To elicit the reflex the skin of the upper and inner aspect of the thigh is stimulated downward from above. In response, the cremasteric muscle contracts with an ipsilateral elevation of the testicle. The nerve innervation is through the ilioinguinal and genitofemoral nerves (L1 and

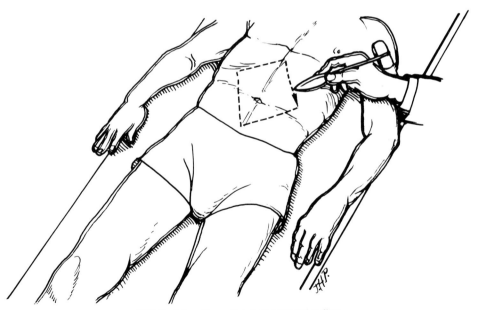

FIG 7–14. Superficial abdominal reflex.

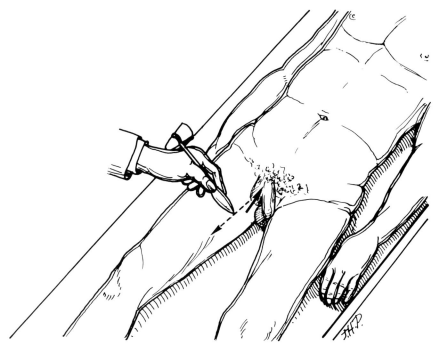

FIG 7–15. Cremasteric reflex.

L2). This reflex should not be confused with the scrotal reflex. In this latter reflex, the dartos of the scrotal sac contracts on stroking or applying a cold object.

Plantar Reflex. When the skin of the posterior and lateral portions of the plantar surface of the foot is stimulated, plantar flexion occurs. When the anterior and medial aspects of the foot are stimulated, especially the ball of the big toe, there is a brief extension of the big toe.

Superficial Anal Reflex. To elicit a response a pin is used to gently and carefully stroke the perianal skin. A positive response is obtained when the external sphincter contracts. The innervation of this muscle is via the inferior hemorrhoidal nerve (S2-S5). This reflex must not be confused with the internal anal sphincter reflex. Here, this latter reflex may be elicited when a gloved finger is inserted into the anus. A response is obtained when the sphincter contracts. This reflex is supplied by postganglionic fibers of the sympathetic division through the hypogastric plexus (presacral plexus). When this reflex is lost the sphincter does not close about the finger.

Pathologic Reflexes

Pyramidal tract responses are more clearly evident in the lower than in the upper extremity. Isolated responses should be carefully interpreted.

Babinski's Sign. It is elicited by stimulating the plantar skin of the foot with a blunt point such as a broken tongue blade. The stimulus is directed from the heel forward. When the toes flex or do not respond the response is negative. However, if the lateral four toes flex and fan while the big toe extends, the test is positive and may indicate an upper motor neuron lesion.

Chaddock's Sign. This is elicited by stimulating the lateral aspect of the foot beneath the lateral malleolus with a dull-pointed object. The response is similar to a positive Babinski test.

Oppenheim's Test. Heavy pressure is applied to the anterior surface of the tibia by the thumb and index finger and by firmly stroking downward from the infrapatellar area to the ankle. The response is the same as in the positive Babinski test.

Rossolimo's Sign. It is elicited when the examiner taps the ball of the foot on the plantar surface of the great toe. The test is performed with the patient supine. An abnormal response consists of a quick plantar flexion of the toes. It also indicates pyramidal tract disease.

Special Tests:

Hoover's Sign (Fig 7–16). While supine, the patient flexes the thigh and lifts one leg, and there is a downward force or movement of the opposite extremity. The examiner can evaluate this by placing both hands beneath the patient's heels. In true organic disease, as in a hemiplegia, the patient accentuates the downward pressure on the examiner's hand when an effort is made to elevate the paretic limb. In hysteria, this response is absent in the normal extremity. In patients with low back pain, increased downward pressure of the opposite normal extremity may be observed.

Naffziger's Sign. (see Chapter 6).

Valsalva's Maneuver. (see Chapter 6).

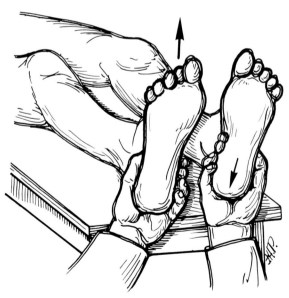

FIG 7–16. Hoover's test.

Brudzinski's Sign. The neck is passively flexed. A positive response occurs when there is flexion of both thighs at the hips. During the test, the chest should be held down. It indicates a painful stretching of the nerves and nerve roots, and is associated with meningeal irritation.

Kernig's Sign. With the patient recumbent the thigh is flexed 90° with the knee flexed 90° to the thigh. The leg is then extended upward. A positive response produces pain, spasm of the hamstring muscles, and resistance to further extension of the knee.

Beevor's Sign (Fig 7–17, A and B). With the patient recumbent, he raises his head against resistance, coughs, or attempts to rise to a sitting position from recumbency with the hands folded on the chest or behind the head. If the abdominal muscles contract equally on both sides of the midline, the umbilicus will remain in the midline (Fig 7–17, A). When there are weakened abdominal muscles on one side, these movements are performed with difficulty. Moreover, if there is paralysis of the abdominal muscles on one side, the umbilicus is pulled to the normal side (Fig 7–17, B). Paralysis of the upper half of one side of the abdominal muscles is associated with a downward movement of the umbilicus when the abdominal wall is tense, while there is upward movement of the umbilicus with paralysis of the lower half. This is termed Beevor's sign. When both sides of the abdominal muscles are paralyzed the umbilicus will bulge during coughing.

Patrick's Test. (see Chapter 8).

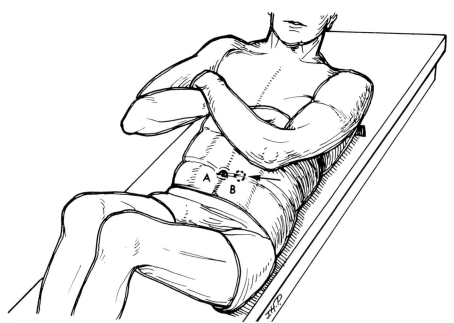

FIG 7–17. Beevor's sign: normal position of umbilicus (*A*); displaced umbilicus to normal side due to paralysis of abdominal muscles of opposite side (*B*).

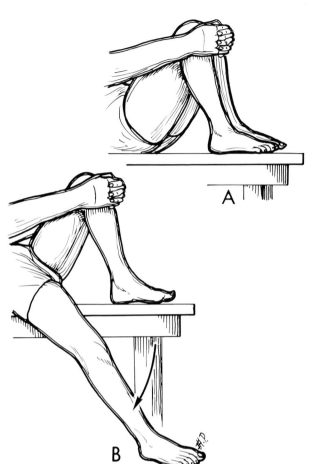

FIG 7–18. Gaenslen's test. See text for further description.

Ober's Test. (see Chapter 8).

Thomas's Test. The Thomas test is present when one thigh is flexed on the abdomen to flatten lumbar lordosis. Any flexion of the opposite thigh represents a fixed contracture of that hip.

Gaenslen's Test (Fig 7–18). This is a helpful test in differentiating between a sacroiliac and lumbosacral lesion. With the patient recumbent and relaxed (Fig 7–18, A) one hip is forcibly hyperextended with the pelvis and lumbar spine fixed by means of extreme flexion of the opposite hip (Fig 7–18, B). In this test, pain is present in sacroiliac and absent in lumbosacral lesions.

Straight Leg Raising Test (Fig 7–19). Normally, the leg can be raised to 90° without discomfort with the patient supine. By raising the lower extremity with the patient supine pain is produced. The examiner should determine if the pain is in the low back or related to hamstring tightness only. Does the pain relate to stretching of the sciatic nerve? If one extremity is elevated and the pain is produced on the same side it is termed a positive ipsilateral straight leg raising

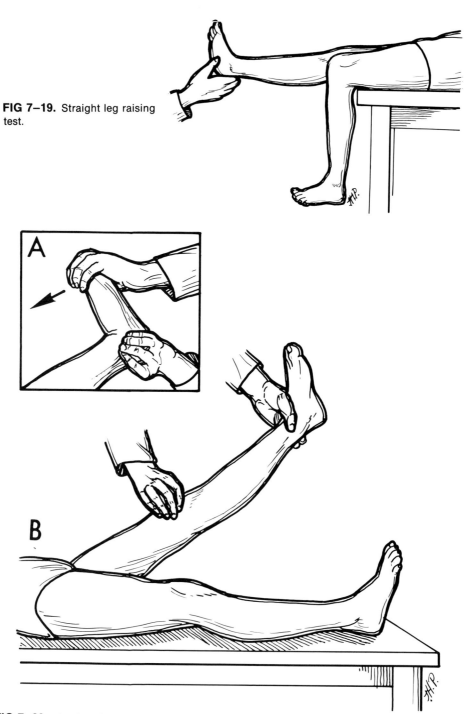

FIG 7–19. Straight leg raising test.

FIG 7–20. Lasègue's test: inset (*A*), dorsiflexing the foot may stretch the sciatic nerve and increase pain.

test. If raising the same leg causes pain in the opposite leg it is termed a positive contralateral straight leg raising test. The number of degrees that the extremity is elevated and produces pain should be recorded. This latter test has been called the well leg straight leg raising test and a positive response may indicate a tumor or herniated disk in the lumbar area.

Lasègue's Sign (Fig 7–20). When the hip is flexed with the knee extended, as in performing the straight leg raising test, not only is there referred pain in the leg but there is resistance to leg raising due to hamstring spasm. A positive response should be recorded as an ipsilateral or contralateral and the degrees of elevation recorded when pain is first produced.

When there is calf tenderness it should be differentiated from thrombophlebitis of the calf (Fig 7–21, B). When the foot is dorsiflexed, calf pain is increased (Homan's sign) (Fig 7–21, A). However, similar pain can be exacerbated by dorsiflexing the foot during the performance of the Lasègue test (see Fig 7–20, A).

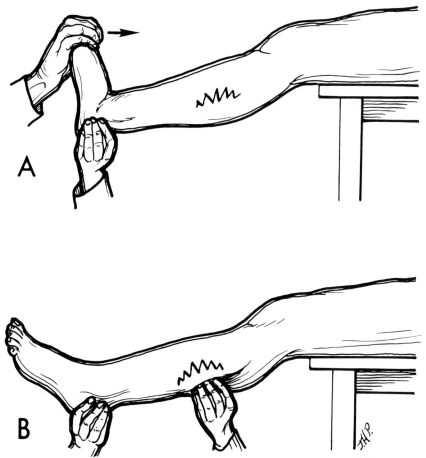

FIG 7–21. Test for thrombophlebis: Homans' sign (A); compression of calf (B).

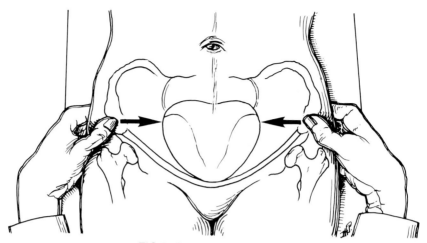

FIG 7–22. Pelvis rock test.

Pelvic Rock Test (Fig 7–22). With the patient supine, the examiner's hands compress the pelvis by pressing the hands together at the superior anterior iliac spines. Pain is produced in the sacroiliac articulation if there is localized pathology.

References

1. DeJong RN: *The Neurologic Examinations: Incorporating the Fundamentals of Neuroanatomy and Neurophysiology,* ed 4. Hagerstown, Md, Harper & Row Publishers Inc, 1979.
2. Gaenslen FJ: Sacroiliac arthrodesis. *JAMA* 1927; 89:2031–2035.
3. Hoover CF: A new sign for the detection of malingering and functional paralysis of the lower extremities. *JAMA* 1908; 51:746–749.

CHAPTER 8

Physical Examination of the Adult Hip Joint

Glenn C. Landon, M.D.
Jorge O. Galante, M.D.

Whether one is treating the acutely injured patient in the emergency setting or the patient with a chronic problem in the office setting, the physical examination of the hip is an essential element of the clinician's thought process in arriving at a diagnosis and formulating a plan for treatment. The physician's examination must be guided by a carefully taken history and supplemented by roentgenologic and laboratory evaluations as needed. However, one must not allow laboratory or roentgenologic studies to supplant a carefully performed physical examination. Those who gloss over the physical examination of the patient and rely on roentgenologic examination to arrive at a diagnosis may sooner or later commit a serious error in diagnosis.

By using a systematic approach to the physical examination, the physician will be less likely to miss an important clinical finding and arrive at an improper diagnosis. An orderly step-by-step examination will be presented and it is suggested that the physician establish a logical sequence in his mind and adhere to this so as to avoid any omissions.

Gait

In the office setting the physical examination often begins by observing the patient's gait as he walks into the examining room. One should immediately begin observation to detect a limp, deformity, or leg length discrepancy. Examination of gait will be aided as the patient disrobes and is placed in a dressing gown that exposes the lower extremities.

A basic understanding of the mechanics of gait is needed to understand pathologic disturbances in gait and is useful in making a diagnosis based on the physical examination of gait.

Gait may be divided into two phases: stance phase, during which time the foot is in contact with the ground, and swing phase, when the opposite foot is in contact with the ground (Fig 8–1). Inman has categorized the important determinants of gait; familiarity with these aids in understanding the analysis of locomotion and the crucial role the hip joint plays in the determinants of gait.

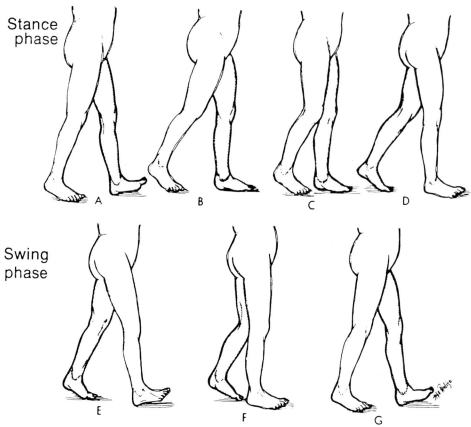

FIG 8–1. Stance *A–D* and swing *E–G* phases of gait (limb in contact with ground is shaded).

The first element of gait is pelvic rotation (Fig 8–2). This serves to flatten the arch of the center of the mass as it moves through space. The second determinant is pelvic list (Fig 8–3). In normal walking, the pelvis lists downward in the coronal plane on the side opposite to the limb in contact with the ground. Pelvic list at normal speeds measures 5°, and this displacement occurs at the hip joint, producing a relative adduction of the stance limb and abduction of the swing-phase limb. The third element of gait is stance-phase knee flexion (Fig 8–4). This is typically 15° in magnitude. This again serves to decrease the oscillation of the center of mass as it passes over the weight-bearing limb. Another important determinant of gait is the lateral displacement of the body (Fig 8–5). Normally the body is shifted slightly over the weight-bearing limb with each step. Approximately 4 to 5 cm of total lateral displacement of the body from side to side occurs with each complete stride. Rotations also occur at the shoulder and thorax.

With a familiarity of normal gait patterns, one may then observe pathologic gaits as an important clinical sign of disease of the hip joint. Certain pathologic gaits are quite characteristic and should be recognized by the clinician.

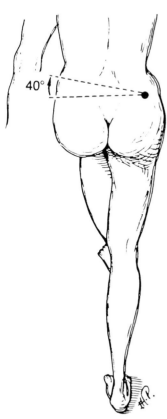

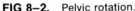

FIG 8–2. Pelvic rotation.

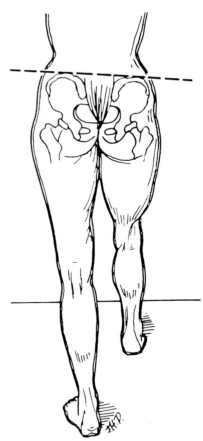

FIG 8–3. Pelvic list.

A Gluteus Medius or Abductor Gait. Patients with weakness or paralysis of the gluteus medius may have an abductor lurch (Fig 8–6). In this gait, because of weakness of the hip abductors the normal pelvic list is exaggerated and the pelvis will list downward on the side opposite to the stance phase limb. The patient will compensate with an exaggerated shift of the trunk to attempt to maintain the center of gravity of the trunk closer to the stance phase limb.

The Antalgic Gait. This is very often seen in painful conditions about the hip (Fig 8–7). The cause of this type of gait is pain in the hip during the stance phase. In an attempt to relieve this pain, the patient tries to shorten the stance phase as much as possible and will shorten the time of stance on the involved hip compared with the normal uninvolved limb.

After examination of the patient's gait one may then perform the Trendelenburg test. This extremely useful clinical test is designed to evaluate the strength of the hip abductors, specifically the gluteus medius and minimus. The examiner typically stands behind the patient and then asks the patient to alternately raise one leg and then the other. Normally, with the patient standing on the left limb, the left gluteus medius will contract and elevate the pelvis on the right side.

In case of weakness or paralysis of the gluteus medius, the pelvis on the opposite side will sink and the patient will shift the trunk over the stance in an attempt to move the center of gravity closer to the involved limb (Fig 8–8). Numerous pathologic conditions may cause weakness of the gluteus maximus. These include fractures, deformities of the femoral neck, such as coxa vara or dislocations of the hip, avulsions of the greater trochanter in total hip replacement, and neurologic involvement with paralysis of the superior gluteal nerve. Although the Trendelenburg test is not specific for any one pathologic condition, it is extremely useful and the presence of a positive or negative Trendelenburg's test should always be noted in the patient's record.

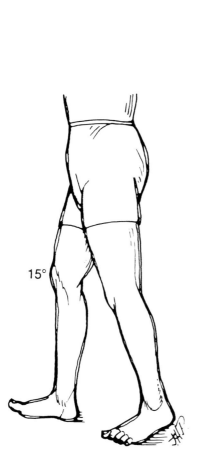

FIG 8–4. Knee flexion during stance phase.

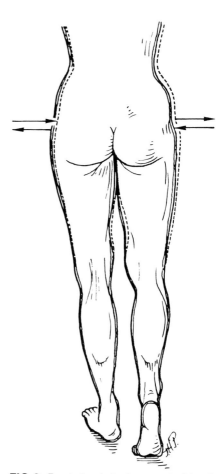

FIG 8–5. Lateral displacement of trunk.

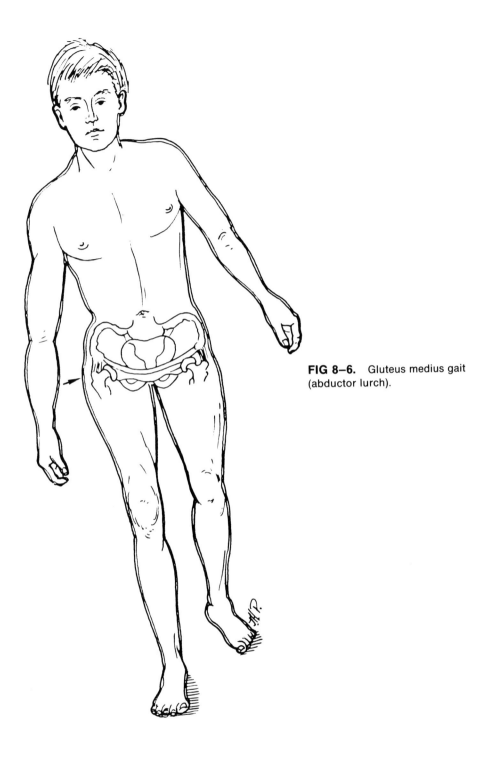

FIG 8–6. Gluteus medius gait (abductor lurch).

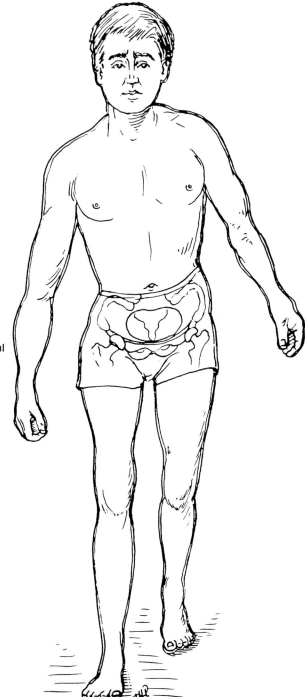

FIG 8–7. Antalgic gait (painful right hip).

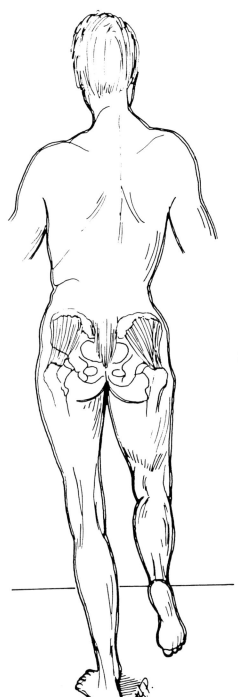

FIG 8–8. Positive Trendelenburg's test.

Inspection

The inspection portion of the examination has already begun with examination of the patient's gait. The skin about the hip should be examined and search for birth marks, discoloration, abrasion, erythema, sinus tracts, or swelling. The presence of previous incisions should be checked as an indication of the type of surgical approach used.

With the patient standing, one notices the position of the pelvis, trunk and limbs. The presence or absence of pelvic obliquity is noted as a clue to leg length discrepancy or contracture of the hip joint (Fig 8–9). The contour of the pelvis should be noted; for example, a patient with long-standing bilateral congenital dislocation of the hip has a very broad-appearing pelvis due to the lateral prominence of the greater trochanter (Fig 8–10).

Presence of angular deformity of the limb should be noted. The contour of the muscles should be examined and the presence of any atrophy noted.

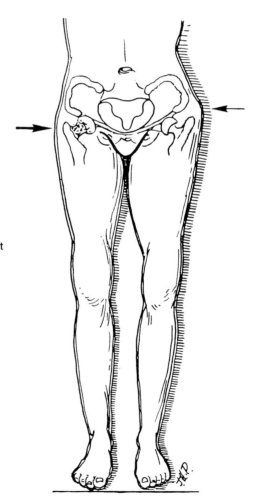

FIG 8–9. Pelvic obliquity noted with patient standing.

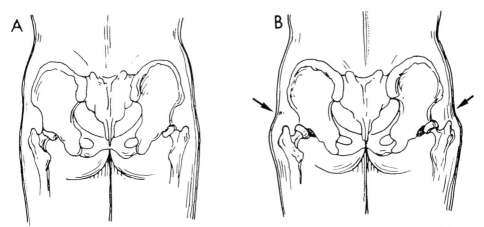

FIG 8–10. Normal contour of hip (*A*) compared to patient with bilateral congenital dislocation (*B*).

Palpation

With the patient standing facing the physician, the iliac crest should be palpated and any pelvic obliquity should be noted. The anterior superior iliac spine can be easily palpated in all but the most obese patients (Fig 8–11). Palpation of the greater trochanter is next performed. The trochanter should normally be at

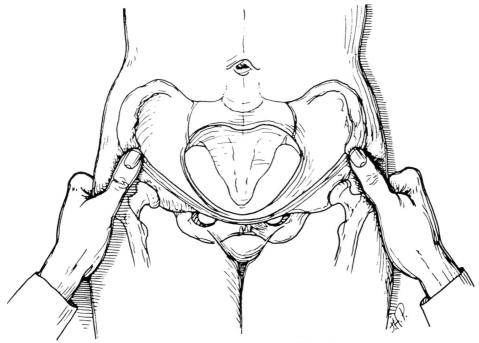

FIG 8–11. Palpation of anterior superior iliac spines.

the same level. With dislocation of the hip, the affected trochanter will be palpated more cephalad than normal. Tenderness over the greater trochanter is indicative of the commonly seen entity of trochanteric bursitis. The pubic symphysis should be palpated as the presence of pain at the symphysis is an indication of the possibility of osteitis pubis or fractures of the pubic rami.

Examination of the posterior aspects of the hip should include the posterior aspects of the greater trochanter, the posterior superior iliac spines, and the ischial tuberosity (Fig 8–12). The ischial tuberosity may be the site of a painful bursitis and one should attempt to elicit pain on palpation of this area.

In addition to the bony prominences and their overlying bursae, important soft tissue structure should be palpated in examination of the hip. In the anterior aspect of the hip, the femoral triangle area should be palpated (Fig 8–13). The femoral triangle is bordered superiorly by the inguinal ligament, medially by the adductor longus, and laterally by the sartorius muscle. The structures in the femoral triangle include the femoral nerve, artery, and vein, and the inguinal lymph nodes. The femoral nerve is most lateral, but is ordinarily not palpable. The femoral artery is palpable just inferior to inguinal ligament and the femoral vein is located just medial to the artery. One should be able to locate the vein as it is useful in certain cases for venous access. The adductor longus muscle is usually palpable when contracted. One should be familiar with the anatomy of the origin of the adductor muscles as percutaneous adductor tenotomy is often performed in children's hip surgery. The presence of lymphadenopathy in the

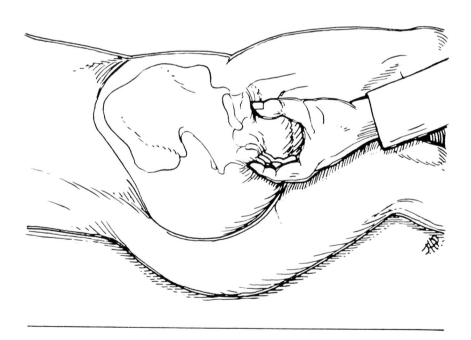

FIG 8–12. Palpation of ischial tuberosity and greater trochanter.

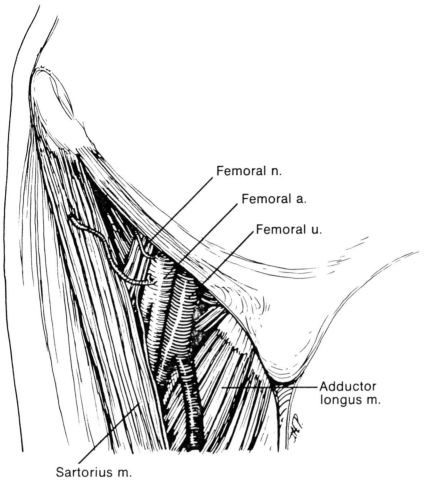

FIG 8–13. Femoral triangle (right hip).

femoral triangle should be noted as a clue to possibility of infection or malignancy.

The course of the sciatic nerve should be familiar to the examiner. The sciatic nerve exits below the pyriformus and then crosses between the ischial tuberosity and the greater trochanter. In thin people it may be easily palpated and one should notice a close proximity to the posterior aspect of the hip joint (Fig 8–14).

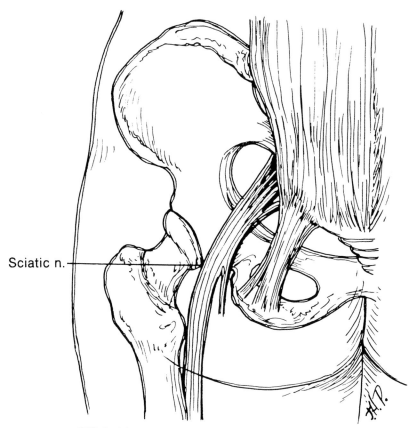

Sciatic n.

FIG 8–14. Sciatic nerve (viewed from posterior).

Physical Examination of the Hip in the Trauma Patient

Certain special considerations deserve mention in the physical examination of the hip in the trauma victim. Normally the patient is unable to walk and the examination must be conducted with the patient supine on emergency room cart. Clothing should be gently removed or cut off in case of obvious fracture or dislocation.

Inspection of the patient should be performed to detect abrasion, swelling, or ecchymosis. The position of the limb should be noted and can be indicative of fracture or dislocation. With a traumatic posterior dislocation of the hip, the involved extremity is found in a characteristic position of shortening, adduction, and internal rotation (Fig 8–15). The greater trochanter will be unduly prominent. If the limb appears abducted, externally rotated with cyanosis, or has swelling of the extremity, one should suspect traumatic anterior dislocation of the hip (Fig 8–16), where the dislocated femoral head can cause pressure on the femoral vein causing venous congestion.

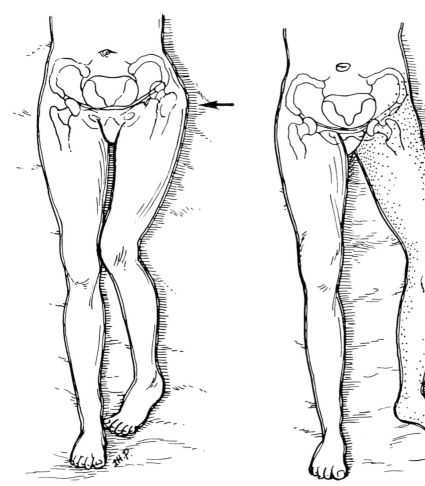

FIG 8–15. Traumatic posterior dislocation with the limb shortened, adducted, and internally rotated.

FIG 8–16. Traumatic anterior dislocation with limb externally rotated.

Fracture of the hip is an extremely common entity especially in the elderly. The antecedent trauma may be extremely trivial in the patient with osteoporosis and often one will hear a history of sudden pain in the hip when the patient is arising from a chair or turning suddenly. The patient with a displaced femoral neck or intertrochanteric fracture will characteristically be in pain lying supine with the extremity shortened and externally rotated. One may easily differentiate between an intracapsular or subcapital fracture or an extracapsular or intertrochanteric fracture by the position of the foot. With an intracapsular fracture the intact capsule usually prevents external rotation of the foot beyond 45° (Fig 8–17), as compared with an extracapsular fracture in which the foot typically lies externally rotated 90° against the bed (Fig 8–18).

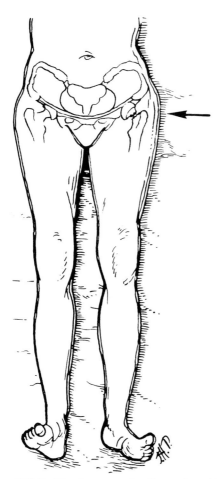

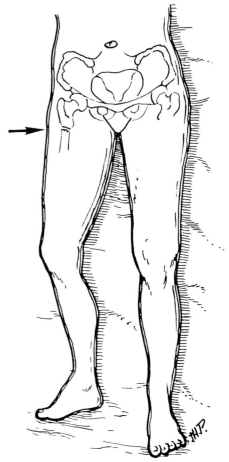

FIG 8–17. Intrascapular (femoral neck) fracture, limb is externally rotated at 45°.

FIG 8–18. Extracapsular fracture (intertrochanteric or subtrochanteric) foot will be externally rotated at 90°.

The pelvic crest, the anterior superior iliac spine, and the pelvic rim should be palpated and compressed, and crepitus or pain noted as a sign of underlying fracture.

It is extremely important to examine the hip area in patients with femoral fractures. Femoral fractures may be associated with ipsilateral dislocation of the hip, and this can be easily missed if the joint is not examined and appropriate roentgenograms taken. As in any examination of the trauma patient, careful notation is made of the neurovascular status of the extremity involved.

Range of Motion Measurement

Range of motion is normally performed with patient supine on examining table. Flexion of the hip is commonly measured first. This is performed coincidental with the Thomas test (Fig 8–19). The Thomas test is designed to detect

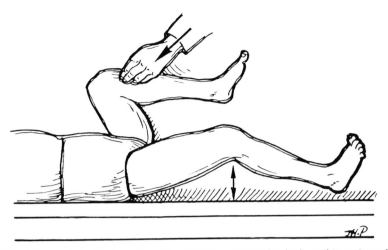

FIG 8–19. Thomas's test (hip is flexed to eliminate lumbar lordosis and to note residual flexion in opposite hip).

the presence of flexion contracture of the hip. One stabilizes the pelvis by placing the hand under the patient's lumbar spine and then flexes the opposite hip, bringing the thigh up. As the hip is flexed in the near maximum position, the lumbar lordosis is flattened. Once this is done the presence of any residual flexion in the opposite hip is noted and the amount is recorded as flexion contracture. The hip should continue to be flexed to its maximum range. The normal range of hip flexion is 120° (Fig 8–20). Extension past the zero position may be possible to 30°. To measure extension, the patient needs to lie prone on the examining table (Fig 8–21). This test is normally not particularly useful in the examination of the adult hip.

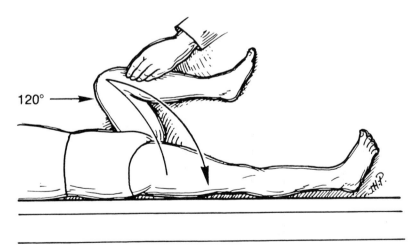

120°

FIG 8–20. Range of flexion of hip.

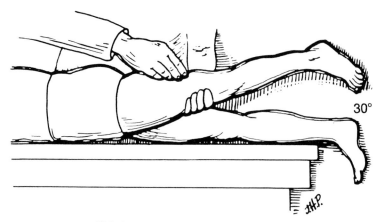

FIG 8–21. Extension of hip joint.

Abduction

Abduction is normally measured with the hip in extension. With the patient supine on the examining table, the examiner places one hand on the iliac crest and grasps the ankle with the other, and then moves the limb from the midline until the pelvis is felt to move. Normally, abduction is present to approximately 45°. Abduction is commonly decreased in arthritic conditions of the hip. An additional useful method for recording hip abduction is measuring the distance between the medial malleoli when both hips are maximally abducted. This is an easy-to-perform and reproducible test.

Adduction

Adduction is normally present to 20° or 30° past the midline. Again this test is performed with the patient supine and the examiner's hand on one iliac crest and then on the ankle. The leg is moved until the pelvis begins to move and the angle past the zero position noted.

Rotation

Rotation may be measured both in flexion and extension. It is a particularly sensitive measurement and is one of the first motions lost early in arthritic conditions about the hip. With the hips in extension and the patient supine, there is normally 35° of internal rotation and 45° of external rotation possible. One may judge the amount of rotation by noting the position of the patella from the neutral position (Fig 8–22). A somewhat more accurate way of measuring is to place the patient supine and flex the knees with the hips in extension. One may then rotate the hip internally and externally and note the position of the leg in relation to zero position (Fig 8–23). Rotation may be also measured with the hip in 90° flexion. In this case the examiner will flex the hip and knee to 90° with the thigh perpendicular to a transverse plane across the anterior superior iliac spines. Internal rotation is measured by rotation of the leg away from the mid-

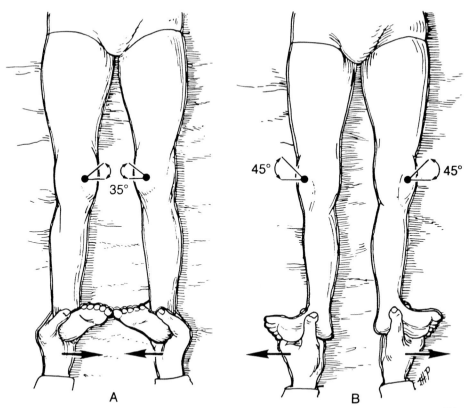

FIG 8–22. Rotation of hip joint in extension: internal rotation (**A**), external rotation (**B**).

line of the trunk and upward, and external rotation measured by rotating the leg toward the midthigh of the trunk.

Neurologic Examination

The neurologic examination about the hip is important in determining the strength of the muscles and also differentiating between the hip joint as the source of pain compared with referred sources of pain from nerve root compression. The neurologic examination about the hip usually consists of muscle testing sensation, and reflex testing.

Muscle Testing

Muscle testing is indirectly performed in the examination of gait and the performance of the Trendelenburg's test. Additional testing of flexors, extensors, abductors, and adductors can be performed.

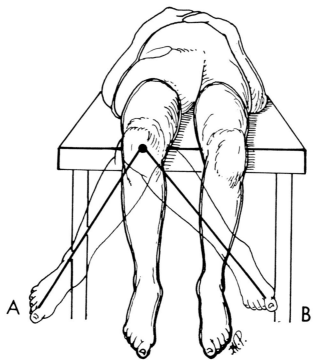

FIG 8–23. Rotation of hip joint with knees flexed: internal rotation (**A**), external rotation (**B**).

Hip Flexors

The iliopsoas is the primary flexor of the hip. It is innovated by the femoral nerve and usually comprises the L1, L2 and L3 nerve roots. To test the strength of the iliopsoas, the patient is examined seated on the examining table and is asked to flex the hip around 90° against manual resistance (Fig 8–24).

Hip Extensors

The primary hip extensor is the gluteus maximus, which is innovated by the inferior gluteal nerve consisting primarily of the S1 nerve root. Secondary hip extensors are the hamstring muscles. To measure the strength of the gluteus maximus, the patient is placed prone on the examining table and is asked to extend the hip against the examiner's hand placed on the thigh and pelvis (Fig 8–25).

Hip Abductors

Primary hip abductors are the gluteus medius and minimus innervated by the superior gluteal nerve of the L5 nerve root. The strength of these has already been tested with observation of gait and the Trendelenburg test. An additional

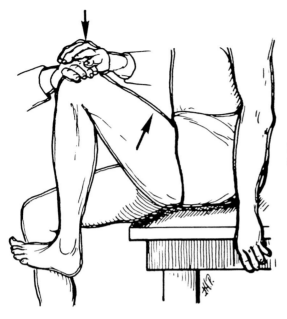

FIG 8–24. Testing hip flexor strength.

test can be performed by placing the patient in the lateral position on the examining table and then having him abduct the hip against resistance (Fig 8–26).

Hip Adductors

The primary adductors are the adductor longus, brevis, and magnus, which are innervated chiefly by the obturator nerve (the L2, L3 and L4 nerve roots). One may test the strength of these muscles by having the patient lie supine with the legs abducted. He is then asked to adduct his legs while the examiner places his hands over the medial malleoli and resists the patient (Fig 8–27).

Sensation

Sensory dermatomes on the hip are illustrated (Chapter 1, Fig 1–1). There are certain cutaneous nerves of importance in pathologic conditions. The lateral femoral cutaneous nerve can be located just distal to the anterior-superior iliac crest. Compression of this nerve causes a painful entity known as meralgia paresthetica. The clunial nerves are the posterior primary divisions of L1, L2, and L3. They cross the iliac crest and can be irritated by incisions placed over this area for bone grafts.

In addition to the examination of sensation around the hips, the patellar and Achilles reflexes should be tested and noted. It is also important to note the presence of ankle and foot dorsiflexion strength, especially when one is dealing with fractures, dislocations, and surgery around the hip. The sciatic nerve is close to the posterior aspect of the hip joint and can be injured in trauma or surgery to the hip. One should be very careful to note the function of the sciatic nerve and especially its perineal branch after any hip surgery.

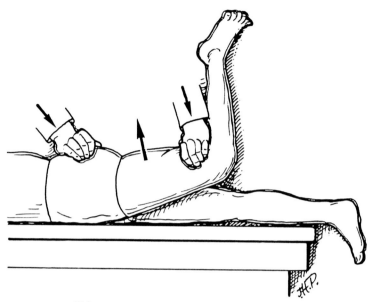

FIG 8–25. Testing hip extensor strength.

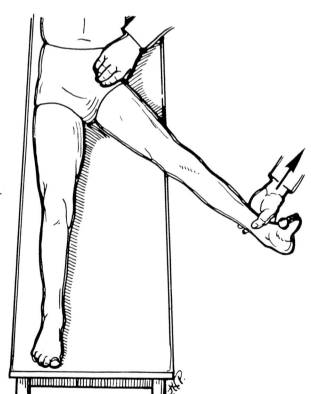

FIG 8–26. Testing hip abductor strength.

180   *G.C. Landon, J.O. Galante*

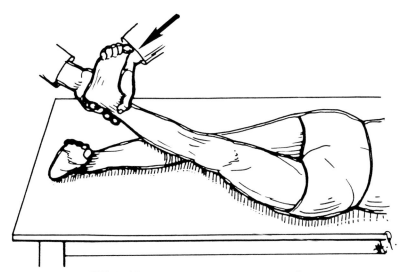

FIG 8–27. Testing hip adductor strength.

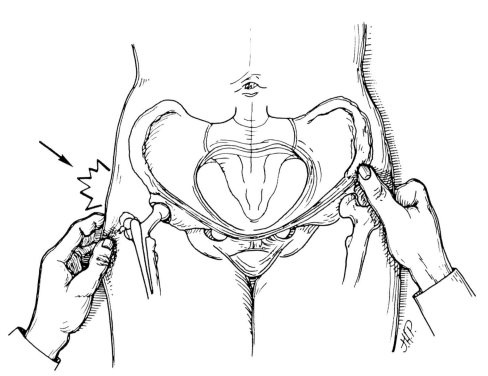

FIG 8–28. Trochanteric bursitis in patient with wire fixation of trochanteric osteotomy for total hip arthroplasty.

Examination of the Patient with Total Hip Replacement

Certain special considerations are important in examination of the patient with prior hip-replacement surgery. One should note the position of the incision as an indication of the type of surgical approach used. Posterior incisions associated with the posterior approach to the hip are known to be associated with a higher incidence of postoperative dislocation. One should search for any signs of erythema or drainage about the previous hip incision. Palpate the area of the incision and over the greater trochanter. In patients who have had trochanteric osteotomy with wire fixation of the trochanter, there is frequently a painful bursitis over the prominence of the greater trochanter (Fig 8–28). Examination of gait in the patient with hip replacement adheres to the same principles already mentioned. The Trendelenburg sign should be noted. The range of motion examination must be performed carefully in the patient with prior hip-replacement surgery, as one should avoid flexion adduction and lateral rotation which

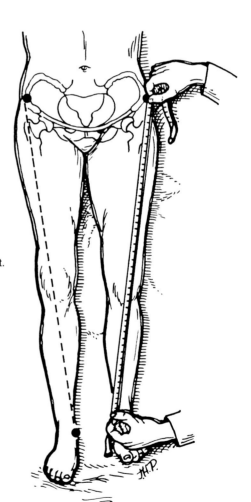

FIG 8–29. True leg length measurement.

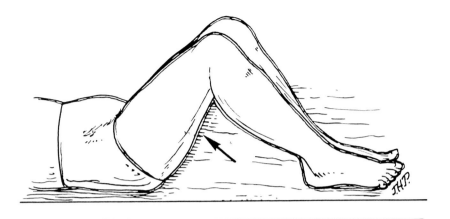

FIG 8–30. Observation of unequal limb length due to short femur.

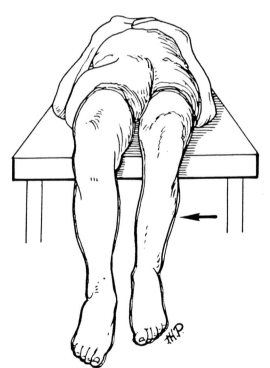

FIG 8–31. Observation of unequal limb length due to short tibia.

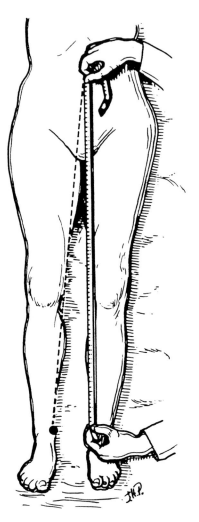

FIG 8–32. Measurement of apparent leg length.

might provoke a dislocation. Leg length discrepancy should be measured and recorded in the patient record. Serial loss of leg length is a reliable clinical sign of loosening and subsidence of the femoral prosthesis.

Leg Length

Measurement of leg length is an important indicator of serious disease of the hip joint and is essential in planning reconstructive surgical procedures.

True Leg Length Discrepancy

With the patient supine on the examining table, the distance between the anterior iliac spine and medial malleolus of the ipsilateral ankle is measured and then compared with the opposite side. The difference is the true leg length discrepancy (Fig 8–29).

One may easily determine whether the discrepancy comes from the femur or the tibia by observing the legs in profile with the hips flexed and the legs off the table compared with the hips and knees flexed with the legs on the table (Figs 8–30 and 8–31).

Apparent Leg Length Discrepancy

Often in pathologic conditions of the hip the patient may appear to have leg length discrepancy, but when measurements are made of true leg length there is no difference. This apparent shortening of one leg may stem from adduction, or abduction or flexion deformities of the hip, or fixed pelvic obliquity. Apparent leg length discrepancy is measured again with the patient supine on the examining table. The reference is taken in the midline by using the umbilicus and the distance measured to a fixed bony landmark such as the medial malleolus (Fig 8–32). If there is an apparent leg length discrepancy with no difference in true leg length, one may then conclude that there is a fixed deformity of the hip.

CHAPTER 9

Examination of the Lower Extremities in the Child, Part 1

Lorin M. Brown, M.D.
W. John Sharrard, M.D. Ch.M., F.R.C.S.

An examination of the infant or child is quite different from that of the adult. Simple observation of the child plays a much more important role in the diagnosis. The diagnostician must be aware of the limitations imposed by youth, and the patient must be treated tenderly. First, observe the gait pattern. Motion will be limited by normal developmental stages. Normal muscle strength testing is not reliable until 5 years of age. Sensory testing other than gross reaction to a stimulus, such as pinprick for a total sensory loss, is not reliable until 9 or 10 years of age. For a variety of reasons, it may take multiple visits to determine what the patient's parents have routinely observed. After the child is examined clothed and reassured, undress the child in a warm room. The young patient should remain on the parent's lap for as long as possible. If the child cannot or will not respond to verbal commands, then sensory stimulation, deep-tendon reflexes, or percussion must be substituted to obtain the desired motion. Observation for asymmetry and differences from the norm can be the first sign of significant underlying pathology.

The Foot and Ankle

The neonatal foot and ankle may exhibit five basic variations from the normal neutral accepted position. The first of these is equinus, where the foot is plantar flexed completely through both the hindfoot and forefoot (Fig 9–1). The second is equinovarus deformity (clubfoot). In this position, in addition to plantar flexion and equinus, the forefoot is pulled into adduction (Fig 9–2). The foot is especially smaller with hindfoot varus, forefoot adductus, supination, and plantar flexion. Laterally, the head of the talus is palpable and elevated. The tibia is not in internal torsion. In the older and neglected cases there may even be lateral torsion present. In milder forms of clubfoot, the heel is wider and less elevated. These cases will often correct well. However, in the more severe cases the heel is elevated and small and usually associated with a "wasted" calf (Fig 9–3).

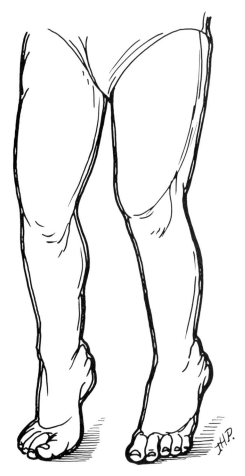

FIG 9–1. Feet in equinus.

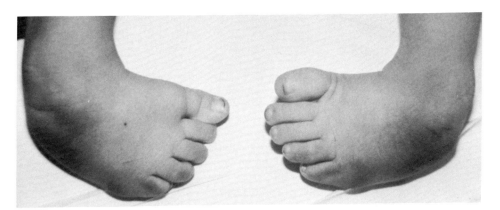

FIG 9–2. Hindfeet in plantar flexion and equinus with the forefeet in adduction (clubfeet).

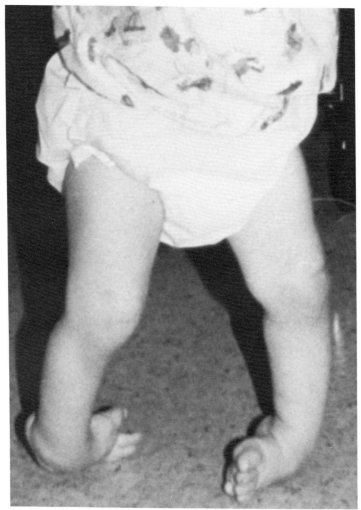

FIG 9–3. Complete congenital clubfeet deformity with wasted calves and full equinovarus adducted foot.

A third variation is cavovarus. The cavovarus foot has a pronated forefoot, a supinated hindfoot, and cavus in the longitudinal arch. There may be a claw toe configuration with contracture of the plantar structures as well. In addition, the forefoot is brought into the adducted position (Fig 9–4). Calcaneus is the fourth position. In this condition the entire foot, both forefoot and hindfoot, is in complete dorsiflexion (Fig 9–5). Calcaneus due to the position of the fetus in utero usually corrects rapidly and easily except when it is associated with a paralytic lesion such as spina bifida. There is a high correlation with hip dysplasia. The fifth posture is that of simple forefoot adduction (metatarsus adductus) in which the hindfoot is in neutral position, but the forefoot is in pure adduction usually at the talonavicular joints or in a combination of the metatarsal cunei-

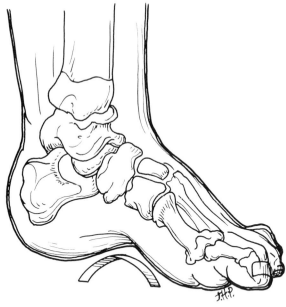

FIG 9–4. Cavovarus foot—foot in cavus with forefoot in varus with high arch.

form and cuneonavicular joints (Fig 9–6). A variation of the equinus foot is the equinovalgus foot, which is found at birth and is usually associated with congenital absence of the fibula or defects of the tibia.

In the clubfoot and metatarsus adductus conditions there is a deep transverse medial arch crease. In the clubfoot, this crease is positioned over the medial plantar surface and marks the start of forefoot drop. The permanency of these positions varies in degree from the flexible residual of intrauterine molding to the rigid neuromuscularly imbalanced deformities requiring treatment. Flexibility must also be distinguished from the "floppiness" of a neuromuscularly imbalanced infant.

Between the ages of 1 and 2 years the child begins to stand, and while the foot is in a stance phase, the forefoot, hindfoot, and arch variations can be observed.

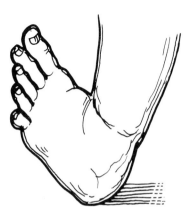

FIG 9–5. Calcaneous foot.

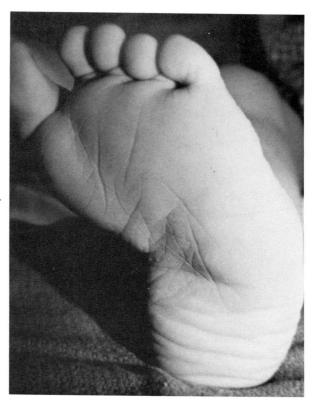

FIG 9–6. Metatarsus adductus.

In the hypermobile child there are lax ligaments in the child's foot that with weight-bearing give the appearance of a flattened medial arch. This may be attributed to a splaying of the medial foot with normal weight-bearing and excessive joint laxity. With this physiologic flatfoot one can observe that with the child on tiptoes the heel goes into slight inversion and the arch is well restored. An ominous sign occurs when the foot stays in valgus in the position of toe standing as this may indicate underlying pathology. It is important to remember that when evaluating the foot, the heel and sole of the shoe should be observed for a corresponding wear.

The forefoot grows first during adolescence and therefore the adolescent child may appear to have a prominent base of the fifth metatarsal. This is not pathologic. A swelling of the posterior lateral aspect of the heel may represent an early calcaneal exostosis. There may also be thickening of the skin and swelling of the bursa. Another abnormality that may be noted is that of dorsal exostosis, especially over the base of the first metatarsal. This usually represents a thickening in the ligaments rather than the bone or bony prominences. When evaluating foot posture, related spinal and cerebral problems must be considered, as the deformity may primarily be related to an underlying pathology such as spina bifida, cerebral palsy (Fig 9–7, A), or muscular dystrophy (Fig 9–7, B) rather than to an anatomic local problem. The main concern is that of progression. There is no progression in the case of arthrogryposis (Fig 9–7, C). Hip adduction contractures associated with subluxation or even dislocation may also occur with these conditions (Figs 9–7, D and E).

A medial prominence over the navicular bone on the foot usually represents an accessory navicular bone. When this is quite prominent, this condition may be painful and even inflamed at times.

A painfully everted foot occasionally occurs as a result of a tarsal bridge or coalition. This results in a peroneal spastic flatfoot. There is some valgus deformity at the midfoot that varies by the location of the coalition. There is spasm in the peroneal muscles and even in the extensor digitorum longus. Three other conditions lead to pain with related deformity of the foot. The first of these is

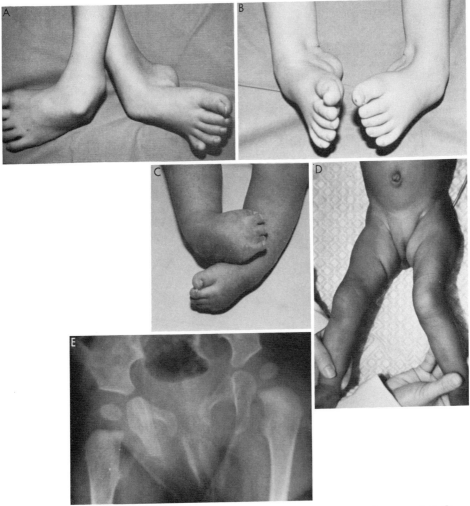

FIG 9–7. **A,** cerebral palsy, equinovarus feet. **B,** muscular dystrophy equinovarus feet. **C,** arthrogrypotic equinovarus feet. **D,** adduction contractures of the hip secondary to cerebral palsy. **E,** windblown pelvis of cerebral palsy causing subluxation of left hip.

that of osteochondritis of the navicular, commonly known as Köhler's disease. It is found in the young. There is pain and swelling in the foot, with palpable tenderness over the navicular joint. The second is apophysitis of the calcaneus, commonly known as Sever's disease. There is pain in the heel and over the insertion of the Achilles tendon. Most of the problem is caused by an Achilles tendon contracture but there may also be an inflammation of the apophysis of the os calcis posterior ossification center. This most commonly occurs in 8- to 10-year-old children. Another cause of pain in the foot is apophysitis of the base of the fifth metatarsal. This is seen in the older child, and there is tenderness and pain over this area. All three conditions are diagnosed on the primarily clinical examination.

There are multiple congenital deformities of the toes. The first of these is congenital varus of the toes. In this condition the "curly toes" fall usually under the adjacent toe. When the toes do not touch there is no significant deformity but when one toe is under the other problems will arise. The deforming force is a partial aplasia of the intrinsic muscles of the toe. Congenital "hammer toes" are seen with flexion at the proximal interphalangeal joint and extension at the metatarsophalangeal and distal interphalangeal joints of the toe. In this deformed position, corns and pressure sores may develop. Congenitally flexed or claw toe is a deformity that differs from the hammer toe in that there is flexion rather than extension at the distal interphalangeal joint. The painful corns and calluses that develop are the main problems. The deforming force here is the long flexor tendon in the face of a weakened extensor tendon. Congenital dorsiflexion of the toes is seen when the proximal phalanx articulates more dorsally. When present in the fifth toe there is also medial deviation and lateral rotation of the toe. There is also a permanent web medially connecting it to the fourth toe.

Vertical talus is a combination of hindfoot equinus and forefoot dorsiflexion (Figs 9–8, A and B). The vertical talus foot, like the clubfoot, is smaller than normal, with a smaller calf resulting from atrophy of the muscle bellies. In this condition the forefoot is positioned from neutral to abduction, the hindfoot in valgus, and a convex plantar aspect creating a rocker-bottom effect on the lateral

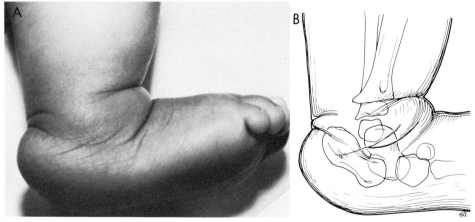

FIG 9–8. **A,** vertical talus (rocker-bottom) foot deformity. **B,** vertical talus skeletal configuration.

view of the foot may be present. The talus is in a vertical position with the calcaneus positioned in equinus, while the forefoot distal to the navicular is dorsiflexed.

Primitive reflexes are retained during the first year of a child's life. Motor power is evaluated by testing the range of strength in the older child using the standard 0 through 5 classification system discussed in Chapter 1 of this text.

All active ranges of motion described are not able to be rated in the young. Simply seeing active motion must suffice. A part of the examination that is often

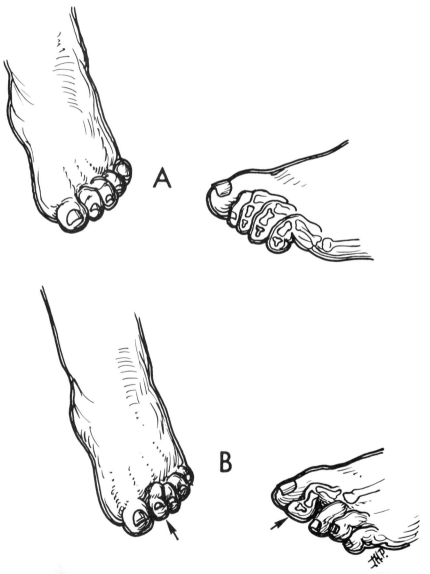

FIG 9–9. Claw toe configuration (**A**), hammer toe configuration (**B**).

overlooked is testing of the intrinsic power of the toes. While pressing in a dorsal and proximal direction on the proximal phalanges of the toes, lack of active resistive power in the cooperative child is indicative of absent or weakened intrinsic musculature of the foot for the motor innervation derived from the S-2, S-3 level. In the infant this may be one of the first signs of a neurologic deficit at this level, especially in conditions such as spina bifida or spinal agenesis. Clawing of the toes may also be one of the first signs seen (Fig 9–9, A). Figure 9–9, B shows hammer toes, which, as discussed before, are a nonpathologic entity.

Bilateral foot deformity that develops after age 5 years may be attributed to Charcot-Marie-Tooth disease. Atrophy of the intrinsic muscles of the foot is found, as well as weakness of the foot progressing to involve the peroneal muscles at a later age. Later involvement of the tibialis anterior muscle is also observed and a forefoot drop may develop. Therefore, the picture of the foot is

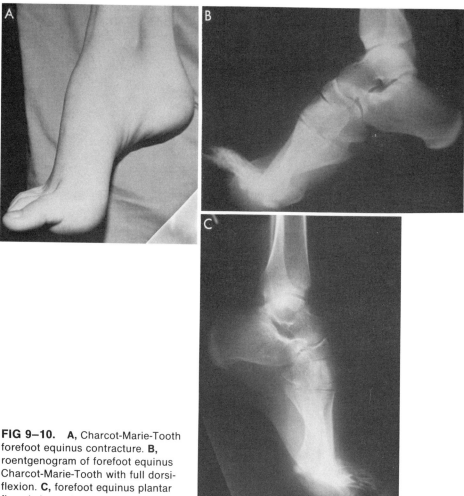

FIG 9–10. **A,** Charcot-Marie-Tooth forefoot equinus contracture. **B,** roentgenogram of forefoot equinus Charcot-Marie-Tooth with full dorsiflexion. **C,** forefoot equinus plantar flexed view—Charcot-Marie-Tooth.

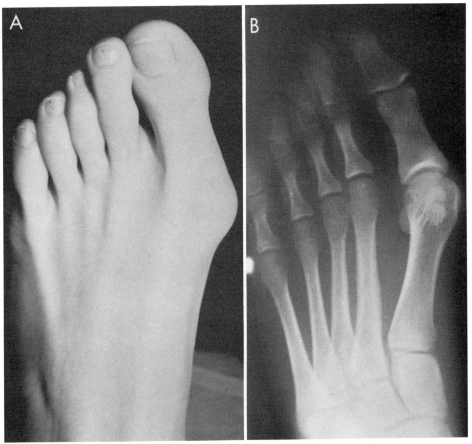

FIG 9–11. **A,** bunion configuration. **B,** roentgenogram of mild bunion.

that of some equinus of the hindfoot and massive equinus of the midfoot (Figs 9–10, A–C). At a later date, muscle atrophy can also be found more proximal in the leg as well as in the hands and forearms. Deep-tendon reflexes of the knee usually subside as well. Clawing of the toes is also seen because of the muscle imbalance with weak or absent intrinsic muscles (Fig 9–9, A). Because the peroneal muscles are involved, the foot will tend to fall into a varus deformity as well.

Deformity of the first metatarsal of the child's or adolescent's foot into varus is seen in metatarsus primus varus with an associated hallux valgus. This is usually found in early adolescence with or without the development of pain and irritation of the first metatarsal head. In addition to the lateral deviation of the great toe off of the medially deviated first metatarsal, there may be rotation of the great toe (Figs 9–11, A and B). There is also the possibility of hallux rigidus of the first metacarpal phalangeal joint. In this case, the joint becomes warm, swollen, and usually painful. Roentgenograms will likewise reveal thinning of the epiphysis of the proximal phalanx.

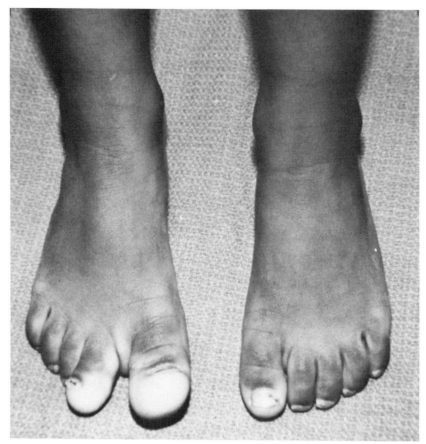

FIG 9–12. Congenital macrodactyly.

Congenital deformities such as macrodactyly (Fig 9–12) and congenital bands (Fig 9–13) are also responsible for varying deformities. In congenital macrodactyly, there is an obvious deformity with random hypertrophy of differing portions of the toes and feet.

Lower Limb Variants

With the knee extended, the tibia normally rotates outward about 45° and inward about 45° (Fig 9–14, A and B). This varies over the child's life as tibial torsion changes with growth. After 8 years of age, further changes are usually minimal.

With infants younger than 1 year, most tibial torsion is associated with bowing of the legs (Fig 9–15). This occurs because with the tibiae rotated inward, the normal anterior medial contour of the bone is projected medially, causing an exaggerated bowed appearance from the front (Fig 9–16). The older child must be examined to determine whether the rotation is from the foot, tibia, or secondary to femoral torsion. The diagnosis of internal femoral torsion can be made either by itself or in addition to that of internal tibial torsion. Both deformities together, of course, result in greater in-toeing during gait than either alone. As a child grows, in response to either tibial or femoral torsion that is not resolving, the foot may go into valgus due to the constant eversion and abduction of the foot. Commonly, the feet are in some degree of varus from the child sitting in the "squaw" position with the feet turned under the buttocks (Figs 9–17, A and C). Lateral tibial torsion may likewise be present with excessive external rotation of the legs at birth, which may or may not regress.

Rotation of the hip may vary from child to child. With extension of the hip, there is greater internal torsion or rotation in the child who in-toes and, conversely, more lateral torsion or rotation in a child who excessively out-toes. Internal (medial) femoral torsion, which includes anteversion of the femoral neck, will produce an in-toed gait (Fig 9–17, D) with 80° of medial rotation and 10° of lateral rotation. This is maintained and exaggerated by the child sitting in the "W" posture (Fig 9–17, B). More than 15° of lateral rotation is considered normal and should not result in an abnormal-appearing in-toed gait. External femoral torsion is physiologically the opposite. With the legs in extension, the patellae can be rotated 90° outward with 0° of medial rotation.

On examining the bowed leg, the examiner must look for the components of internal tibial torsion and varus of the tibia. These are the most likely causes of the clinically observed bow deformity. Observe the silhouette of the tibia. The varus deformities starting below the knee joint may represent Blount's disease (Figs 9–18, A–C). Varus of either the femur, the tibia, or both, may be of rachitic origin, or from other metabolic or paralytic conditions. Anterior bowing of the tibia in infancy may well be caused by congenital pseudoarthrosis or pre-

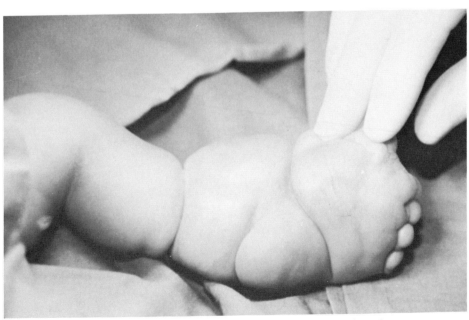

FIG 9–13. Lymphedema associated with congenital band syndrome.

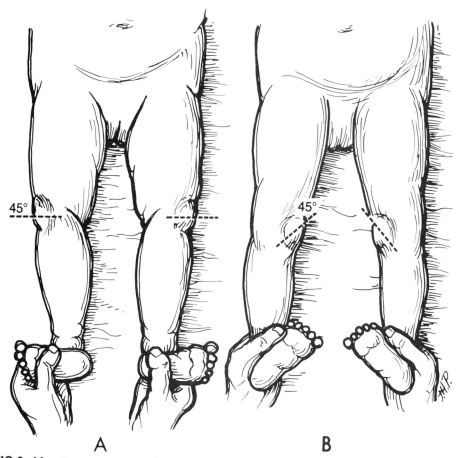

FIG 9–14. External rotation of legs with hips extended (**A**). Internal rotation of legs with hips extended (**B**).

pseudoarthrosis of the tibia. These etiologies must be differentiated when establishing the correct diagnosis that is causing the deformity.

Physiologic varus of the tibia resolves after age 18 months. By the approximate age of 3 years, the child may develop physiologic "knock-knee" or valgus deformity to the legs. Following this, by ages 5 to 7 years, the child should have straightened to the normal adult configuration. Measurements should be taken between the medial malleoli, and should be followed at routine intervals. Again, with abnormal valgus, growth arrest or rachitic deformity must be considered in the differential diagnosis.

The Knee

The child's knee, like the adult's, is not only the articulation between the femur and the tibial plateau but also between the patella and the distal femur. Examination of the infant may reveal a lax joint, which often accounts for a clicking sound that is referred to the hip during the examination of the newborn. The cruciate and collateral ligaments are lax. The first sign of knee pathology may be an effusion. This may be very subtle and only detectable when all the knee fluid is forced into the suprapatellar pouch on the lateral side of the patellar ligament. Then the fluid-filled medial side is gently percussed and the depressed lateral areas are observed for a fluid wave on refilling (Fig 9–19). Large amounts of fluid will produce the so-called ballotable patella (Fig 9–20, A and B). When the patella is compressed into its femoral groove, it bounces back upward if the child can hold the quadriceps relaxed. A long-standing problem will result in atrophy of the thigh and calf. The leg should be measured in circumference and compared with the opposite side at equal distances from either the joint line or another palpable anatomical structure (Fig 9–21). Swelling observed in the anterior knee will be localized to three basic areas. The swelling between the patella and skin is usually that of a prepatellar bursitis. This is usually seen in addition to induration, erythema, and tenderness. The second point is at the patellar ligament's insertion on the tibial tubercle. This is found with induration, erythema, and tenderness of the infrapatellar bursa. Finally, swelling around the patellar

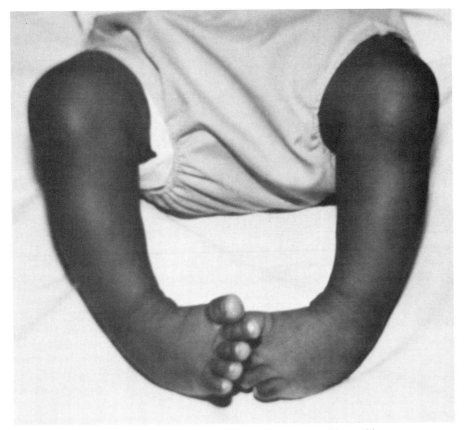

FIG 9–15. Normal tibial torsion with associated bowed legs.

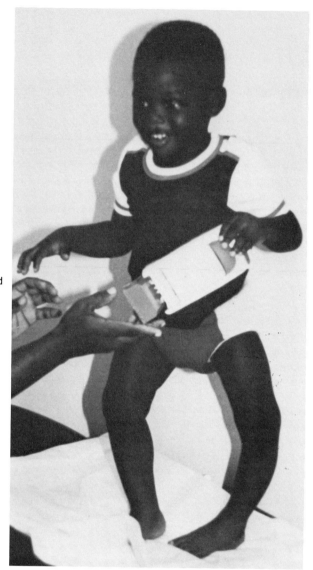

FIG 9–16. Exaggerated physiologic bowed leg.

ligament with induration and erythema is that of infrapatellar fat-pad inflammation.

Another common site of swelling around the knee is the area over the tibial tubercle. This is usually found in Osgood-Schlatter disease. The apophysitis of Osgood-Schlatter disease causes swelling and pain over the tibial tubercle. Radiologic evaluation of the area should be done to eliminate a neoplastic, infectious, or traumatic process in this area. The diagnosis is usually a clinical one. In the older child, the bursa that is soft over the tibial tubercle is replaced by a hard

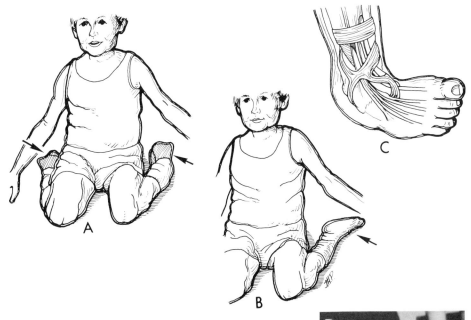

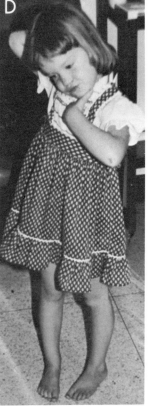

FIG 9–17. **A,** "squaw" posture. **B,** "W" sitting posture. **C,** foot stretched into varus by "squaw" posture. **D,** in-toed stance of internal femoral torsion.

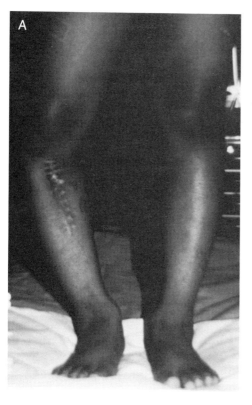

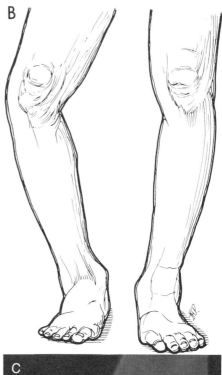

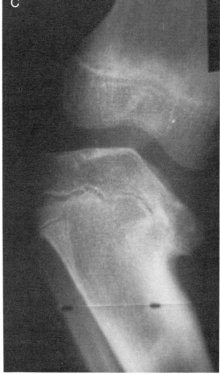

FIG 9–18. **A,** Blount's disease malformation. **B,** Blount's disease malformation. **C,** roentgenogram of Blount's disease.

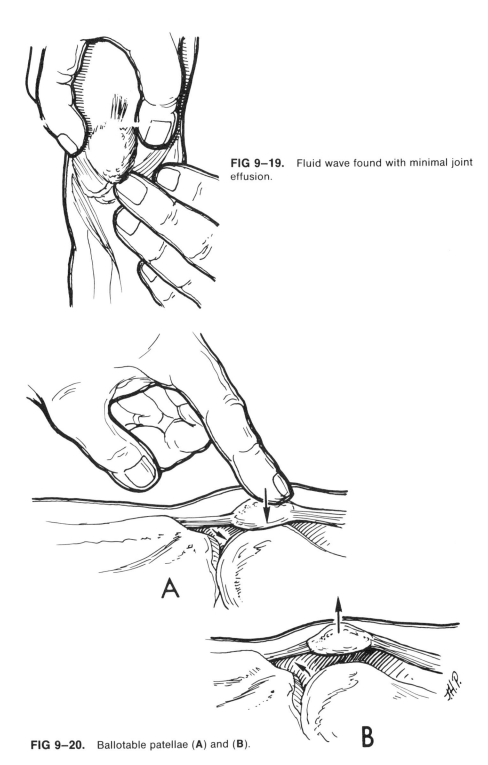

FIG 9–19. Fluid wave found with minimal joint effusion.

FIG 9–20. Ballotable patellae (**A**) and (**B**).

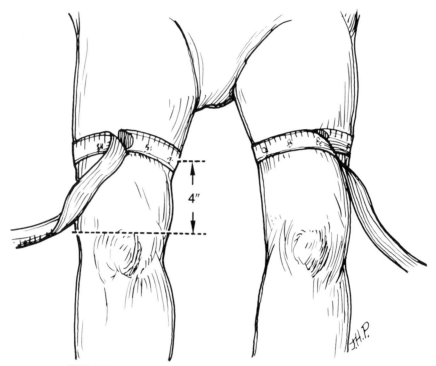

FIG 9–21. Thigh measurement for atrophy of quadriceps.

underlying exostosis of the residual hyperostotic bone. The bursa over the tubercle is more prominent when the knee is in extension.

There are many causes of cystic bulging masses. A Baker's cyst is found in the midline, ballooning posteriorly from swelling into a pouch in the torn posterior capsule. There may be complaints of dull pain. This is worse when the knee is in extension. A popliteal aneurysm is pulsatile in nature while an arteriovenous malformation is not. However, popliteal aneurysms are never found in children. Medial knee swelling over the pes anserinus may be caused by swelling beneath the conjoined tendons of the sartorius, gastrocnemius, and semitendinosus. A cyst of the lateral meniscus may be congenital and appears anterior as well as posterior to the lateral collateral ligament at the level of the knee joint. Finally, a medial meniscal cyst is a developmentally cystic anomaly present anterior or posterior to the medial collateral ligament at the joint line. This problem is made more prominent with the knee in flexion.

Inspection of the child's knee may show diffuse swelling. Aspiration will most likely show a hemarthrosis if there is a fracture of the distal femoral epiphysis, proximal tibial epiphysis, tibial spine, or torn internal structure of the knee. Palpation of the patella may reveal either a fracture line or a complete separation of the fracture. A child, unlike an adult, is unlikely to rupture the quadriceps muscle proximal to the patella. Avulsion of the tibial tubercle or of the inferior patellar pole are equivalent injuries. Symptoms consist of inability to extend the knee and/or a palpable defect over the tibial tubercle area, with swelling and pain.

Complaints of pain either deep in the knee or under the patella may be attributed to degenerative process of the articular surface of the patella, termed the patellofemoral syndrome, or chondromalacia. The complaints will vary with the patient's pain tolerance level. The child may complain of pain and pressure with climbing stairs, squatting, and after long periods of flexed-knee sitting. Deep or rotatory compression of the patella will elicit pain or discomfort. With flexion and extension of the knee, crepitation is often heard by both the observer and the patient. The amount of crepitation has no relationship to the degree of pain expressed. A slight effusion may also be present, as well as erythema and warmth. Due to the lax ligaments of childhood, the patella may be pushed laterally and then medially (Fig 9–22) and almost the entire undersurface may be palpated directly. Also, the femoral articular surface can be palpated for tenderness of its surface, as well as the inflamed synovial tissue that is interposed between the skin and cartilage. Initially, a child who has had patellar dislocation will show a positive "apprehension sign" on examination (Fig 9–23). As most dislocations displace to the lateral side, attempting to redislocate the patella in this direction with laterally directed medial patellar pressure will cause the child to try to prevent the maneuver. This causes pain and discomfort, especially in the medial retinaculum that has been recently torn. Diagnosis is usually confirmed by history and roentgenograms taken at the time of the dislocation.

Further examination is required to determine whether there is any internal derangement of the knee after a detailed history is taken of the exact location and mechanism of injury.

It is recommended that a routine roentgenologic examination be performed before the physical examination to rule out a nondisplaced fracture of the tibial spine, epiphyseal plate, or the articular surface, which may be displaced by

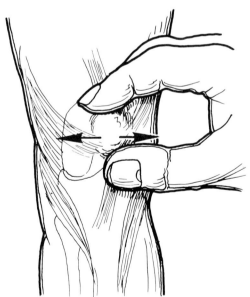

FIG 9–22. Hypermobile patella of childhood.

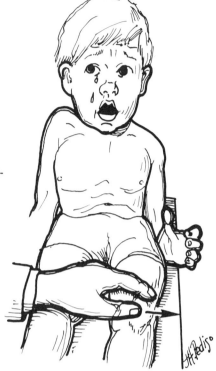

FIG 9–23. Apprehension test for dislocatable patella.

manipulation. Laxity to varus or valgus stress, with the knee in extension, or 30° of flexion in the juvenile, is usually associated with epiphyseal fracture. In the immature skeleton, the ligaments are much stronger than the cartilaginous epiphyseal plates, which will separate first. After plate closure near the end of growth, disruption occurs through the ligaments and capsule as in the adult. Anterior to posterior instability of the knee is exhibited by either the drawer sign or the Lachman test. More extensive description of the ligament examination may be obtained in Chapter 10 on examination of the adult knee. For the child's examination, the patient is placed supine and the knee is placed at 90° of flexion and pulled forward on the proximal tibia in both internal and external tibial rotation. As previously noted, young persons will exhibit a normal increase in the play of motion and the affected knee must be compared with the normal one. However, greater than 1 cm of forward motion of the tibia on the femur should be considered abnormal. The Lachman test for instability of the knee is the same, but is performed with the knee in 30° of flexion.

As with the collateral ligaments, the cruciate ligaments are stronger than the bone of the anterior or posterior tibial spines. They usually will avulse in the immature skeleton before rupture of the ligament. In the older adolescent, the adult pattern will be found with greater laxity of the cruciate ligament either signifying a partial or complete tear of the cruciate. Greater laxity is related to a combined injury of the cruciates and medial collateral ligament. With the leg externally rotated, the posterior capsule and structures should tighten and reduce the amount of laxity even if the cruciate is torn. If the drawer sign is not lessened by external rotation, it can be assumed that both sets of structures are torn to some degree. Likewise, internal rotation tightens the posterolateral structures and should reduce anterior motion unless they are also torn. The posterior drawer sign is posterior displacement of the tibia on the distal femur. A partial or complete posterior cruciate lesion is the adult analogue of an epiphyseal plate injury in the immature skeleton, which is usually a Salter-Harris type I or II injury.

Meniscal injury is rare in the young child but should be looked for and tested for as the possible cause of an effusion. A loose body or torn meniscus will often prevent the lax knee from either passively or actively being fully extended. In the young, if a tear is present, there is an increased incidence of anterior horn tears. These are usually a peripheral detachment at either the anterior or medial corner of the meniscus. A tear will elicit pain to palpation at the coinciding joint line. Also, a solid end point to knee extension will not be felt, but rather a rubbery bumper-like effect will be felt short of full extension. If the meniscus is

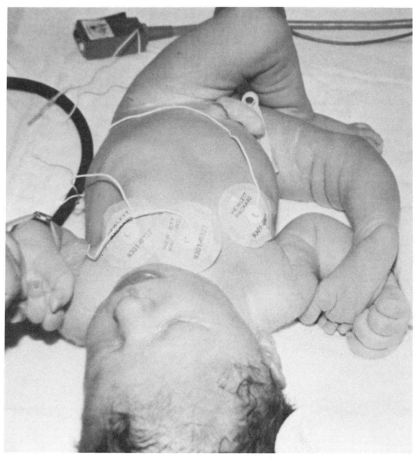

FIG 9–24. Hyperextended knees from birth posture.

torn, either passive or active range of motion, with the tibia externally and internally rotated, may reveal a clunklike sound and vibration caused by the femoral condyle moving over the derangement of a rubbery displaced meniscus. This is termed the McMurray test.

When examining the newborn, a hyperextended knee may signal either a simple hyperextension deformity caused by the breech position or another intrauterine posture where the leg is held anteriorly hyperextended (Fig 9–24). This is the result of stretching of the hamstring muscles as well as the posterior capsule, which results in the child being unable to flex its leg at birth. A rare complication is that of complete dislocation of the tibia anteriorly on the femur (Fig 9–25). In this condition, the tibia plateau is palpable completely proximal to the distal femoral epiphysis. It is not easily reducible as is the hyperextended knee. It may not be reducible at all without significant traction or surgery. Confirmation of a dislocation is made on lateral roentgenologic examination of the knee. In the newborn, an arthrogram may also be required to delineate the actual extent of the cartilagenous end of the bones. Note that the patella is present but is in extreme alta position due to shortening of the quadricep muscles.

The patella usually dislocates to the lateral side. With a full congenital dislocation of the patella there is a swelling seen over the lateral side of the knee. In children younger than the age of 4 or 5 years who have congenital dislocation, the patella is almost impossible to feel. There is a depression over the femoral condyles where the absent patella should be. The knee is held in flexion at birth and the leg is laterally rotated at the knee. The patella most likely will not be reducible. Roentgenograms will confirm the condition when the patella ossifies. This is usually delayed as well. Before the patella appears, the diagnosis can be made when an anterior to posterior roentgenogram of the femur reveals a lateral view of the tibia. For the best treatment results it is essential that the

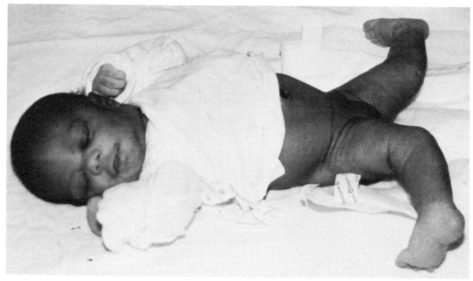

FIG 9–25. Hyperextended knees from congenital dislocations.

diagnosis be made before age 3 or 4 years, before ossification of the patella occurs.

Findings in a child of clicking or clunking may be attributed to a congenital discoid meniscus. This is an abnormally formed lateral meniscus. It is shaped like a disk rather than the normal C shape, and is also thicker, with the posterior horn not attached to the tibia. For this reason, when the child walks there may even be an audible sound present. The child may present with a history of an old injury of the knee, having had an effusion, or an acute episode of trauma. There may be instability in the knee and pain on the outer aspect, just as with medial meniscal tears. Normal examination of the knee should be performed, although in this instance the problem is in the lateral compartment rather than the usual medial compartment.

Suggested Readings

1. Hesinger RN, Jones ET: *Neonatal Orthopaedics.* New York, Grune & Stratton Inc, 1981.
2. Hoppenfeld S: *Physical Examination of the Spine and Extremities.* New York, Appleton-Century-Crofts, 1976.
3. Lovell WW, Winter RB: *Pediatric Orthopaedics.* Philadelphia, JB Lippincott Co, 1978.
4. Salter RB: *Textbook of Disorders and Injuries of the Musculoskeletal System,* ed 2. Baltimore, Williams & Wilkins Co, 1983.
5. Sharrard WJW: *Pediatric Orthopaedics and Fractures.* Oxford, England, Blackwell Scientific Publications, 1979.

CHAPTER 10

Examination of the Lower Extremities in the Child, Part 2

Lorin M. Brown, M.D.
Robert B. Salter, M.D.

The Neonatal Hip Examination

The hip joints are constantly flexed throughout intrauterine life, and consequently the newborn infant exhibits between 50 to 90 degrees of hip-flexion deformity or contracture. There is an increase in the external rotation of the hip joint, which is also the result of fetal posture. The infant's femoral neck-shaft angle starts at about 150° and will decrease with growth, until in the adult the angle lies at about 127°. Therefore, a child has an increase in the lateral deviation of the femoral shaft to the pelvis relative to that of an infant. The range of motion of the hips is assessed by first moving them from maximum adduction to maximum abduction (Fig 10–1). In the coronal plane, flexion to extension is then tested with the lumbar spine flat on the examination table (Fig 10–2, A). A hip-flexion contracture is identified by a positive Thomas's test (Fig 10–2, B). With the normal hip held in maximum flexion of 135° the contracted hip will be held off the table by the flexor muscle and tendon contraction. Figure 10–3, A, demonstrates the amount of normal internal and external rotation possible in the supine extended hip, while Figure 10–3, B, shows the same range of rotation when tested in the prone position. The normal supine range of internal and external rotation of the hip is also tested for with 90° of flexion at the hip and knee (Fig 10–4). Figure 10–5, A and B, demonstrate the normal internal and external rotation possible with the hip and knee in extension in the supine position.

Variations in the original intrauterine positions must be taken into account when examining the patient. Examination of the infant is done with certain disorders in mind. Congenital dislocation and subluxation of the hip joint are two of the most common conditions found in the newborn. During early life, from birth until age 3 months, it is of great importance to diagnose these conditions because of the relative simplicity of treatment. The Ortolani maneuver

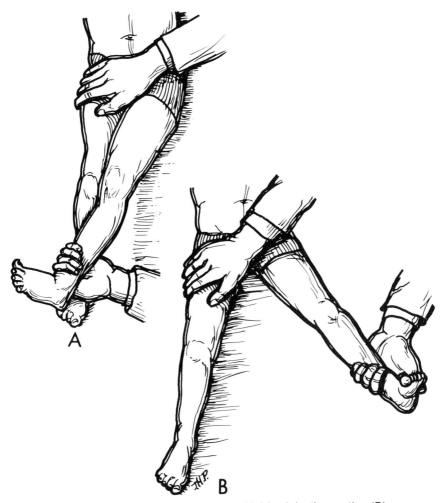

FIG 10–1. Hip adduction motion (**A**); hip abduction motion (**B**).

is used to examine the baby for a congenitally dislocated hip. The hips are held in 90° of flexion and each side is tested independently while the opposite side of the pelvis is stabilized. The hip is first abducted, and when maximum abduction without force is reached, forward pressure is placed on the greater trochanter to push the femoral head into the acetabulum. The sound is a "thump" rather than the popularly described "click." This is illustrated in Figure 10–6 by going from the broken line figure of the femoral head and neck to the solid line figure of the hip. When the hip capsule is unduly lax and the femoral head can be pushed out of the acetabulum, but at rest the hip is in the located position, the hip is termed "dislocatable." The Barlow maneuver, which detects a dislocatable hip, reverses the Ortolani test and allows the hip to be pushed out of its joint. This is illustrated in Figure 10–6 by going from the solid line drawing of the hip to the broken line femoral head and neck drawing. The thigh is held in the flexed

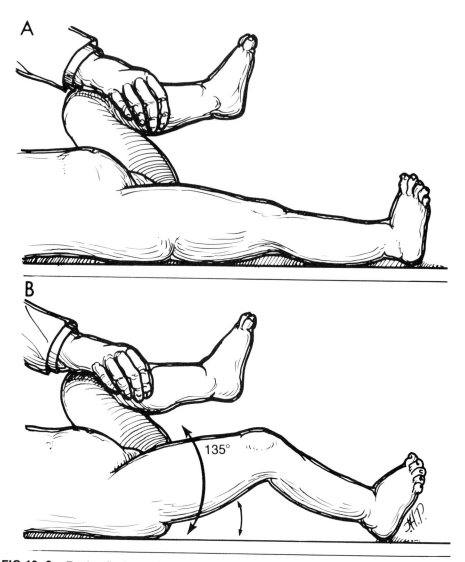

FIG 10–2. Testing flexion and extension in coronal plane (**A**); positive Thomas's test for hip flexion contracture (**B**).

position and then is adducted and pressure applied posteriorly on the medial proximal thigh. Usually the dislocatable hip becomes located again with simple abduction of the thigh.

If an infant is lying flat on its back on the examining table, with the anterior superior spines level, and with the legs held in extension the skin creases can be observed. A common finding, with a complete congenital dislocation of the hip, will be that of asymmetrical skin creases of the thighs (Fig 10–7). This can also be assessed with the child lying in the prone position (Fig 10–8). However, without any other supportive data this finding is not indicative of hip pathology. A more significant indication of a unilateral dislocation is the Galeazzi sign (Fig 10–9). With the child lying supine, the hips flexed to about 90° and the knees completely flexed, there is unequal height to the knee joints with the shortening being on the dislocated side. This is due to the femoral head being dislocated posteriorly, thereby causing the thigh to appear shorter. If the child is not held

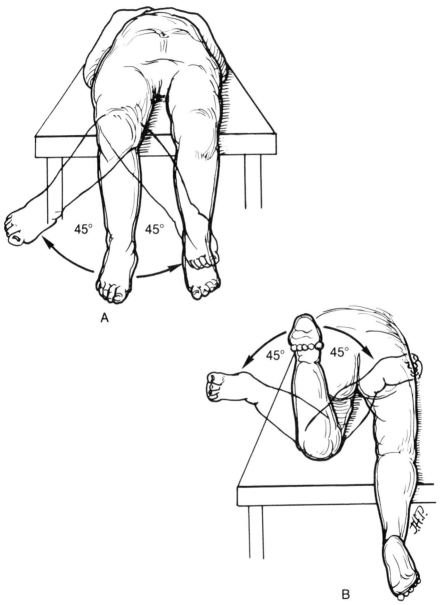

FIG 10–3. Normal range of internal/external rotation motion possible in supine, extended hip (**A**); normal range of internal/external motion possible in prone extended hip (**B**).

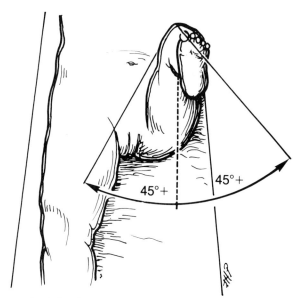

FIG 10–4. Range of rotation is shown with patient in supine position with hip flexed 90° and knee flexed 90°.

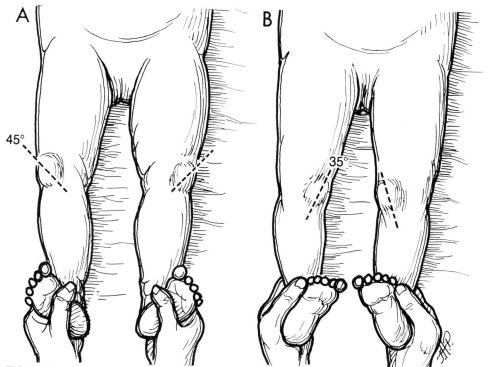

FIG 10–5. Normal external rotation (**A**) and internal rotation (**B**) possible with hip in extension in supine position.

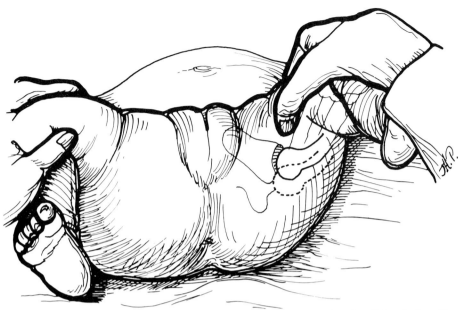

FIG 10–6. Positive Barlow's maneuver with dotted hip representing the dislocated position.

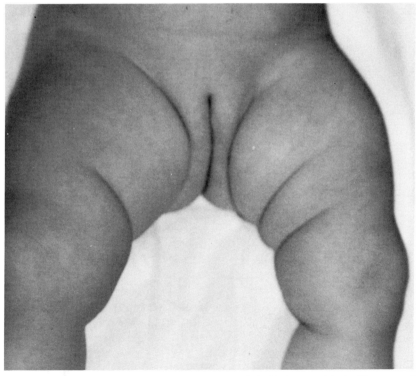

FIG 10–7. Anterior view of extra fat creases of the left thigh associated with congenital dislocation of the left hip.

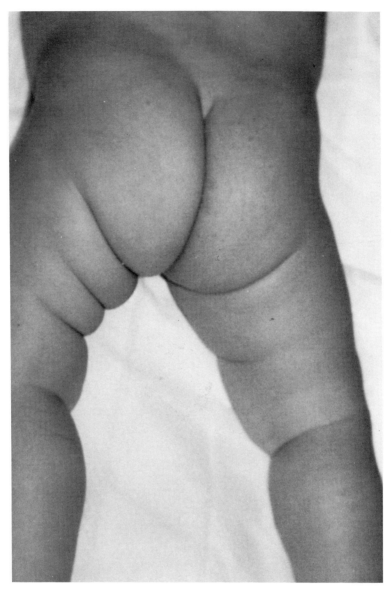

FIG 10–8. Posterior view of extra fat creases of the left thigh associated with congenital dislocation of the left hip.

in a symmetrical fashion with the pelvis square to the table, this test is invalid. After age 3 months, the ligaments, as well as the capsular tissue, become tighter and another sign appears, namely limited abduction of the hip (Fig 10–10). This is usually due to the dislocated hip being held in flexion and adduction, allowing secondary shortening of the adductor tendons. Absence of this sign in the younger child is not reason to rule out congenital dislocation or subluxation of the hip. As the hip becomes tighter and firmer, the Ortolani and Barlow signs

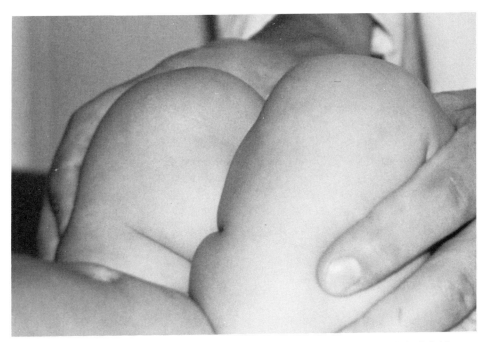

FIG 10–9. Positive Galeazzi's sign associated with congenital dislocation of the left hip. Note that the left knee is at a lower level than the right.

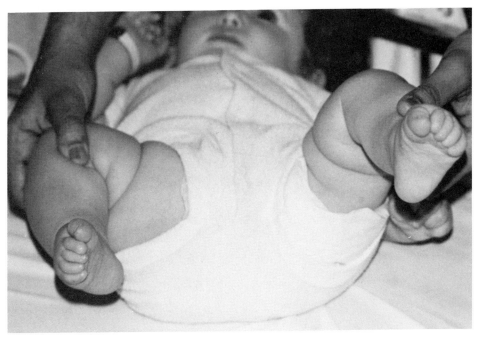

FIG 10–10. Limited abduction of the left hip associated with congenital dislocation of this hip.

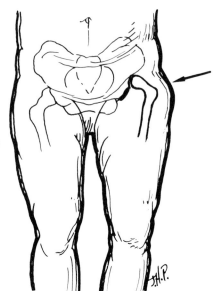

FIG 10–11. Skeletal representation of complete congenital dislocation of the left hip.

disappear. At this point, the hip is constantly dislocated (Fig. 10–11) or subluxated.

In the subluxated hip, the femoral head is still in contact with the true acetabulum, but is not seated in the desired concentric location (Fig 10–12). There is secondary acetabular dysplasia, with the roof or superior surface of the acetabulum being maldirected.

Another physical sign that can also be seen with a congenital dislocation is "telescoping" of the hip. This is found in the presence of a complete dislocation.

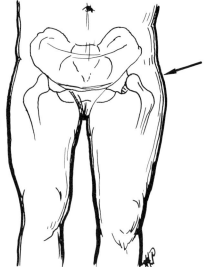

FIG 10–12. Skeletal representation of congenital subluxation of the left hip.

With the involved hip flexed to 90°, the femur can be pushed posteriorly and pulled anteriorly (telescoped) because the femoral head is dislocated from the acetabulum.

In the young patient, dislocation can be detected by checking for hamstring tightness. With this test the hips are flexed, abducted, and externally rotated (Fig 10–13, A). Then as the infant's knees are passively extended, tightness of the

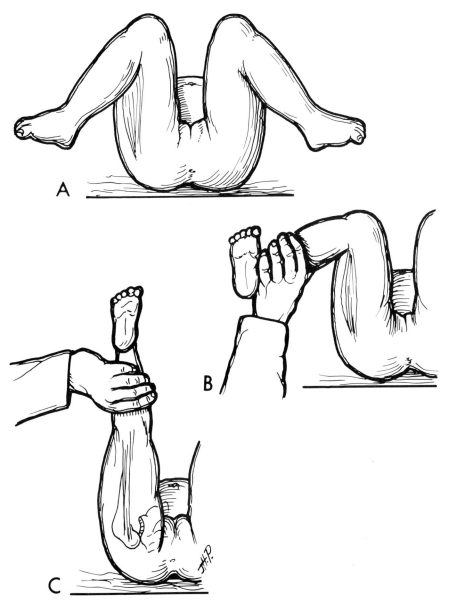

FIG 10–13. Lower limbs held with the hip and knees in flexion (**A**); extension of knee checked by firm tone of hamstring muscles when hip is in acetabulum (**B**); extension of knee unchecked due to lax hamstrings when femoral head is dislocated (**C**).

hamstring muscles prevents complete extension (Fig 10–13, B). If the knee can be completely extended when the hip is in this position, it strongly suggests that the hip is dislocated (Fig 10–13, C).

Over the age of 18 months, the child with a dislocated hip is most likely walking. Limping can be observed clinically. There is a positive Trendelenburg sign (Fig 10–14). This is due to loss of the normal fulcrum of the hip joint and consequent ineffectiveness of the abduction muscles on the dislocated side. This allows the pelvis to drop downward on the opposite side when the child stands on the involved lower limb. This sign can be elicited even in a child at a very young age, as long as the child is able to stand. By having the parent hold the child's hands, and then observing the child from behind and lifting one foot from the floor a positive Trendelenburg sign can be observed. During gait the Trendelenburg limp is combined with a short limb limp. When both hips are

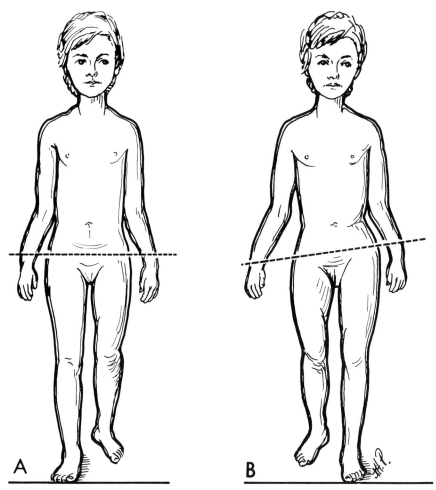

FIG 10–14. Normal negative Trendelenburg's sign (**A**); positive Trendelenburg's sign (**B**) from problem on the child's left side.

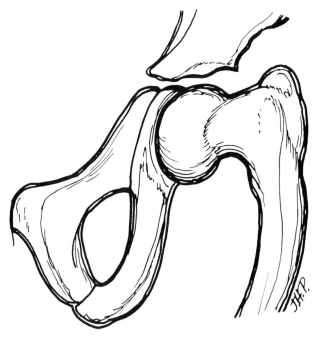

FIG 10–15. Coxa vara.

dislocated there are bilateral Trendelenburg's signs that result in a waddling duck–type gait. Significant congenital subluxation will cause the Trendelenburg gait, although less noticeable, to be present, particularly when the child becomes tired at the end of the day.

Any abnormal finding in the child's physical examination of the hip is an indication for radiographic examination.

Coxa Vara Deformity

In the congenital malformation of coxa vara, (Fig 10–15) the child exhibits a positive Trendelenburg sign due to elevation of the greater trochanter, and hence, loss of the normal tension in the abductor muscles. There is no pain associated with this condition. Other forms of femoral dysplasia, such as hypoplasia (proximal femoral focal deficiency), must be ruled out by roentgenograms. Shortening of the femur and limitation of abduction may also be seen.

Painful Hip

Pain in the child's hip can be caused by a variety of disorders. Physical examination includes the detection of local tenderness and the assessment of any limitation of hip joint motion caused by muscle spasm. An additional sign is elicited by the FABERE maneuver (FABERE is the acronym for Flexion, Abduction, External Rotation, and Extension). With the hip placed in this position, the knee is passively extended. This compresses the hip joint with tightening of the hamstring muscles and should cause pain if the pathology is located within the hip joint itself rather than in the periarticular tissues. With conditions such as Legg-Perthes disease, osteochondritis dissecans of the hip joint, septic hip, sympathetic effusion of adjacent osteomyelitis, intra-articular fracture, acute juvenile rheumatoid arthritis, and transient toxic synovitis of the hip joint, in which there is an excessive buildup of intracapsular fluid, there will be pain elicited by this sign. An antalgic gait is associated with painful disorders of the hip. This is a "quick step" limping gait that lessens the patient's pain, by decreasing the time of weight-bearing on the affected limb.

Other more serious congenital afflictions can also deform the child's hip, for example, spina bifida with myelomeningocele, cerebral palsy, and arthrogryposis. Most of these progress in severity as the child grows. The same features are present as are found in a congenital dislocation of the hip, as the neuromuscular imbalance of these conditions leads to a paralytic dislocation of the hip either at birth or shortly thereafter. The arthrogrypotic child is often born with the hips dislocated and in a rigid fixed position with limited range of motion as the child grows. The infant with myelomeningocele may be born with dislocated hips, although more often the hips dislocate after birth, secondary to the permanent muscle imbalance. In the child with cerebral palsy, the hips may not dislocate secondary to the muscle imbalance until after age 2 years.

Congenital muscular dystrophy may not be obvious at birth but is usually detectable by the time the child reaches walking age and it is progressive thereafter.

The sudden onset of restricted motion of the hip joint that may occur throughout infancy and childhood is the result of acute inflammation. The child becomes irritable and is unwilling to move the affected hip that is held in flexion, external rotation, and abduction. The child will resist any passive movement of the hip. There may be erythema of the overlying skin. Differential diagnosis includes a septic hip joint, juvenile rheumatoid arthritis, or osteomyelitis of the neck of the femur. Another similar but less serious painful disorder of the hips is transient toxic synovitis. This condition is usually seen from age 3 to 10 years. There is pain in the area of the hip joint along with an antalgic limp and varying restricted motion of the hip joint.

Avulsion of the Anterior/Superior Iliac Spine

Another cause of pain in the area of the child's hip is trauma. If the child falls on the extended hip, the sartorius muscle can avulse the apophysis of the anterior superior iliac spine. Pain is felt in the anterior aspect of the pelvis over this prominent bony prominence. The child usually resists passive motion. The only positive clinical findings are local tenderness and pain that is aggravated by extending the hip while the knee is flexed. Other fractures about the hip joint must be ruled out by radiograph at this time.

Avulsion of the Adductors From the Adductor Tubercle

In this condition the only significant symptom may be pain in the groin area of the child. Abduction of the affected hip causes pain and direct palpation of the adductor tubercle will confirm local tenderness. Roentgenograms made at a later date will reveal exuberant callus formed by reattachment of this avulsion fracture.

Slipped Capital Femoral Epiphysis

Chronic slipped capital femoral epiphysis usually occurs between the age of 8 years and the cessation of growth. The epiphysis can slip at any age from an acute episode of trauma, but in the chronic slowly slipping epiphysis, the problem is obviously more insidious in onset. The child usually presents with either pain in the hip or pain in the anterior-medial side of the knee. This is because the referred pain of the hip pathology radiates downward through the obturator nerve. There is an associated antalgic gait. The lower extremity is held in external rotation. The child usually lacks some active and passive internal rotation particularly with the hip in extension. Depending on the severity of the slipped epiphysis, the time interval, and speed of progression, there may be an associated synovitis of the hip. This, of course, would cause pain in the region of the hip joint itself and cause a more marked limitation of rotation. Diagnosis is confirmed by anterior posterior and frog position radiographs of the pelvis. Since the capital femoral epiphysis slips mostly posteriorly, a minimal slip is most readily detected in the frog position or lateral radiograph.

Suggested Readings

1. Hesinger RN, Jones ET: *Neonatal Orthopaedics*. New York, Grune & Stratton Inc, 1981.
2. Hoppenfeld S: *Physical Examination of the Spine and Extremities*. New York, Appleton-Century-Crofts, 1976.
3. Lovell WW, Winter RB: *Pediatric Orthopaedics*. Philadelphia, JB Lippincott Co, 1978.
4. Salter RB: *Textbook of Disorders and Injuries of the Musculoskeletal System*, ed 2. Baltimore, Williams & Wilkins Co, 1983.
5. Sharrard WJW: *Pediatric Orthopaedics and Fractures*. Oxford, England, Blackwell Scientific Publications, 1979.

CHAPTER 11

Physical Diagnosis of the Knee

Russell F. Warren, M.D.

Complaints referable to the knee, as well as injuries of the knee, constitute the most common problem for which orthopaedic care is sought. Unfortunately, many physicians are content to make a simplified diagnosis of the "internal knee derangement." This diagnosis is used to cover all possible ills related to the knee and does little more than signify that the knee is the source of the patient's complaint(s). Generally, patients relate that they surmised as much. In the past 15 years the increased use of arthrography and, in particular, arthroscopy has resulted in less reliance on the clinical examination, with the result that this most important skill is in danger of being lost. While these tests are helpful and at times imperative in confirming a diagnosis, we still find that arthroscopy as a diagnostic tool provides few surprises and is reserved for treatment, as well as confirming our clinical impression. A careful clinical examination is still essential in establishing a highly accurate diagnosis from which a meaningful program of treatment can be developed.

As in diagnosing any problem one must have a sound understanding of the ranges of normal variation as well as an explicit knowledge of the regional anatomy. Without these tools the examination will have little value regardless of the level of training.

General Examination and Gait

When examining a patient with a knee problem, a careful history will generally raise a certain index of suspicion regarding a specific diagnosis. It generally suggests whether the problem is chronic or acute and if it is systemic or local. In addition, it provides data as to whether the origin is ligamentous, patellar, meniscal, or arthritic. With this in mind, it is helpful to leave the knee examination for last, less other significant problems that relate to the knee are overlooked. Thus, the patient is asked to stand and walk. It is best for the patient to be dressed in gym shorts and in bare feet for a proper knee examination as it avoids embarrassment for the patient and provides an excellent view of the lower extremities. When standing, the patient is observed from the front and back and then while walking. Foot alignment is noted. Is the arch normal or is there pes planus? Is

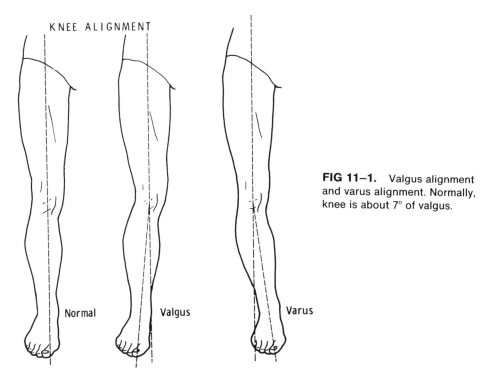

KNEE ALIGNMENT

Normal   Valgus   Varus

FIG 11–1. Valgus alignment and varus alignment. Normally, knee is about 7° of valgus.

the heel in neutral or is there calcaneal valgus or varus position, which may alter the forces on the knee. The overall alignment of the leg should be noted. Does the patient stand with the knee(s) in valgus or varus? Normally, there is about 7° of knee valgus (Fig 11–1). During stance, is the pelvis level or is one lower extremity truly shorter than the other? If there is real shortening is it in the femur or tibia? The presence of atrophy can often be seen by inspection, as well as by comparing the contour of the muscles of each extremity. Next, the patient is asked to ambulate. The gait pattern is ascertained as being normal or as pathologic. If there is significant pain an antalgic gait will be seen. This occurs when the patient experiences pain of a level that requires him to quickly remove the weight from the affected leg. In this manner he will spend less time in the stance phase on the involved side compared with the uninvolved side. The pelvis should be carefully noted for an abductor lurch, which will indicate that the hip is involved with attendant knee pain, possibly representing only a referred pain pattern. In this type gait, the pelvis will drop on the side opposite the weakened gluteus medius muscle, which has failed to stabilize the pelvis and keep it level during single stance phase. If this is noted, a Trendelenburg test is performed to confirm the impression of hip pathology. While observing gait, the patient is asked to walk directly toward the examiner to note the presence or absence of a knee thrust. This may be medial or lateral (Fig 11–2). Sudden instability occurs as the patient enters single-limb stance phase on an arthritic knee.[1] It consists of a collapse of the medial compartment in a varus knee secondary to destruction of the medial compartment, with the thrust directed in a lateral direction as the medial condyle and plateau come together.

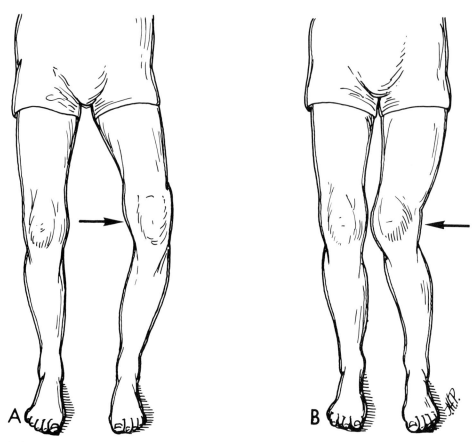

FIG 11–2. Lateral thrust is created if there is medial osteoarthritis (**A**). This occurs as medial compartment suddenly collapses during stance phase. Conversely medial thrust occurs during stance phase in lateral compartment osteoarthritis (**B**).

Conversely, in lateral compartment arthritis with a valgus deformity, a medial thrust will be seen. As the patient walks, view the knee from the side. During heel strike does the knee go into hyperextension or recurvatum, as may be seen in patients with grossly insufficient quadriceps? In addition, the patient is asked to perform a deep knee bend. Note the production of pain in relation to site and timing during the deep knee bend, as well as while arising from a knee bend. A full squat may induce the pain associated with a torn meniscus at the posterior horn, with the pain noted at the deepest point of the squat. Pain of patellar origin often will be noted as the patient arises from the squatting position as the quadriceps is maximally contracted and forces are increased at the patellofemoral articulation. Obviously, severe pain, an effusion, or an acute injury will prevent the performance of this test.

Inspection

Next, the patient is asked to sit on the examining table and lie first in the supine and then in the prone positions. While supine, the lower extremities are inspected. In chronic problems, the skin color, texture, and the presence or absence of hair are noted as indicating possible vascular insufficiency or reflex sympathetic dystrophy. Before focusing on the knee, the thighs and calves should be examined. Have the patient contract the muscles isometrically while noting the contour of the muscles, the tone, or the presence of atrophy. Also, it is helpful to measure for atrophy at a prescribed point proximal to the patella (12.5 cm), noting and recording the circumferences of the thighs and the calves. In palpating the muscles, defects from a previous muscle tear may be appreciated.

While inspecting the knee as well as the leg, any swelling is carefully recorded as to size, shape, and location. This should be done in the prone as well as supine positions. The knee, if flexed, may easily conceal a mass in the popliteal fossa; while commonly a popliteal cyst, uncommon lesions such as synovial sarcoma or a popliteal aneurysm may develop in the popliteal space. Inspection about the knee may disclose abrasions, lacerations, or areas of localized redness and swelling, which may suggest an infectious origin for the patient's problem. The classic signs of infection should be noted. If a swelling is seen about the anterior surface of the knee, note its exact location and decide if it communicates with the joint or is outside the joint. A localized swelling over the patella may represent a prepatella bursitis or an infected prepatella bursa (Fig 11–3). It is easily differentiated from a joint effusion. In the former condition, swelling is precisely located over the front of the patella while in the latter, swelling is diffuse and associated with a

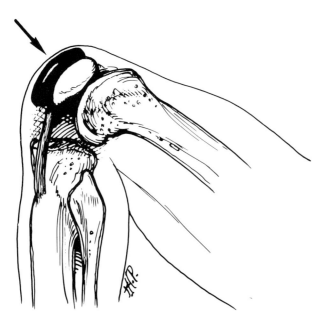

FIG 11–3. Prepatellar bursa may be quite swollen, causing examiner to mistakenly assume that fluid is within joint.

loss of the contour of the knee. Note any swelling over the tibial tubercle, which is common in teenagers with Osgood-Schlatter disease. Medial and, in particular, lateral prominence should be sought both visually and by palpation as cystic degeneration of menisci may present a cyst of varying size at or near the joint line. They usually feel firm and are slightly compressible. Aspiration will often confirm the presence of gelatinous clear fluid within the cyst, which may be colorless or tinged slightly yellow. Diffuse swelling about the knee implies an effusion that can easily be proved by ballottement of the patella or noting a fluid wave (see Fig 11–10) and compared with the opposite normal knee. In large, heavy patients inspection is more difficult, and findings can easily be missed. Once the inspection part of the examination is finished, the examiner should record the hip ranges of motion bilaterally, the neurocirculatory status of the lower extremities, and at the completion of the examination of the opposite, hopefully, control knee.

In performing the examination of the hips, the tightness of the hamstrings should be noted by performing a straight-leg raising maneuver. Normally, most patients can tolerate leg elevation to 90° with minimal complaint. If there is tightness, there may be a neurologic cause or simply a hamstring contracture that may have developed, as frequently seen in runners. These contractures can result in injury to the muscle tendon unit or, in a more subtle condition, may alter the forces at the knee so that greater forces are required of the quadriceps mechanism while running, resulting in patellar pain syndromes. Often, hamstring stretching will aid in correcting this problem. In children, hamstring contractures often suggest neurologic dysfunction secondary to spondylolisthesis, disk disease, or tumor.

The neurocirculatory component of a knee examination is critical. Its details are dependent on one's clinical suspicions. Lumbar disk herniation may cause localized leg pain that may be associated with local tenderness. Thus, the examiner can easily be misled by believing that it is local rather than a referrred distant problem that is the cause of the patient's complaint. While this appears to be more common in upper extremity pain patterns, it should be considered in lower extremity complaints as well. Similar consideration for neurologic etiology in young patients may prove that spondylolisthesis is responsible for the complaint, while older patients with spinal stenosis often will complain of thigh pain, weakness, and possibly some leg pain associated with activity. In any event, with muscle weakness and atrophy a differential diagnosis should include a variety of neurologic conditions that may manifest initially with pain or weakness about the knee. Hip complaints will often present with pain referred to the inner knee because the sensory innervation of the hip and skin over the medial knee are by the obturator nerve. At times knee pain will be the chief complaint and can be associated with vague thigh discomfort. This may be seen in young children with Legg-Perthes disease, in the adolescent with a slipped capital femoral epiphysis, or in the middle-aged or elderly patient who presents with a degenerative arthritis of the hip. Thus, the hip should be routinely examined as a possible cause of the knee pain. The gait pattern will often provide a clue if an abductor lurch is demonstrated. The range of motion of the hip must be noted and any limitation of rotation recorded, as well as any evidence of flexion contracture.

Similarly, the initial complaint may relate to pathology of the vascular system about the knee. Intermittent claudication secondary to vascular occlusion is relatively easy to determine, while entrapment of the popliteal artery from an anomalous medial head of the gastrocnemius or a mucous cyst in the wall of the popliteal artery is more difficult to diagnose in the young patient. A condition of popliteal aneurysm may occur and must be exluded. An examination of the patient's peripheral pulses as well as the reflexes is important in order to exclude a neurovascular cause of a problem. Finally, before starting an examination of the involved knee it is best to initially evaluate the opposite knee. This will accomplish several things, including gaining the patient's confidence to provide him with some insight, and to provide a comparison in assessing ligament and patellar dysfunction.

Motions

Prior to palpating the knee, the examiner should record the patient's active and passive knee motions bilaterally. Normally, there is full extension and 140° to 150° of flexion. Active knee extension is best tested with the patient sitting, noting the power of the quadriceps and palpating the tone of the muscles as this is performed. With atrophy, the muscles become soft and lose their normal firm quality. In addition, the quadriceps and infrapatellar tendons are palpated, noting any defects as in a rupture or local tenderness secondary to an inflammatory process. If the patient cannot actively fully extend the knee, but full passive extension is possible, this is termed an extensor lag (Fig 11–4).

This implies damage to the muscle-tendon unit as in a rupture of the quadriceps at its patellar insertion or of the patellar tendon from the tibial tubercle. It is surprising how often major quadriceps tendon ruptures are missed. This most often occurs when the examiner is fooled by the presence of some active, but weakened, knee extension despite a large tear in the tendon. The quadriceps mechanism can extend the knee to within 20° of full extension, despite a large tear within the quadriceps tendon, by a transmitted pull through the patellar retinaculum that surrounds the patella. The examiner should palpate the ten-

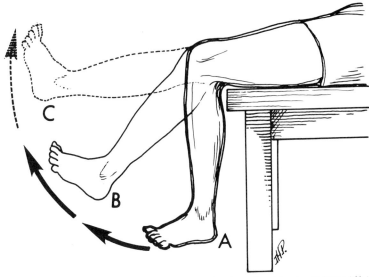

FIG 11–4. Extension lag: with active knee extension leg should extend from (A) to (C). If extension is possible only to point B but pressure extension to C is present, then an extension lag exists. This is often seen in quadriceps tendon ruptures.

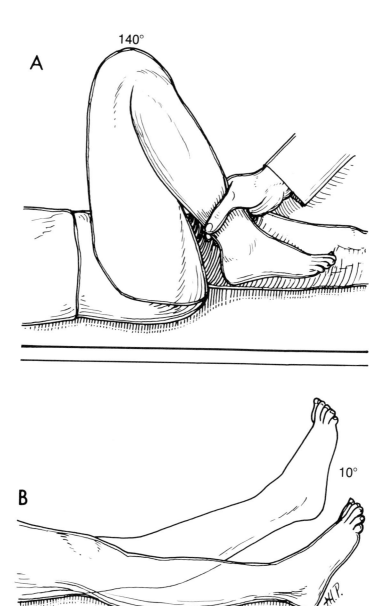

FIG 11–5. Full flexion (*A*); position of knee recurvatum of 10°, which may be normal (*B*).

don as active extension is attempted. Hamstring strength should also be tested for distal ruptures, which are uncommon or often occur in the middle or proximal regions. Knee motion is recorded, with 0° representing the knee when it is straight. Flexion represents the arc of motion from 0° to the point of maximum flexion, and is generally about 140° to 150° (Fig 11–5, A). Recurvatum is measured as positive extension and is recorded in plus (+) degrees (Fig 11–5, B).

Passive knee extension is noted with the patient lying supine, with the examiner facing the patient while holding the heels. The knee is viewed from the side and may extend beyond a straight line and into a position of recurvatum (Fig 11–6, A). If it is bilateral, it may be normal even up to 20°, or pathologic if observed to be unilateral, as seen in knee ligament injuries. In ruptures of the

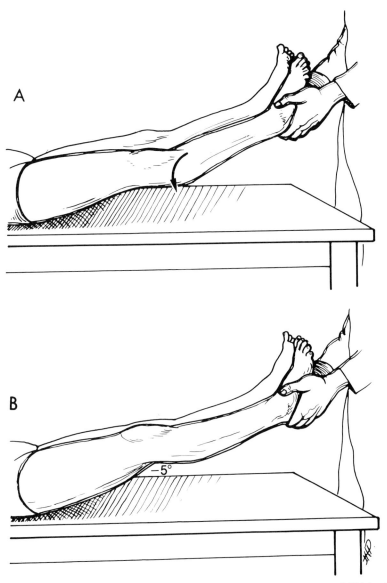

FIG 11–6. While holding heel, note degree of knee extension and external tibial rotation that occurs (A). If excessive, this indicates injury to the anterior cruciate ligament and posterior lateral corner of the knee. Bounce test is performed by holding heel and allowing knee to snap into extension (B). If there is a mechanical block to extension, "snap" into extension will become soft gradual stop.

anterior or posterior cruciate ligament, the leg should be held in the position described and it should be noted if the tibia rotates externally (Fig 11–6, A) as it sags into hyperextension. This indicates an anterior cruciate, and popliteus tendon injury. Conversely, a deficit of extension is considered a flexion contracture and measured as negative degrees from zero position. Often, in meniscus injury, a deficit of full extension may be seen and is termed a "locked knee." In testing for this condition, a "bounce test" is performed. In a normal knee, as the knee sags into extension, a firm stop is noted by the examiner, whereas in a locked knee a more gradual, rubbery, or soft stop to extension is palpated (Fig 11–6, B). An extension deficit may be secondary to a mechanical problem, as in a torn meniscus, but is often the result of a patella pain syndrome that we term "pseudolocking." In this situation, an examination under general anesthesia will demonstrate a full range of knee motion. While a mechanical problem may cause a deficit of extension as in a torn meniscus or loose body, Frankel et al.[4] have demonstrated that often it is similarly an alteration of the instant center of motion secondary to the pathology that has created a lack of extension. In addition, joint contractures from intra-articular or extra-articular adhesions, or a joint effusion will prevent the knee from achieving full extension or flexion.

A deficit of flexion is measured with the patient supine and flexing the hips and knees. It is measured in degrees, although it may be helpful for the examiner to note how far the heel is from the buttocks and record this distance as well (see Fig 11–5, A). Lack of normal flexion motion may occur from a variety of intra-articular or extra-articular pathologic conditions. It may occur secondary to problems intrinsic to the knee, with a resulting effusion preventing flexion, or extrinsic to the knee, where there has been soft tissue injury preventing the normal glide of the capsular envelope about the knee, as in femoral fractures. Once the function of the joint and its range of motion are recorded, the specific knee examination may begin.

Palpation

In palpating the joint, an organized examination is necessary to avoid missing significant findings. The warmth of the skin should be compared with the opposite knee. Palpation about the patella is performed first, noting sites of tenderness in the retinaculum, the quadriceps tendon, and the patellar tendon, both proximally and distally.

Tenderness at the inferior pole of the patella is frequently seen in basketball players where microavulsions and inflammation within the tendon frequently develop. Distally, the tibial tubercle is appreciated and tenderness as well as swelling is noted. Osgood-Schlatter disease develops here with inflammation secondary to partial avulsions of the apophysis at this site. In evaluating patella problems the patella is moved side to side, noting the amount of movement, crepitation, and pain production. The knee is then crossed over the opposite leg, with the examiner exerting pressure on the patella in a lateral direction (Figs 11–7, A and B). While performing this maneuver, the examiner should note the patient's facial expression. Marked apprehension suggests that patella instability is present. In some patients the patella may slide completely out of the femoral groove. In addition, the Q angle should be noted. This term refers to the angle of the quadriceps and the patellar tendons. To measure the Q angle, the knees

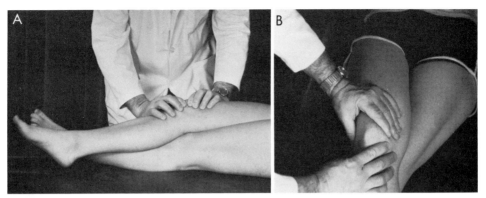

FIG 11–7. **A,** position for testing patella mobility while applying a lateral and then a medial force. **B,** note the patient's response.

are extended and a line is drawn along the axis of the quadriceps tendon to the anterior superior iliac spine, while a second line is drawn for the tibial tubercle through the patella intersecting the first line. The normal Q angle range is 15° to 20° (Fig 11–8). High and low Q angles may be seen. With patellar dislocation, the patella will move laterally in some patients, resulting in a low Q angle (< 10°), while in other patients it will remain in the femoral groove and the angle will be high in the 25° to 30° range. In completing this part of the examination, it is wise to note the patient's active patellar tracking during knee extension. This is performed with the patient sitting and observing how the patella tracks during knee extension. As the knee extends, the patella will generally move in a straight manner proximally followed by a small terminal lateral deviation. In dislocation this may be significantly exaggerated, with a marked lateral terminal deviation or even dislocation on full extension (Figs 11–9, A and B). During this maneuver, the size and tone of the vastus medialis are noted. There is considerable variation; some patients have a hypertrophied vastus medialis while others are grossly deficient, with a hollow area seen medially with a very high vastus medialis insertion site. This condition is known as quadriceps dysplasia as described by Fox[3] and is felt to play a role in patella instability and pain syndromes. Finally, in evaluating the patella, it should be moved in a medial and lateral direction with the knee extended and the muscle relaxed. A recording of up to 2 cm of mobility is normal. It is significantly increased with patella instability problems and diminished in patellofemoral arthritis, or if adhesions are present, about the patella, as in a knee with limited motion.

In palpating about the patella, any swelling or tenderness superficial to the patella should be noted. Prepatella swelling may be the result of chronic irritation, trauma, or infection. If infection is suspected aspiration is performed, with care being taken to avoid contaminating the joint.

A joint effusion is suspected if there is diffuse swelling about the knee; however, this latter finding may be missed if a small effusion is present. In noting the presence of an effusion it appears easiest to try to trap the fluid in the suprapatellar pouch. This is done by using one hand to force the fluid into the pouch and palpating it with the opposite hand, or balloting the patella, noting any soft resistance as the patella is lifted from the femur (Fig. 11–10). If a large effusion

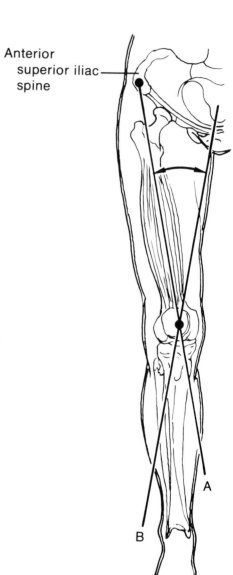

Anterior
superior iliac
spine

FIG 11–8. Measurement of the "Q" angle.
A, a line is drawn from the anterior superior
iliac spine to the patella, intersecting with line
B, which is drawn from the tibial tubercle to
the patella. The arc formed represents the "Q"
angle.

is present, then a fluid wave may be transmitted across the joint and palpated
with the opposite hand.

Palpation of the knee for sites of tenderness and swelling is then performed
about the joint margins. Usually, flexing the knee to 90° facilitates exploration of
the joint line. Tender sites should be precisely located and identified as being
specifically at the joint line or positioned more diffuse proximally or distally to
the joint (Figs 11–11 and 11–12). In seeking joint line tenderness, palpate well
posterior to the posteromedial and posterolateral corners. With a torn meniscus,

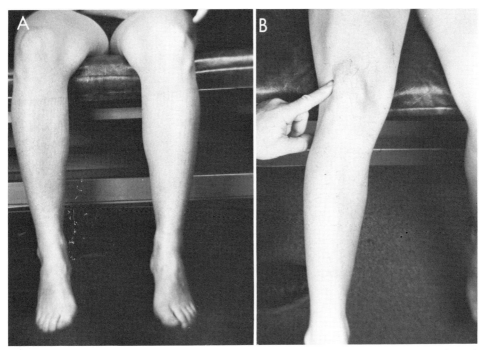

FIG 11–9. A, knee flexed to 90°. Note position of patella. **B,** as knee extends there is lateral tracking of patella.

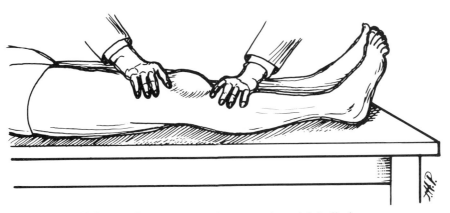

FIG 11–10. Method for demonstrating a joint effusion.

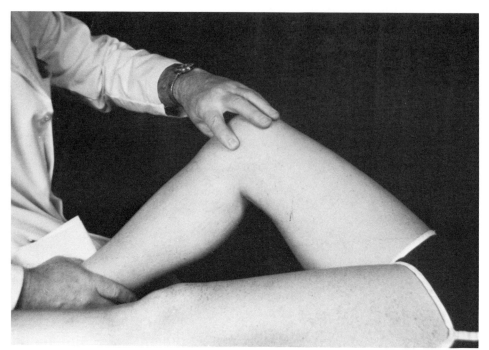

FIG 11–11. Palpating medial joint line for tenderness.

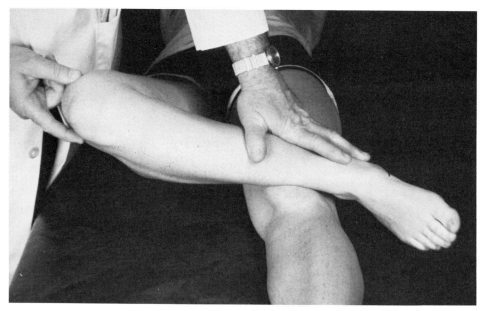

FIG 11–12. Figure-of-four position to evaluate lateral collateral ligament and joint line for tenderness.

joint line tenderness may be the only finding. Unfortunately, referred pain to the joint line is very common with patella pain syndromes that are associated with or without chondromalacia of the patella. These referral patterns are more common medially (60%) than laterally (30%), and occur posteriorly in 8% of the cases.[11] In palpating along the joint line, small cysts communicating with degenerative meniscal lesions should be sought. These may be proximal or distal to the joint line and not directly over the meniscus. They often vary in size with activity and will feel quite firm on palpation. Generally, they are lateral, but on occasion will be seen medially. In laterally palpating about the knee for local tenderness it is helpful to use the figure-of-4 position (see Fig. 11–12) to examine the lateral joint line and lateral collateral ligament. This maneuver will open the lateral compartment, allowing the lateral collateral ligament to be easily palpated and will allow the examiner to be able to note any tenderness along the meniscus and the popliteal tendon.

In examining the knee, the examiner should appreciate a variety of bursae that exist (Fig 11–13). One of the common bursa lies deep to the pes anserinus. These structures can be irritated, resulting in local tenderness secondary to inflammation along the hamstring tendons. A fairly common condition that will present as medial pain mimicking a torn medial meniscus is the result of inflammation about the semimembranous tendon. If a local injection of novocaine eliminates the pain, the clinical impression may be confirmed.

Laterally, a common clinical diagnosis that is frequently made in runners is the "iliotibial band syndrome" wherein inflammation develops deep to the iliotibial band as it passes over the lateral femoral condyle. Usually, some local tenderness at the femoral condyle is observed. The popliteus tendon may become inflamed posterolaterally, and is associated with pain often noted while running downhill. Local tenderness over the tendon attachment site at the femur is found and increases with internal tibial rotation. In palpating the knee, the specific

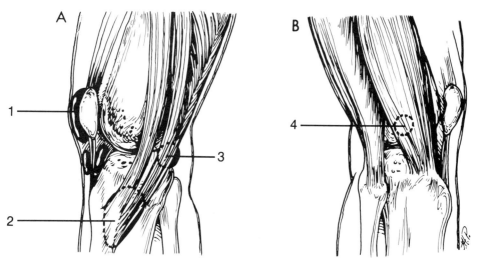

FIG 11–13. Common bursal sites of local tenderness: (*A*) medial view (1) prepatellar, (2) pes anserinus, (3) semimembranoses, and (*B*) lateral view (4) lateral femoral condyle deep to iliotibial band.

attachment sites of the ligaments are important to note, as acute sprains of the ligament will generally have sites of well-localized tenderness. Medially, the medial collateral ligament may tear proximally, in its middle portion, or distally, deep to the pes anserinus tendons. If a grade I sprain of the medial collateral ligament is present, it is often exacerbated by valgus stress placed on the knee. Laterally again, the lateral collateral ligament is evaluated in the figure-of-4 position if possible, or in an acute injury with the knee extended. Tenderness along the fibular head is seen with avulsion injuries, and if it is along the tibial plateau or femoral condyle, bone pathology may be indicated. This is frequently seen in stress fractures or in a variety of bone lesions. In evaluating patients with knee complaints, the possibility of a bone tumor should be considered. Although the knee may show an effusion with local atrophy, even when the lesion is extra-articular, the patient may still present with knee pain. Often, when these patients have some complaint of pain relating to the patella and secondary localized muscle atrophy, the examiner must avoid the error of making a diagnosis of "patellar pain syndrome" solely on the basis of the patient's complaints and perhaps missing an underlying bony lesion that is the cause.

Inspection and palpation of the posterior aspect of the knee is often ignored. This area of the knee should be examined for swelling and local tenderness. Popliteal cysts are common and may be quite large. In young children they are generally not associated with intra-articular pathology and will often disappear with observation. In adults the converse is true. Interestingly, these cysts may dissect downward into the calf, particularly in patients with rheumatoid arthritis, and present with sudden pain mimicking thrombophlebitis. In palpating posteriorly, the popliteal pulse should be noted and if a mass is present, auscultation for an aneurysm may reveal a bruit.

Synovial sarcomas may present in this location and are difficult to diagnose, particularly if a flexion contracture is present. Arthrography aids greatly in the evaluation of a popliteal mass as the leakage of dye into the mass will confirm the presence of a popliteal cyst.

In examining the knee, a variety of tests have been described. Some are helpful and others less so. Usually, they are used in conjunction with each other to arrive at a diagnosis of meniscal or ligament dysfunction.

Examination of the Meniscus

Previously, much of the attention concerning the examination of the knee has been directed toward diagnosing injuries of the meniscus. Tests such as Mc-Murray's,[12] Apley's,[1] and Steinmann's[14] have received considerable attention and before arthrography and arthroscopy were solely relied on to establish the diagnosis. Unfortunately, these tests are not infallible and occasionally, normal menisci have been removed based on a reliance on them alone. Depending on the availability, arthrography for medial menisci pathology is highly accurate (98%); that of lateral menisci is less so (85%). In addition, the use of arthroscopy and the surgical treatment of torn menisci with the arthroscope has improved the diagnostic level greatly, to the point where with experience, an experienced arthroscopist will rarely misdiagnose a meniscus lesion. Even without these techniques, the clinician in chronic cases can still arrive at a correct diagnosis with a high degree of accuracy and then use these techniques to decide on the type of lesion present and perform appropriate surgical treatment if needed.

In evaluating a patient before examining the knee, the examiner will already have a diagnosis in mind particularly if the patient gives a history of a specific incident; for example, often involving a twist of the body with the foot fixed. Other common mechanisms include forced flexion, such as a fall in which tibial rotation is either prevented or exaggerated.

Meniscal tears are frequently seen in association with acute anterior cruciate ligament injuries (30%) or in chronic injuries (90%). The medial meniscus plays a role in joint stability. Experimentally, we have found that after excising the anterior cruciate ligament, the medial meniscus acts as a doorstop to prevent further anterior tibial translation on the femur[11] (Fig 11–14). With the knee in extension, the increment of anteroposterior movement in the anterior cruciate ligament–insufficient knee after meniscectomy is 18%, increasing to 58% at 90° of flexion. This accounts for the high number of meniscus tears in chronic anterior cruciate ligament injuries. Mechanisms that produce an internal tibial rotation associated with a "pop" and rapid swelling suggest a previous anterior cruciate ligament injury, while a valgus and external rotation force will result in medial collateral ligament and anterior cruciate ligament trauma that may include a medial meniscus tear.

In older patients, the meniscus may undergo a process of degeneration that

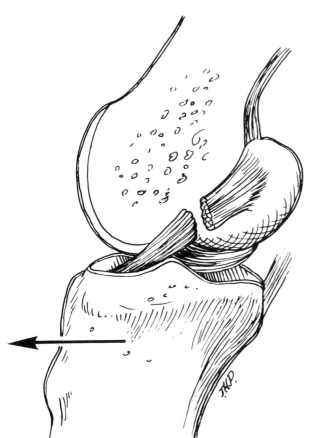

FIG 11–14. In ruptures of anterior cruciate ligament, medial meniscus acts to prevent further anterior tibial displacement.

can fully develop a progressive horizontal cleavage or a radial tear without a specific traumatic incident being evident. In younger patients, a history of locking is frequent. This is a result of a meniscus tear displacing into the joint. The patient may note that certain specific maneuvers unlock the joint. This supports the suspicion of meniscus injury. The locking may result from a true locking or be secondary to pain produced when the knee is brought into extension as the patient resists this motion. There may be an alteration in the instant center of motion preventing full extension.

A history of joint pain associated with rotation is often noted when pain is produced by a deep knee bend. Swelling is common and supports the impression of meniscal injury in contrast to patellofemoral pain syndromes, which are less likely to cause an effusion. Often, meniscal symptoms are intermittent and relieved by rest.

The examiner should note any abnormal gait that can vary with the acuteness of the condition. Ask the patient to point with one finger to the area of pain. Generally, meniscal complaints are well localized medially or laterally and occasionally posteriorly and anteriorly, but rarely in more than one area. Ask the patient to perform a deep knee bend and note any pain produced and its site. Duck walking will be quite painful in patients with posterior horn tears of the medial meniscus.

Have the patient first lie down supine and then prone with the knee hanging from the table edge (Fig 11–15). This will allow the examiner to record any subtle loss of knee extension. With the patient supine, the examiner performs a bounce test by holding each heel and snapping the knee into extension (see Fig 11–6, B). An effusion or meniscal tear will produce a soft bounce, possibly causing some pain on extension. A normal knee will snap into full extension without pain. Carefully palpate for an effusion and then for local joint line tenderness. Meniscal pathology will usually produce localized tenderness along the joint line over the site of the tear. For lateral meniscal lesions, the figure-of-4 position is excellent for locating the joint line and noting tenderness behind, anterior, or over the lateral collateral ligament (see Fig 11–12).

In evaluating a meniscal tear, the examiner must recall that the patellar pain syndrome commonly causes referred pain and local tenderness to the medial joint line in two thirds, and laterally in one third, of the cases. Local tenderness or pain over a meniscus alone is insufficient to make a diagnosis of meniscal pathology although the diagnosis should be considered.

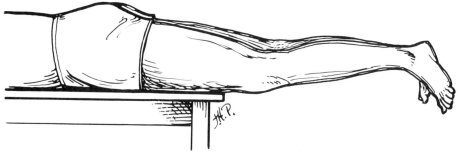

FIG 11–15. Prone test for knee extension. Method for determining subtle losses of knee extension.

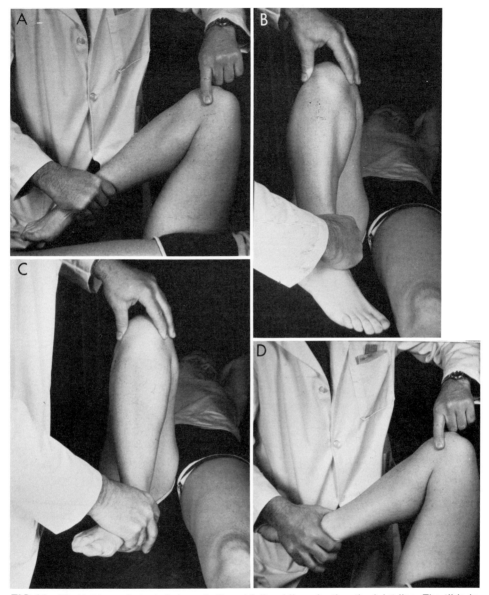

FIG 11–16. McMurray's test. **A,** knee is flexed fully while palpating the joint line. The tibia is internally rotated as the tibia is slowly extended. **B,** anterior view of internal rotation. Externally rotate (**C**) the tibia while fully flexed and slowly extend (**D**) the knee while palpating medially.

McMurray's Test

Rotational tests are helpful in supporting the diagnosis, the best known of which is the McMurray test.[12] This test is basically a rotational test performed with the knee in full flexion and then gradually extended to a right angle while holding the foot fully internally rotated or externally rotated.

To perform this test, the patient lies supine and the examiner palpates the joint margin with the index finger and thumb of one hand while acutely flexing the knee and with the other hand holding the ankle or distal tibia (Figs 11–16, A–D). In performing this maneuver, any snap or click should be noted and its location discerned if possible. Isolated patella clicks, and in particular transmitted or innocuous clicks in the hip, should be excluded. If a segment of torn cartilage is caught during this maneuver a snap and pain may be induced.

McMurray believed that internal rotation (see Fig 11–16, B) would test the posterior half of the lateral meniscus while external rotation would test the posterior half of the medial meniscus (see Fig 11–16, C). He did not think it was helpful for tears of the anterior horn of either meniscus. This test is useful if it is positive but frequently is falsely negative. In addition, patellar clicks can be difficult to exclude. Often loose-jointed patients will demonstrate clicks in both knees that occur during the rotation and flexion secondary to movement of the meniscus without a tear being present.

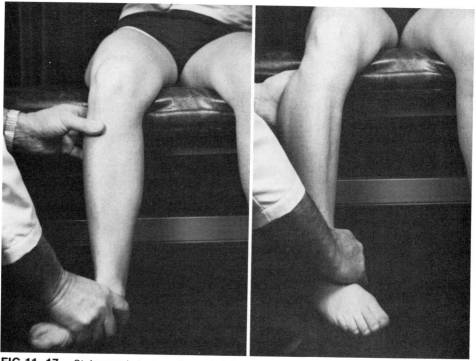

FIG 11–17. Steinmann's test: performed sitting or supine with knee at 90° of flexion. **A,** forceful external and **B,** internal rotation are applied, noting production of pain.

Steinmann's Test

Additional rotational tests may be helpful in differentiating meniscal from patellar complaints because rotation will not ordinarily increase pain secondary to patella pathology, while acute rotation even without full flexion will often increase pain related to a meniscus.[14]

The Steinmann test is performed at 90° of flexion (Fig 11–17, A) with the patient sitting with his legs off the table or lying supine. The tibia is grasped and forcefully externally (see Fig. 11–17, A) or internally rotated (Fig 11–17, B). In meniscal tears this will frequently result in pain production. This test if positive is quite helpful but false negatives may occur.

Apley's Test (GRIND TEST)

In 1946, Apley published his article on the diagnosis of meniscal injuries. He felt that the click noted in the McMurray test was often unreliable. He offered an alternative solution. To perform this test, the patient is prone and the knee flexed to 90°. The couch should be low so that the examiner can use his knee to hold the patient's thighs to the couch while applying distraction (Fig 11–18).

Initially, both feet are grasped and fully internally and externally rotated with the knee at 90° of flexion. One foot is then grasped with both hands while the examiner's knee is on the patient's posterior thigh. The patient's knee is flexed to

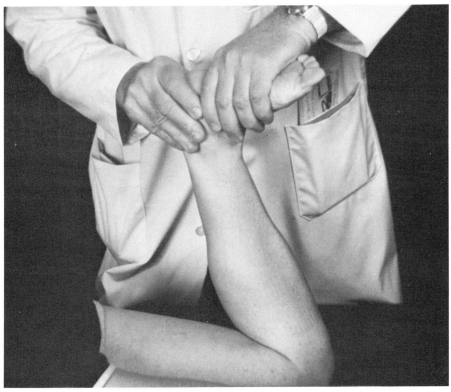

FIG 11–18. Apley's grind test.

90° before a nonviolent sudden external rotation is applied. Any pain elicited is noted. Next the patient's knee is distracted by applying an upward force while the examiner's knee holds the patient's thigh on the couch. Again, external rotation motion is applied and pain is noted. If the pain is increased by the maneuver then a rotational sprain is suggested.

Following this portion of the test, the compression test is performed by using the examiner's body weight to compress the tibia on the femur again during external rotation. If compression produces an increase in pain, then the grind test is positive and a torn meniscus suggested. To diagnose a torn lateral meniscus, the knee is forcefully externally rotated while more internal rotation is used for a suspected medial tear. Unfortunately, the grinding or compression also compresses the patella and may confuse the examiner as to the source of the patient's pain.

The distraction test is not useful since there are better ways to diagnose sprains about the knee, while the compression test may be helpful. The rotational component is probably the most important aspect and is actually a Steinmann test in a prone position.

While these tests are helpful, no one test is perfect, and false negative as well as occasional false positive results are possible. Overall, the simple rotation test at 90° of flexion probably represents the most helpful test, as well as the occurrence of localized joint line tenderness in the absence of patella complaints.

Arthrography in present-day use is helpful and, if not available, then arthroscopy will greatly aid in the diagnostic acumen of the examiner, although the clinical examination alone permits a high percentage of these tears to be correctly diagnosed in the nonacute state.

Patella

Problems referable to the patella are probably the most common complaints the examiner will hear when examining patients with knee complaints.

The patella is essentially a sesamoid bone that lies within the quadriceps tendon and acts to increase the length of the moment arm for the quadriceps tendon (Fig 11–19). The patella has several facets, including a large lateral, a

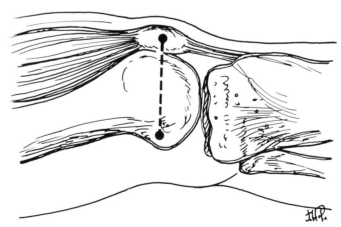

FIG 11–19. Patella acts to increase moment arm of quadriceps tendon by displacing tendon away from center of knee rotation.

smaller medial facet, and a vertically oriented odd facet. Their contact with the femoral groove will vary with knee flexion. The patella has the thickest cartilage of any bone and as a result of high pressures or the lack of pressure will undergo degeneration resulting in chondromalacia. Many patients with complaints of patellar pain will have chondromalacia of some degree, while others with similar complaints have no apparent chondromalacia. A diagnosis of chondromalacia should be reserved for direct observation and a diagnosis of patella pain syndrome used until a more precise diagnosis is established. The patella tracks in its groove as the knee is extended and normally there is a mild degree of terminal lateral deviation. If this is excessive, the patella may subluxate or dislocate completely from the femur on knee extension. Diagnostic problems referable to the patella will be discussed. They include patella pain syndromes, patella subluxation, and dislocation.

First, in taking a history, the patient's complaints will be fairly typical. The onset is generally gradual in the patellar pain syndrome without a specific history of injury. However, the patellar pain syndrome may occur as a result of a sudden high load being applied to the patella, as in striking the knee on the dashboard of the car as it suddenly decelerates. Most complaints are gradual in onset and related to repetitive use, as in runners or activities that require many deep knee bends. The pain is medially located in two thirds of patients, it is lateral in a third, and posterior in about 8%. It is often diffuse. It is increased by climbing and particularly when descending stairs, squatting, and kneeling. Sitting for prolonged periods, as in a car or movie, results in stiffness and increased pain. Arising from a chair is often painful. The complaint of swelling is generally mild and an effusion is uncommon in patellar pain syndrome but can be seen in traumatic dislocations.

First note the position of the patient's knees while standing. Is there genu varus or valgus? Do the patellae point inward? This suggests femoral neck anteversion, which is frequently seen in these patients. Next, the patient is asked to perform a deep knee bend. If pain occurs on arising from the bend rather than at the full point of flexion it suggests a patella origin for the pain.

The patient is then seated and the position of the patella noted. Does it face outward as in patellar instability? The patient slowly extends one knee and then the other while the examiner notes the motion of the patella (see Figs 11–9, A and B). Normally, it tracks straight with a minimal amount of deviation laterally. In some patients with patella instability, the examiner may observe it sliding off the femur in the last 30° of extension.

Next, the patella is palpated for tenderness and mobility (see Fig 11–7). An effusion is uncommon in cases of patellar pain syndrome. Maximum tenderness is often present along the medial joint line (see Fig 11–11), but may also be present laterally. In this event, a meniscus tear may easily be mimicked. Tenderness may be present proximal or distal along the quadriceps tendon but is generally more exquisite at the medial or lateral facet. This is best tested by flexing the patient's knee 30°, crossing it over the opposite knee, and then palpating the deep medial and lateral surfaces (see Fig 11–7, B).

Tests for Patellar Injuries

The patellar compression test is performed by forcefully compressing the patella on the femur as the knee is extended, noting any pain production.

The patellar apprehension test is performed in the cross-legged position by using both hands to force the patella laterally, noting the patient's response as well as the patellar motion (see Fig 11–7, B). Normally, a patella will move less than 2 cm. In subluxation, mobility is increased and apprehension is frequently noted. In some loose-jointed patients the patella can be pushed completely off the femur. Guarding may prevent dislocation because of apprehension and may be the only finding associated in patella dislocation.

Next, the knee is fully flexed and any pain production noted (see Fig 11–5). Patients with patellar pain syndrome will usually feel discomfort with this maneuver while patients with dislocation may not protest at all. The rotational tests mentioned earlier should be negative. But the Apley grind test may give a false positive test because of patella compression.

In general, careful history taking may cause one to suspect a patellar problem so that the examination will merely confirm this impression. In observing a patient's knee a variety of abnormalities may be noted, including a deficiency of the vastus medialis, lateral bands or patella alta, genu valgum, and tibial torsion. All these findings may be seen in patients with quadriceps dysplasia and may be a factor in patients who develop patellar pain.

Ligament

The examination of the static stability of the knee has become a muddled topic for many surgeons. A wide variety of tests and concepts that have evolved over the past decade have been misunderstood and have confused the subject without allowing the establishment of a precise anatomical diagnosis that permits an organized treatment program to be established.

For purposes of discussion, straight plane instabilities of the knee will be reviewed first. When rotational instabilities occur, they are generally the result of a combination of straight plane instabilities. In examining for an acute knee injury the rotational tests, including the pivot shift test, are often of no value when the patient is awake because pain prevents relaxation. Nevertheless, for a diagnosis of an anterior cruciate ligament injury in both the acute and chronic states, the examiner should already have some impression of injury to a specific ligament based on the vectors of the forces involved, the presence or absence of a "pop" at the time of injury, and the patient's sense of movement between the femur and tibia, with the patient often using a two-fist sign to describe his sense of giving way (Fig 11–20). The physical examination will then confirm the suspicion and may give additional valuable information. For the acutely injured knee, the examination method should be altered slightly from that performed for chronic problems, as the production of pain will preclude a complete clinical evaluation. Often, the knee is markedly swollen, distorting normal landmarks. If abrasions are present, they should be noted and may indicate the direction of the forces involved and help in deciding treatment. With large effusions, the joint will usually be held flexed. While pain may be significant, in complete ruptures of ligaments it may be surprisingly mild. Similarly, a joint effusion may be small if the fluid has leaked through significant capsular tears.

Having completed an inspection and palpation of the knee, a specific examination of the ligaments is performed. In evaluating the anterior cruciate ligament, a variety of tests are used and include the anterior drawer sign, Lachman's test (Fig 11–21), and pivot shift test. In the past, the anterior drawer sign was the standard test for diagnosing anterior cruciate ligament injuries. It is positive in 94% of chronic anterior cruciate ligament injuries but positive in only 54% of

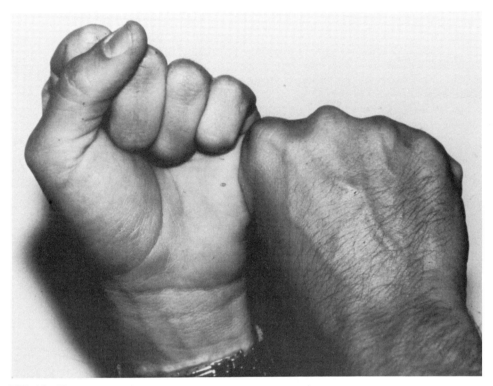

FIG 11–20. Two fist sign. This is often used by the patient to describe his sense of knee instability. It is nearly always associated with anterior cruciate ligament injury rather than meniscus injury.

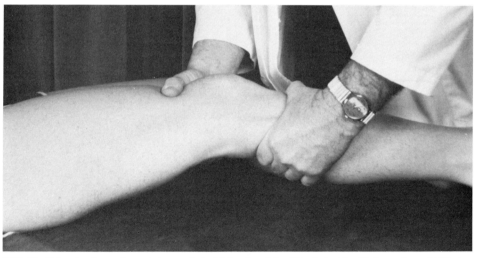

FIG 11–21. Lachman's test: femur is held firmly while tibia is held with knee flexed 30°. An anterior force is applied to tibia, noting the excursion and end point.

acute anterior cruciate ligament injuries when the secondary restraints (meniscus, and medial collateral ligament) are intact (Fig 11–22). In a recent study of acute anterior cruciate ligament injuries, the anterior drawer sign was positive in 54% of isolated anterior cruciate ligament injuries, increasing to 69% with medial meniscus tear, 89% with lateral meniscus injury, and 100% when both menisci were torn along with the anterior cruciate ligament. Conversely, the Lachman test is positive in 99% of acute anterior cruciate ligament injuries, regardless of associated injury. Why does this difference exist? In a study of tibial displacement following cruciate resection, it was observed that tibial translation is maximum at 30° and considerably reduced at 90°.[5] The Lachman test as described by Torg[16] is simply an anterior drawer test performed in a position of 20° to 30° of knee flexion (Fig 11–21). In performing this test, three observations are required. First, the excursion of the tibia on the femur is observed; second,

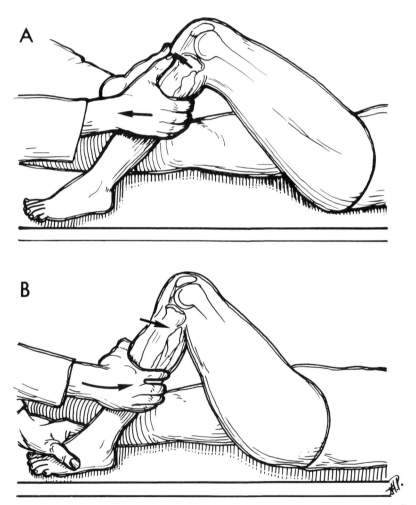

FIG 11–22. Anterior drawer sign performed by applying force to tibia while knee is flexed 90° (A). Posterior drawer sign is performed by applying posterior force to tibia with knee flexed 90° (B).

248   R. Warren

the presence of an end point is noted, and finally, the obliteration of the sulcus anterior to the infrapatellar tendon is observed. If the knee is placed in a position of less than 20° of flexion, the excursion secondary to anterior cruciate ligament rupture will be diminished and a false negative may occur. The end point is a term used to describe the sensation as the tibial excursion suddenly stops. In essence, it represents the sudden rise in stiffness within the anterior cruciate ligament as a load is applied and the strain suddenly decreases. The lack of an end point, if present in the control knee, is the most sensitive sign of an injured anterior cruciate ligament. Rarely, a torn meniscus forced into the joint may minimize the excursion or eliminate the end point. Additional tests for anterior cruciate ligament injury exist as noted. The drawer test is performed next. In the acute knee, if flexion is less than 90°, then the standard drawer test is not possible and aspiration may be required. The drawer test is used to evaluate both for anterior cruciate ligament and posterior cruciate ligament injuries.

The Anterior Drawer Test

In performing an anterior drawer test the knee is flexed 90°, with the examiner facing the patient and supporting the foot (see Fig 11–22, A). Prior to performing the test, the position of the tibia on the femur should be noted and any drop back, however subtle, should be looked for. Partial tears of the posterior cruciate ligament may lack a drop-back sign but complete tears will generally allow some posterior displacement.

When performing the anterior drawer test the hamstrings must be completely relaxed, as any spasm here will prevent forward displacement of the tibia. Both hands are placed posterior to the proximal tibia and pressure is anteriorly exerted slowly and then repeated more forcefully. Again, excursion and end point are noted. Grading is carried out on a 1-to-3 basis, with a 5-mm increase representing a grade of 1+; 5 to 10 mm, 2+; and over 10 mm, 3+. In performing an anterior drawer test and diagnosing anterior cruciate ligament injury, the examiner must be certain that he is not pulling the tibia forward from a posteriorly displaced position to its normal anatomical position, as in a posterior cruciate ligament injury, rather than testing for an anterior cruciate tear. A clue to the diagnosis of posterior cruciate ligament injury may be indicated when performing the Lachman test or the anterior drawer test, if increased excursion is noted, but there is an excellent end point. In this case, a posterior cruciate ligament injury should be suspected, as well as partial injury to the anterior cruciate ligament.

Other Tests

The posterior drawer test is then performed by pushing the tibia in the opposite direction; again the end point and excursion should be noted (see Fig 11–22, B). In acute injuries, the posterior excursion is increased and the end point is soft, while in chronic injuries the excursion is often severe. However, the end point will return as the secondary restraints have failed over time.

Medial and lateral instability are then evaluated. These are performed with the knee positioned at 0° and then at 30°. In extension, the anterior cruciate ligament and posterior cruciate ligament will provide some static stability to valgus or varus stress so that a lesion of the collateral ligament may be missed. At 30° of flexion, the medial collateral ligament is stressed while any opening of the medial compartment is noted (Fig 11–23). Sprains may be graded on a 1-to-3 scale depending on the observed instability. If a mild sprain is suspected by

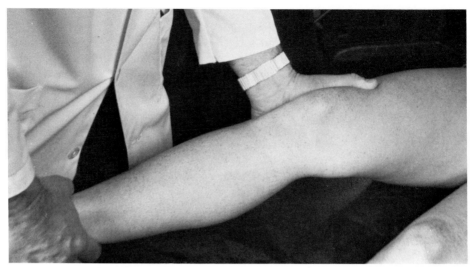

FIG 11–23. Valgus stress for medial lateral collateral injury in 30° of flexion.

history and there is tenderness along the ligament, without the joint opening, this is classified as grade I. A grade III represents a complete disruption with the tibia opening in a "barn door" fashion with no end point being observed. Generally, this is greater than 7 mm of joint opening. This degree of injury to the medial collateral ligament implies concomitant damage to the anterior cruciate ligament. In knee joints with a smaller degree of opening it is classified as 2a or 2b. The former, 2a, represents a minimal opening of less than 3 mm and an aggressive treatment program is used compared with a grade 2b where there is a marked opening but an end point is present. In these patients, a slower recovery program is initiated.

Lateral collateral ligament sprains are similarly evaluated in flexion and extension. Isolated injuries of the lateral collateral ligament are unusual and generally associated with anterior cruciate or posterior cruciate ligament injuries. We have found that an isolated section of the lateral collateral ligament will result in only small increments of varus opening, but combined with a popliteus injury varus rotation will increase to 5–6 mm at 30° of flexion[7] (Fig 11–24).

Rotational Tests for Ligament Injuries

Pivot Shift Test. This test initially described by Palmer[13] and then readdressed by Galway et al[6] is an excellent test for anterior cruciate ligament injury. A variety of tests have subsequently been reported, including the flexion rotation and the jerk tests, but in essence they are all used to demonstrate the same phenomenon.

In performing the pivot shift test, muscle relaxation is critical. Thus, this test was positive in only 38% of 100 patients with an acute anterior cruciate injury on the initial examination in the office. However, this rose to 98% using general anesthesia.[2]

The test is performed with the patient supine and the knee flexed 30° (Figs 11–25, A and B). The foot is held in mild internal rotation that should not be excessive or it will decrease the shift. A valgus force is created on the knee by placing the opposite hand on the tibia as the knee is then extended and as the valgus force is continued, a jump will be noted at about the 20° to 30° position. This is the shift that occurs as the tibia suddenly subluxates forward on the femur indicating a torn anterior cruciate ligament. Often, there is some damage to the lateral capsule, particularly the mid third. This test may be performed in the reverse manner from extension to flexion, again noting the jump on reduction. If difficulty in obtaining the test is noted, particularly in large, heavy patients, a cross-handed technique may facilitate this examination (Fig 11–26).

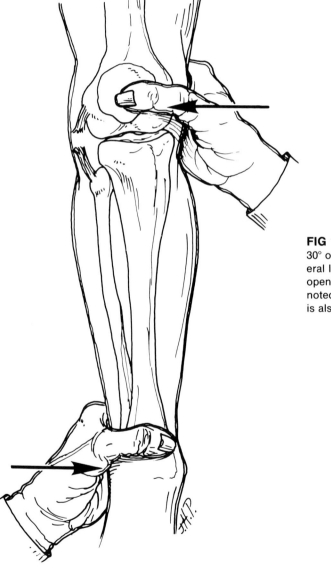

FIG 11–24. Varus stress in 30° of flexion for lateral collateral ligament injury: minimal opening (2 to 3 mm) will be noted unless popliteus tendon is also injured.

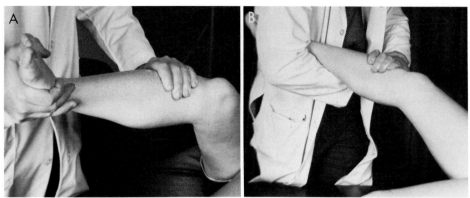

FIG 11–25. A, pivot shift test performed with foot in mild internal rotation and knee flexed. **B,** crossed-hand method to obtain positive shift in large bulky patients.

In other patients, marked guarding will be noted as the patient senses that a slip is about to occur. If the examiner is gentle when administering this test, he will obtain more relaxation and a higher incidence of shifts. When the shift occurs in evaluating a patient with a chronic injury, ask him if this mimics his complaint. If the answer is positive, this strongly suggests that an anterior cruciate ligament rupture is his main problem.

A grade I shift represents a mild grind on the lateral compartment with minimal rotation observed. These shifts are rarely symptomatic, in contrast to a grade II or III shift, which generally causes symptoms. In a grade III shift, the femur and meniscus actively lock in place briefly with a marked sudden jump perceived as subluxation then reduction occurs. A grade II shift has a clear-cut jump, although not to the extreme degree of grade III. Although it is subjective, this grading method is consistent and useful on repeated examination. A pivot shift test is often diminished and occasionally eliminated in patients with acute knee injuries in whom there is gross medial ligament damage. This occurs when the examiner is unable to create significant valgus compression in the lateral compartment. In performing the pivot shift test the magnitude of the shift may be enhanced by placing the tibia in a position of external rotation while obducting the hip. Conversely, in the position of external tibial rotation, a reverse pivot shift may occur if there is posterior lateral instability secondary to a torn popliteus tendon and lateral collateral ligament. This may confuse the examiner into thinking that the anterior cruciate ligament is torn. In fact, posterior lateral instability is rarely seen alone and is generally associated with injury to the posterior cruciate ligament or to the anterior cruciate ligament. Thus, in the same knee one may note a true pivot shift as well as a reverse pivot shift.

Reverse Pivot Shift. This test, described by Jacob and Staubli,[10] is performed similar to the pivot shift except that the tibia is forcefully externally rotated, resulting in a posterior tibial subluxation off the femur in flexion, only to reduce with a sudden jump as the knee is extended. This indicates damage to the posterolateral corner, including the lateral collateral ligament, the popliteus, and arcuate ligament. To correctly diagnose the site of damage, the examiner must

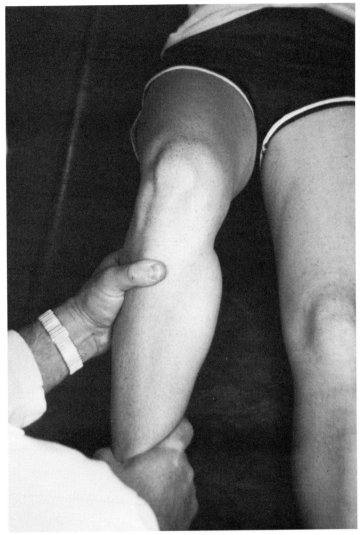

FIG 11–26. Arcuate spin test for posterior lateral instability: force is directed posteriorly and external rotation is applied to tibia, noting degree of rotation of tibia on femur.

note the position of the tibia prior to the sudden jump, while holding the foot externally rotated. This is the jump from a posteriorly displaced position to a reduced one at about 30° of flexion that occurs in posterior lateral instability.

In contrast, a true pivot shift will occur with the foot held in some external rotation as the tibia subluxates forward from a reduced position in flexion to a displaced forward position at about 20° to 30° of flexion. These patients with a pivot shift in external rotation must be separated from those with a reverse shift by noting the position of the tibia on the femur before displacement.

Additional Tests for Posterior Lateral Instability

Hyperextension Recurvatum Test.   In this test, developed by Hughston[8] (see Fig 11–6, A), the examiner holds the leg in extension, noticing the hyperextension varus and external rotation of the tibia on the femur. This is produced by generally massive lateral side injuries involving the lateral collateral ligament, the popliteus, arcuate, and anterior cruciate, and often the posterior cruciate ligaments. Injury restricted to the posterior lateral corner without injury to the anterior cruciate ligament will not produce true hyperextension.

The Arcuate Spin Test.   The name of this test is a term we have used to describe the excessive external rotation observed at 90° of flexion (see Fig 11–26). In performing a posterior drawer maneuver the tibia is forcefully externally rotated. With posterolateral corner damage, as well as anterior cruciate ligament or posterior cruciate ligament injury, the tibia will spin on the femur in this direction. It can best be appreciated by noting the tibial tubercle and head of the fibula as the tibia is forced into external rotation. We have found that cutting the popliteus combined with the lateral collateral ligament will markedly increase this rotation.[7]

The Reverse Lachman Test for Posterolateral Corner Injury.   This test is performed at 30° of flexion, and a force is applied in a posterior direction as well as an anterior one. In performing this test, an excellent end point will be noted as the tibia is brought forward, but an increased excursion is appreciated, indicating that the tibia is starting from a posteriorly displaced position secondary to the posterior cruciate ligament injury, or injury confined to the lateral collateral ligament and popliteus. If the tibia is pushed further posteriorly and rotated externally, a marked increase in the rotation as well as increased excursion will be seen if there is damage to the posterior lateral corner, noting however that a small amount of true posterior tibial translation will be seen (4 mm), despite an intact posterior cruciate ligament. Both this rotation and posterior displacement will increase significantly if additional injury to the posterior cruciate ligament is present.[7]

The Slocum Test.   This is essentially a test performed while carrying out the classic anterior drawer test. It is performed with the foot internally rotated 30°, at neutral, and externally rotated 15°. Normally, in performing an anterior drawer maneuver with the tibia rotated externally or internally, the amount of excursion noted in the neutral position will diminish (Fig 11–27). If it does not, it indicates additional damage at the posterior medial or posterior lateral corner of the knee. When this test is positive, injury to the anterior cruciate ligament is also present.

Finally, in completing the examination, if the complaints are subtle a variety of functional tests may bring out complaints not noted in the previous examination. These include running in place, duck walk, maximum vertical jump, and horizontal jump on one leg. If space allows, agility maneuvers may also be used.

Having completed the examination, a working diagnosis can generally be made, using appropriate roentgenograms and additional studies as indicated. Clinical muscle testing will often miss significant degrees of weakness. In this case Cybex isokinetic testing may be useful. A careful knee examination that is organized to evaluate a variety of pain patterns and exclude systemic causes

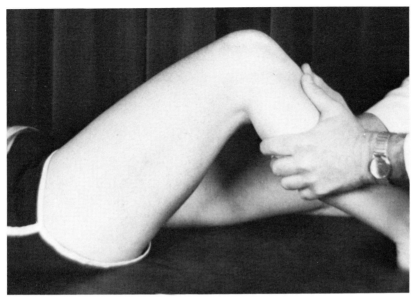

FIG 11–27. Slocum's test: anterior drawer sign performed at 90° of flexion. Drawer sign is performed with the foot internally rotated 30°, at neutral, and externally rotated 15°.

before focusing on the knee will ordinarily enable the examiner to arrive at an accurate diagnosis.

References

1. Apley AG: The diagnosis of meniscus injuries: Some new clinical methods. *J. Bone Joint Surg* 1947; 29:78.
2. Donaldson W, Warren RF: Evaluation of 100 acute tears of the anterior cruciate ligament. Presented at the American Orthopaedic Society of Sports Medicine, Williamsburg, Va, July 1983.
3. Fox T: Dysplasia of the quadriceps mechanism. *Surg Clin N Am* 1975; 55:199.
4. Frankel VH, Burstein AH, Brooks DB: Biomechanics of internal derangement of the knee: Pathomechanics as determined by analysis of the instant center of motion. *J Bone Joint Surg* 1971; 53A:945.
5. Fukubayashi T, Torzilli PA, Sherman MF, et al: An in vitro biomechanical evaluation of anterior-posterior motion of the knee. *J Bone Joint Surg* 1982; 64A:258–264.
6. Galway RD, Beaupre A, MacIntosh DL: Pivot shift: A clinical sign of symptomatic anterior cruciate insufficiency. *J Bone Joint Surg* 1972; 54B:763.
7. Gollehon DL, Warren RF, Torzilli P: Posterior lateral restraints on tibial rotation. In preparation.
8. Hughston JC, Norwood LA Jr: The posterolateral drawer test and external rotational recurvatum test for posterolateral rotatory instability of the knee. *Clin Orthop* 1980; 147:82–87.
9. Insall JN: *Surgery of the Knee.* New York, Churchill Livingston, 1984, p 59.

10. Jacob P, Staubli HU: The reversed pivot shift sign. *Orthop Trans* 1981; 5:487.
11. Levy IM, Trozilli PA, Warren RF: The effect of medial meniscectomy on anterior-posterior motion of the knee. *J Bone Joint Surg* 1982; 64A:883-888.
12. McMurray TP: The semi-lunar cartilages. Br J Surg 1941; 29:407.
13. Palmer I: On the injuries to the ligaments of the knee joint: A clinical study. *Acta Chir Scand Supp* 1938; 53.
14. Ricklin P, Rüttiman A, del Buono MS: *Meniscal Lesions: Diagnosis, Differential Diagnosis and Therapy*. American translation by K. H. Mueller, ed 2. New York, Thieme Stratton, Inc., 1983.
15. Slocum DB, James SL, Larson RL, et al: Clinical test for anterolateral rotary instability of the knee. *Clin Orthop* 1976; 118:63.
16. Torg JS, Conrad W, Kalem V: Clinical diagnosis of anterior cruciate ligament instability in the athlete. *Am J Sports Med* 1976; 4:84.
17. Wickiewicz T, Warren RF: Patella pain syndrome. Review of 100 patients. Unpublished data, 1977.

CHAPTER 12

Physical Diagnosis of the Foot and Ankle

Manmohan Singh, M.D.

Kenneth A. Johnson, M.D.

The foot and ankle area is readily amenable to a full examination by inspection, palpation, and passive manipulation of the joints. However, a systematic approach to a clinical examination is essential when assessing a new patient. The purpose of this chapter is to present a method for examining patients with foot and ankle problems. Obviously, every clinician must develop a routine from personal experience; this material is intended as a starting point for such a venture. The chapter is divided into three parts: Part 1 presents an outline for clinical examination of the foot and ankle; Part 2 describes the clinical diagnosis of localized conditions in the foot and ankle; and Part 3 deals with the involvement of the foot and ankle in systemic disorders.

Clinical Examination

History Taking

When an office visit is scheduled for a foot or ankle problem, the patient is instructed to wear a pair of old shoes, preferably the ones used at work. This presents an opportunity not only to scrutinize the way the shoes wear, but also indicates the patient's preference in footwear. In a well-equipped office, facilities are also available for making footprints, taking weight-bearing roentgenograms, and photographing the clinical appearance of feet.

When obtaining history related to the presenting complaint, the patient is allowed to describe the subjective symptoms in his or her own words. Leading questions may be used only later to clarify relevant details and to exclude a history of generalized diseases such as gout, diabetes, and rheumatoid disorders that commonly involve the foot. When making notes, the date of onset or injury, progression of symptoms, and the treatment received are recorded. It is also important to take note of the patient's professional and leisure-time activities that may cause significant stress on the feet.

Orthopedic foot and ankle problems usually present as obvious deformities, well-defined injuries, or chronic foot pain. If the complaint is a cosmetically unpleasant gait, a frequent problem in children, an exact description of what the parents find unacceptable is obtained. A history of the mother's health during pregnancy, the mode of delivery, birth weight of the child, and milestones in the development of walking are recorded. This not only gains the parents' confidence but may also lead to the discovery of an occasional child with cerebral palsy or other neuromuscular defect.

In cases of injury, the patient is questioned about the exact position of the foot and ankle at the time of injury. This determines the type of injury, especially in cases of ankle fractures. Frequently, the patient is unable to recall the mechanism of injury. Therefore, it is important to know if the patient was able to stand up and walk after the injury. Did swelling develop soon after the injury or several hours later? Was ice or heat applied to the injured area?

If pain is the chief presenting complaint, the patient is asked if it is exacerbated by weight-bearing or activity and relieved by rest. Is the onset of pain related to a recent change in a job or sporting activity? Is the pain present at night or associated with morning stiffness? The relationship of foot pain to shoe wear is extremely important. Is the pain relieved or aggravated by walking barefoot? Did the patient recently buy a new pair of fashionable shoes? Does the patient wear appropriate shoes for the sporting activities practiced? Complaints of localized paresthesias and numbness in addition to pain may be associated with lesions of nerves proximal to the site of symptoms.

Inspection

After taking the history, the patient is requested to remove the footwear and, if necessary, the trousers to expose the lower limbs to above the knees. The patient takes a few steps while the examiner runs through a mental checklist, focusing attention on the hindfoot, midfoot, and forefoot successively: Do the feet toe in or toe out? Do the heels reach the ground for a heel-toe gait? Is there any varus or valgus deformity? Look especially for pronation of the midfoot, which may be more evident during ambulation than while the patient is standing still. In the forefoot, is there restricted rolling of the great toe or accentuation of hallux valgus? Do the toes make contact with the floor? Is there clawing of lesser toes during toe off? The patient is then directed to the examining table while the clinician turns his attention to the shoes the patient was wearing.

Scrutiny of Footwear. Look at the shoes carefully. Hugh Owen Thomas, who once expressed the hope that he would not be remembered merely as an inventor of splints, wrote in 1890, "there are three classes of feet—the excellent, the medium, and the bad. The first wear the outer side of the shoe heels more than the inner side; the medium wear the heels level; the bad ones wear down the inner edge and the posterior curve of the heels." Examine all components of the shoe (Fig 12–1).

A pronated flatfoot wears down the medial border of the sole more than the lateral. Toe deformities, such as hallux valgus and hammer toes, leave telltale marks on the vamp. Heel valgus and varus may distort the counter of the shoe.

Inspection of Feet. When pain is the chief complaint the patient is asked to point to the site of pain. Sometimes the site is so typical as to suggest a diagnosis (Fig 12–2). With the patient sitting on a chair at a convenient height, inspect the dangling foot and compare it with the opposite side. Look for obvious deformities that may suggest a congenital or acquired variation, fracture or sprain, or

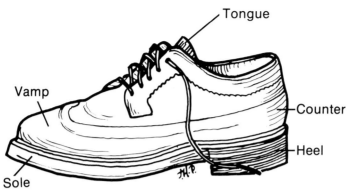

FIG 12–1. Parts of shoe to be examined: Look for heel and sole wear along the lateral and medial edges, obvious distortion of counter and stretched out areas in vamp.

one of the arthritides. The dorsum of the foot may show generalized swelling in inflammatory conditions. Localized soft tissue masses and bony overgrowths may be evident.

Look for obvious deformities of the toes and nails. The big toe may be directed laterally (hallux valgus), and may underride or override the second toe. The lesser toes may show flexion deformities at the distal interphalangeal joint (mallet toe), proximal interphalangeal joint (hammer toe), or at both interphalangeal joints with dorsal subluxation of metatarsophalangeal joint (claw toe). These deformities may result in corns over the dorsum or near the tips of the toes. Overlapping fifth toe, congenital curly toes, and small flail fourth or third toes due to a short metatarsal are fairly common anomalies. The clefts between the toes must be inspected for soft corns or fungus infection.

The patient is next instructed to curl and spread the toes and any limitation is noted. Active dorsiflexion and plantar flexion of the ankle and inversion and eversion of the foot are also tested. Pain and limitation of motion during these maneuvers can result from trauma or inflammation.

With the patient supine, the sole of the foot is inspected for areas of hyperkeratosis or skin breakdown. From a diagnostic standpoint, the sole maintains a log of the weight-bearing history of the foot. The anatomical location of callosities or ulcers is noted. Usual sites of such lesions are the metatarsal heads, the medial side of the big toe and tips of the lesser toes. The nonweight-bearing instep area may occasionally show nodules caused by plantar fibromatosis or rheumatoid disease. The heel area is carefully inspected for swelling or fullness in cases of painful heel conditions.

Applied Anatomy. For descriptive purposes the foot can be divided into three functional segments (Fig 12–3). The posterior segment contains the talus, which lies directly under the tibia and forms a part of the ankle joint, and the calcaneus, which is the hind part of the foot and rests on the ground.

The midfoot includes five tarsal bones: the navicular, the three cuneiform bones, and the cuboid. The forefoot is composed of five metatarsals and 14 phalangeal bones. The big toe has only two phalanges but normally projects the farthest in the foot, followed in sequence by the second to the fifth toes. On the other hand, the second metatarsal projects the longest followed by the third,

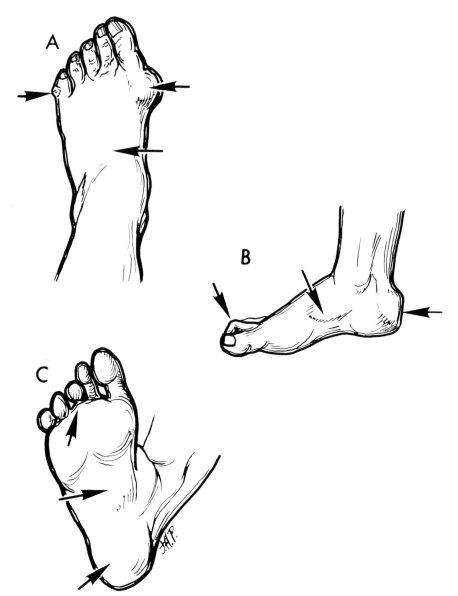

FIG 12–2. Typical sites of pain that suggest a diagnosis: arrows point to corn, bunion, and Sever's osteochondritis on the dorsum (**A**), hammer toe, accessory navicular and calcaneal bursitis in lateral view (**B**), and digital neuroma, chronic foot strain, and subcalcaneal bursitis on sole (**C**).

first, fourth, and fifth in that order. The articular surface over the metatarsal heads extends from the plantar to the dorsal aspects, allowing shallow articulations on the phalanges to glide into excessive dorsiflexion. This motion is essential to normal walking.

Proximally, the tarsometatarsal joints, collectively referred to as Lisfranc's joint, are an uneven border between the midfoot and the forefoot. The longest metatarsal, the second, articulates with the smallest cuneiform, the middle, which forms an indentation between the other two cuneiform bones. The second metatarsal can thus move only in dorsiflexion and plantar flexion. The articulation of the first metatarsal to the medial cuneiform, on the other hand, allows not only flexion and extension but also permits rotation through an arc around the second metatarsal. The third metatarsal articulates with the lateral cuneiform bone, and the fourth and fifth metatarsals with the cuboid. The three lateral metatarsals also possess the ability to rotate around the second, thus "cupping" the sole and increasing the transverse arch of the forefoot.

The anatomical concept of a transverse arch of the foot does not apply to the weight-bearing forefoot. In a normal foot, the five metatarsal heads can be seen

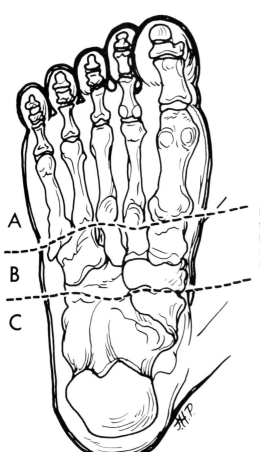

FIG 12–3. Functional segments of foot: forefoot (**A**), midfoot (**B**), and hindfoot (**C**). It is probably more accurate to refer to these as fore-, mid- and hind-parts of foot.

to lie in the same horizontal plane. However, in the midfoot, a rigid transverse arch is formed by the three cuneiforms and the cuboid, and is held together by strong interosseous ligaments. The middle cuneiform acts as the keystone to this arch. The three cuneiforms articulate with the tarsal navicular proximally, forming joints that allow the gliding motion necessary for adaptation to an uneven surface.

The midfoot articulates with the hindfoot through the so-called midtarsal or transverse tarsal joints, namely the talonavicular and the calcaneocuboid. These articulations, sometimes referred to as Chopart's joint, work together to allow rotation of the forefoot around the hindfoot. On the other hand, the talonavicular joint working with the subtalar joint makes the so-called peritalar articulation that permits rotation of the rest of the foot around a stationary talus. The "peritalar joint" is much more mobile than the "midtarsal joint."

The talus is the mechanical keystone at the apex of the foot, which sits astride the calcaneus. The two sides and the superior surface of the talus are "gripped" by the malleoli and the tibial plafond, thus forming the ankle joint. Dorsiflexion and plantar flexion of the ankle occur around a transverse axis through the talus. In dorsiflexion, the fibula glides upward and the ankle mortice "expands" slightly as the wider anterior portion of the body of the talus wedges between the malleoli.

Movements and Range of Motion

For the sake of simplicity, motions are tested along three different axes. Dorsiflexion and plantar flexion are movements at the ankle joint that occur around a transverse axis that passes through the body of the talus. Since the normal foot toes out about 16°, this motion occurs at an angle of 16° to the transverse axis of the body. Inversion and eversion are movements of rotation of the foot along its long axis. Generally, these movements are assigned to the subtalar joint, which forms an axis of about 42° to the ground. Abduction and adduction of the forefoot, occurring along a vertical axis, are movements of the midtarsal joints, but these cannot occur independently of the movements of eversion and inversion. Moreover, inversion usually occurs with plantar flexion and eversion with dorsiflexion of the ankle joint. Further confusion is added by improper use of the terms "pronation" and "supination" as substitutes for "eversion" and "inversion." It should be clearly understood that the terms "pronation" and "supination" refer to the weight-bearing foot, while the complex movements of eversion and inversion indicate changes in the form of the whole foot when it is not bearing weight. With these injunctions in mind, test and record the range of motion of different joints as described below.

Dorsiflexion and Plantar Flexion. To test the dorsiflexion and plantar flexion of the ankle joint, keep the foot in slight inversion and grasp the heel of the foot in the palm of one hand and the midfoot between the thumb and the fingers of the other hand (Fig 12–4). Neutral position for the ankle is the lateral border of the foot at 90° in relation to the leg, with knee in full extension. A normal ankle allows 20° of dorsiflexion and 40° of plantar flexion from this position. Measurements of ankle motion are made by centering the goniometer over the lateral malleolus. With the base of the goniometer lying along the long axis of tibia, readings are taken with the goniometer arm parallel to the sole in the hindfoot area.

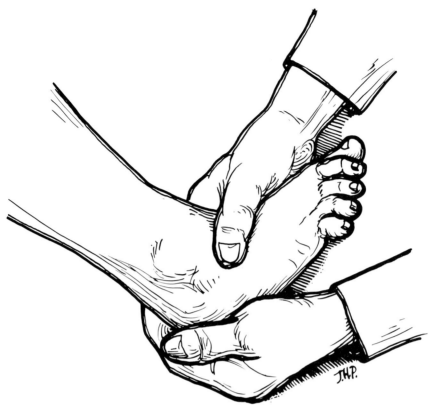

FIG 12–4. Examination for ankle motion: palm of one hand holds heel while other hand secures midfoot. Patient is asked to actively dorsiflex and plantar flex ankle while motions are being tested.

Repeat the measurements of dorsiflexion and plantar flexion with the knee held at 45° of flexion. If the arc of motion is different than the previous reading it indicates presence of heel cord tightness. For all practical purposes, movements of the ankle joint are considered limited to dorsiflexion and plantar flexion, but in some individuals with hypermobility of ankle joint, medial tilt of the talus can occur within the ankle mortice. This is the result of a congenital laxity of the lateral collateral ligaments and predisposes the patient to recurrent ankle sprains.

Inversion and Eversion. Inversion and eversion of the foot occur mainly at the subtalar joint and are tested with the patient supine. The ankle is first dorsiflexed to the neutral position; the calcaneus is then gripped in the palm of one hand while the other holds the midfoot over the top. The foot is then rocked into inversion and eversion while the patient is completely relaxed or actively assisting in the movement. A normal joint allows about 20° of eversion and about 30° of inversion. This movement cannot be accurately measured with a goniometer. Record the range as estimated by the arc described by the plantar surface of the foot as it turns medially (inversion) and laterally (eversion) (Fig 12–5).

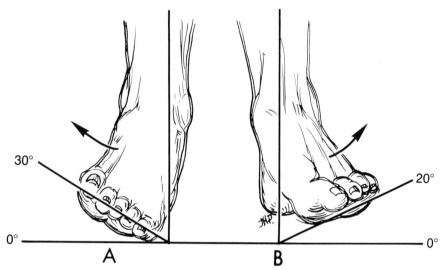

FIG 12–5. Subtalar motion in normal foot: inversion (**A**), and eversion can only be approximately judged during clinical examination (**B**).

Adduction and Abduction. Forefoot adduction and abduction occur mainly at the midtarsal joints and are tested passively. With the patient supine, hold the calcaneus in one hand and the forefoot in the other. Move the forefoot laterally and medially in relation to the calcaneus. Compare the range of motion to the opposite foot. This test is important in children with congenital forefoot deformities. Exact measurements are impossible and it is sufficient to record whether the movements appear normal, abnormally free, or restricted. The direction in which the movement is restricted should be recorded (Fig 12–6). The other tarsal joints allow little more than gliding motion, which is important for the foot to conform to uneven surfaces. This motion cannot be accurately recorded, but a note is made about suppleness or stiffness of the forefoot.

Metatarsophalangeal and Interphalangeal Motion. The other joints that allow significant motion in the forefoot are the metatarsophalangeal and interphalangeal joints. Of particular importance are the joints of the great toe. Place the patient's foot in neutral position, namely 45° flexion at the knee and the foot at 90° to the leg and record the dorsiflexion of the first metatarsophalangeal using a goniometer (Fig 12–7). This maneuver gives smaller values than if the goniometer base is placed along the first metatarsal shaft, but has the advantage of giving reproducible readings. Normal dorsiflexion of the great toe is approximately 50° when measured as described. Plantar flexion of the first metatarsophalangeal and interphalangeal joints of the big toe is measured by placing the goniometer on the dorsum and centering it over the appropriate joint. Normal flexion at these joints is approximately 30°.

Movements of the lesser toes can be similarly measured but clinically it is sufficient to note if there are fixed contractures or if the joints are supple. Restriction of joint motion can be the result of soft tissue contractures, bony abutment, or intra-articular adhesions. Motion may be restricted also due to pain resulting from inflammation or injuries.

Palpation

Successful clinical examination requires accurate knowledge of the anatomy of the region under consideration. The most constant and accurate landmarks are the palpable bony prominences, which lead to other related structures. It is essential to develop an approach that systematically palpates the important bony landmarks in a definite sequence so that no area is missed. Always examine the normal foot first before starting on the involved side.

Surface Anatomy. On the medial side of the foot and ankle look for the medial malleolus. The navicular tuberosity lies anterior to it and is the most prominent structure between the malleolus and the great toe. One can easily palpate the shaft and head of the first metatarsal and the two phalanges of the great toe. The sustentaculum tali lies just below and behind the medial malleolus. The tendo Achillis is easily recognized as is the extensor hallucis longus tendon by active

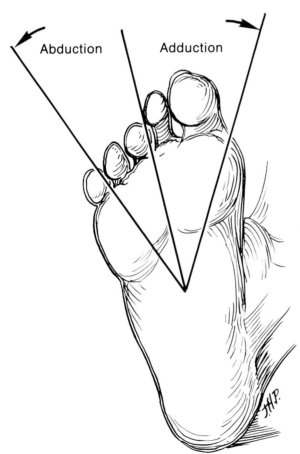

FIG 12–6. Forefoot motion in normal foot: Abduction and adduction of forefoot are tested while stabilizing midfoot. Neutral axis for forefoot and toes passes through second toe.

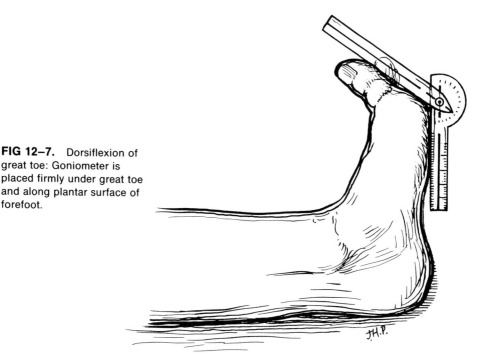

FIG 12–7. Dorsiflexion of great toe: Goniometer is placed firmly under great toe and along plantar surface of forefoot.

dorsiflexion of the great toe. Active inversion of the foot brings the anterior tibial tendon into relief. The posterior tibial tendon is palpable behind the medial malleolus. The flexor hallucis longus tendon covers the sustentaculum tali, which marks the level of the subtalar joint. The talonavicular joint lies just behind the navicular tuberosity. The ankle joint is palpable between the medial malleolus and the tibialis anterior tendon. The pulsations of the posterior tibial artery can be palpated about 2 cm behind the medial malleolus.

On the dorsum of the foot, the tendons of extensor digitorum longus are easily distinguishable. The dorsalis pedis artery can be palpated in the space between the first and the second metatarsals, lying between the tendons of extensor digitorum longus and extensor hallucis longus near the midfoot. The metatarsophalangeal and interphalangeal joints are easily palpated between the dorsal and plantar surfaces of the foot. The sesamoids of the great toe and the medial tubercle of the calcaneus can be palpated on the sole of the foot.

Along the lateral border of the foot, palpate the lateral malleolus. The depression just anterior to this is the sinus tarsi, an important landmark in surgical exposure of the foot. The bony prominence of the base of the fifth metatarsal is easily palpable. The shaft and head of the fifth metatarsal and the phalanges of the little toe can be followed from there. The tendons of the peroneal muscles can be thrown into relief just behind and below the lateral malleolus by active eversion of the foot. The belly of extensor digitorum brevis can be palpated near the base of the sinus tarsi on active dorsiflexion of the toes. The calcaneocuboid joint lies midway between the lateral malleolus and the base of the fifth metatarsal. The three bands of the lateral collateral ligament of the ankle can be palpated anterior, inferior, and posterior to the tip of the lateral malleolus. The anterior tibiofibular ligament lies between the lateral malleolus and the extensor digitorum longus tendons.

Palpation. With the patient lying supine, palpate the bony landmarks and the adjacent soft tissue structures in the sequence outlined above. The purpose of palpation is: (1) to relate areas of swelling or tumoral prominence to their anatomical location in the underlying bone or joint or overlying soft tissue; (2) to locate areas of tenderness and determine the involved structure; and (3) to reproduce the patient's symptoms by various diagnostic maneuvers, such as lateral compression to elicit pain in Morton's neuroma.

The patient is then asked to turn prone and the back of the heel, ankle, and calf are inspected and palpated. An important diagnostic maneuver performed with the patient prone is the Thompson "squeeze" test in cases of suspected tendo Achillis rupture.

The patient is asked to step off the examining table and walk over to stand facing a wall with feet about 6 in. apart. Instruct the patient to rise on the tiptoes. Normally, the patient stands with the foot toeing out slightly so that some of the lesser toes are visible on the lateral side of the ankle. The heels roll into slight varus and the longitudinal arch is accentuated on rising on the tiptoes.

The patient is then asked to turn around and with the patient standing, the forefoot is palpated. Tightness of the adductor hallucis muscle will cause pronation of the great toe and increase any obvious hallux valgus deformity in the upright posture. Attempt to correct any obvious deformities to assess if the soft tissues are supple enough to allow correction. Footprints or clinical photographs are then made, as indicated in an individual case. Roentgenograms form an integral part of the physical diagnosis for foot and ankle problems. Although details of roentgenograms are beyond the scope of this chapter, routine films required for the diagnosis of various foot and ankle problems will be mentioned where necessary.

The Child's Foot

An examination of the child's foot is quite different from that of an adult, and is discussed in detail in Chapter 2. A few basic concepts are repeated here for the sake of clarity. Children usually present with deformities of the foot and ankle region that vary in severity from grotesque changes to mere suspicions in the parents' minds. The clinician is called on, more often than not, merely to decide that the problem is inconsequential. Severe cases of congenital clubfoot or congenital vertical talus are evident in infancy. Milder cases of torsional deformities or flexible flatfeet may be seen only after the child has started walking.

Talipes or Clubfoot. The word talipes derived from Latin talus (meaning ankle) and pes (meaning foot) was originally coined to describe a deformity that makes a person walk on the ankle. It now stands for any variety of clubfoot and is the conventional prefix to descriptive terms that indicate the position of the foot. These terms are: (1) equinus, meaning plantar flexion; (2) calcaneus, meaning dorsiflexion; (3) varus, meaning inversion; (4) valgus, meaning eversion; and (5) cavus, meaning high arched instep. A combination of two or more of these terms after the prefix talipes indicates the deformity observed in an individual case.

Having described the deformity, the clinician has to decide whether the deformity of the child's foot is: (1) postural, due to a cramped intrauterine position; (2) congenital, due to a primary defect in the cartilage analge of the skeleton; or (3) acquired, due to the effects of a paralytic neuromuscular disorder such as myelomeningocele, diastematomyelia, or polio. On physical examination, the postural deformities are usually mild, flexible, and easily corrected by manipulation. On the other hand, congenital talipes usually gives marked, rigid deformities with abnormal skin creases, changed bony relationships, and small heel and calf size. To complete the diagnosis of talipes, it is essential to look for other congenital defects. The mouth should be inspected for cleft palate; the hips examined for congenital dysplasia; and the lumbosacral region scrutinized for indications of spina bifida occulta. In older children, the strength of various muscle groups around the ankle is tested. In an infant, simply observing active motion must suffice. Intrinsic power of the toes is tested by pressing upwards on the proximal phalanges of the toes and feeling the resistance. Weakness of intrinsic muscles of the foot may be the first sign of a neurologic deficit at S1–S2 level.

Torsional Deformities. Rotational variations involving the lower extremities result in an in-toeing or out-toeing gait and are a frequent source of concern to the child's parents. In a vast majority of cases these changes are postural, resulting from intrauterine position, and resolve spontaneously during infancy. Nevertheless, it is important for the clinician to distinguish between "rotational variations" within the wide range of normal and the unusual "torsional deformities" that fall outside the normal range.

After an initial inspection of the gait pattern, a child with a rotational problem is best examined when lying prone on the table. The three limb segments, namely the thigh, the leg, and the foot, are evaluated separately. Femoral torsion is judged from the rotation at the hip joint. With the pelvis fixed flat, the knees are flexed to 90°, and the thighs are rotated to the angle that is maintained by gravity alone. Internal and external rotation at the hips is thus measured. With the knee still flexed, the hips and ankles are fixed in neutral, and the angle between the long axis of the thigh and the long axis of the foot is noted. This relationship shows the presence of any torsional variation in the tibia. Forefoot deformities that affect the rotational profile can also be observed with the child prone and the knee flexed to 90°. The long axis of the foot bisecting the heel should pass through the space between the second and third toes.

In infancy, the rotation profile of the lower extremities shows the influence of intrauterine position in which hips are flexed and externally rotated (hence greater lateral than medial rotation at the hips), and in which the legs and feet are kept internally rotated (hence medial rotation of tibia and sometimes metatarsus adductus). These changes resolve spontaneously during childhood. The forefoot adduction resolves during the second year of life, and the medial tibial torsion resolves in early childhood; the femoral anteversion diminishes during late childhood so that the lateral rotation at the hips decreases. This normal remodeling should be anticipated when treating children with torsional deformities of the lower extremity.

Pes Planus or Flatfoot. "Flatfoot" is a term commonly used loosely to describe a condition in which the longitudinal arch is low or absent. The more esoteric term "pes planus" carries no greater descriptive value. Therefore, it is highly desirable to have the ablity to further qualify the word "pes planus" with adjectives that explain the underlying pathology (Table 12–1). The integrity of the longitudinal arch of the foot is dependent on the configuration of the tarsal bones and the

TABLE 12–1.

Classification of Pes Planus

Rigid
    Congenital vertical talus
    Tarsal coalition
Flexible
    Idiopathic ligamentous laxity
    Talipes calcaneovalgus
    Triceps surae contracture
Acquired
    Myelodysplasia or polio
    Cerebral palsy
    Muscular dystrophy
    Peripheral nerve injury
    Tibialis posterior insufficiency
    Ehlers-Danlos syndrome
    Down's syndrome

strength of the ligaments that bind them together. In a child the pes planus deformity may be: (1) rigid, when it is the result of bony involvement (tarsal coalition) or joint dislocation (congenital vertical talus); (2) flexible, when it results from excessive laxity of ligaments supporting the longitudinal arch; and (3) acquired, when the underlying pathology is muscle weakness and imbalance, tendinous contracture, or generalized abnormality of collagen such as Ehlers-Danlos, Marfan's, or Down's syndrome.

Examination for pes planus is best conducted with the child standing. By making prints of the weight-bearing foot, three degrees of severity are recognized: (1) mild or first degree, in which the longitudinal arch, although depressed, is still visible; (2) moderate or second degree, when the longitudinal arch is completely absent; and (3) severe or third degree, where the longitudinal arch is absent and medial border of the foot is convex because weight is borne on the subluxated head of talus presenting below and anterior to the medial malleolus.

The next step in examination is to decide if the flattening of the longitudinal arch is present constantly (rigid flatfoot) or if the foot assumes an arch when nonweight-bearing (flexible flatfoot). The patient is asked to walk with the back toward the examiner and to rise on the tiptoes so that the calf muscles can be evaluated. Then, facing the clinician, the patient stands on the back of the heel so the tibialis anterior can be evaluated. Last, the patient rolls the feet into pronation and supination to allow observation of subtalar motion. With the patient still standing, the big toe is pushed into dorsiflexion by the examiner. If the longitudinal arch forms during this maneuver, it indicates a sag at the naviculocuneiform joint. The arch is not restored in cases of talonavicular sag. This test is not reliable in cases of contracture of the tendo Achillis.

The foot is next examined with the patient reclining. Note to see if the arch forms during nonweight-bearing and measure the range of motion in different directions. Dorsiflexion is limited by a tight tendo Achillis, a not too infrequent cause of acquired flexible flatfoot. Plantar flexion is sometimes limited because of a short tibialis anterior tendon, which is an occasional cause of acquired flexible flatfoot. Inversion alone is limited in spastic flatfoot because of tarsal coalition and spasm of peroneal muscles. Eversion is free in a flexible flatfoot but a rigid everted flatfoot allows very little further eversion.

Pes Cavus. A high-arched foot is usually an acquired deformity, but idiopathic cases in which no neurologic deficit is evident are sometimes seen. Examine the foot carefully to determine if the cavus is due to plantar flexed metatarsals and forefoot equinus (i.e., cavus); elevation of the midfoot with hindfoot varus (i.e., cavovarus); or due to calcaneus of the heel, with compensatory forefoot plantar flexion (i.e., calcaneocavus). Details of neurologic conditions involving the foot are discussed later in this chapter.

Localized Conditions

The Great Toe

Deformities of the great toe can be completely symptom-free or they can occasion great distress. These include: (1) Hallux valgus or lateral deviation of the great toe at the metatarsophalangeal joint with a medial prominence. The commonly used term "bunion" is synonymous with this deformity, which is the most common cause of pain in the great toe in women. (2) Hallux rigidus or limitation of motion at the first metatarsophalangeal joint usually presents with painful "dorsal bunion" or exostosis over the first metatarsal head. It is a common cause of pain in the great toe, particularly in men. (3) Hallux varus or medial deviation of the great toe is usually iatrogenic.

Hallux Valgus. Most commonly seen in middle-aged women, hallux valgus is usually bilateral. As an acquired condition, hallux valgus has been attributed to the forcing of a wide forefoot into a pointed shoe with high heels; it may also be hereditary or it can be congenital. The congenital variety may result from varus of the first metatarsal due to an abnormal medial obliquity of the first cuneiform-metatarsal joint. The great toe then goes into valgus and rotates into pronation so that its plantar aspect looks laterally. These patients seldom have associated second toe deformity. Even in acquired hallux valgus certain predisposing causes can be present. These may include one or more of the following: (1) residual metatarsus primus varus; (2) abnormally long great toe; or (3) unusual convexity of the first metatarsal head. When such a foot is forced into pointed shoes, the great toe moves into valgus, and secondary muscle imbalance develops over several years. The adductor hallucis becomes tight, pulling the great toe into further valgus. The sesamoids shift into the space between first and second metatarsals, the long flexor and extensor tendons shift lateral to the long axis of the great toe and progressive deformity becomes established.

The term "bunion" in common use refers to the medial prominence at the level of the first metatarsophalangeal joint. This deformity is the result of three components: (1) valgus angulation of the great toe at the metatarsophalangeal joint; (2) enlargement of medial portion of the first metatarsal head by bone apposition; and (3) development of a bursa over this medial bony prominence. Asymptomatic hallux valgus is frequently seen on routine examination of the feet for other conditions. In progressive cases, pain eventually develops because of one or more of the following causes: (1) local irritation, redness, and bursitis over the medial bony prominence caused by tight shoe wear; (2) an associated hammer toe deformity; and (3) generalized metatarsalgia due to wide splaying of the forefoot. The underlying cause of pain must be sought during clinical examination.

With the patient standing, inspect the feet for pes planus or heel valgus. In the forefoot, note the severity of hallux valgus, which can be subjectively described as mild when there is medial prominence but only minimal lateral deviation; moderate when there is significant lateral deviation with medial prominence; and severe when the lateral deviation is severe enough to overlap or underlap the second toe or cause hammer toe deformity (Fig 12–8). In some instances, the lateral deviation of the great toe may be distal to the metatarsophalangeal joint (hallux valgus interphalangeus). As the patient takes a few steps, look for exaggeration of toe pronation and note if the second toe reaches the floor. Ask the patient to spread the toes actively and note the competence of abductor hallucis. Now try to passively move the great toe into alignment with first metatarsal. This tests for tightness of the adductor hallucis muscle. When you repeat this maneuver with the patient supine, it will distinguish adductor tightness from contracture of the medial joint capsule. If the contracture of the first metatarsophalangeal joint is the limiting factor, the great toe cannot be brought into alignment even with the patient seated.

With the patient resting, look for plantar callosities and dorsal corns. Usual sites for hyperkeratosis in cases of hallux valgus are medial side of the great toe, the lateral border of the fifth metatarsal head, and the second and third metatarsal heads. In advanced cases of hallux valgus, the weight-bearing is shifted to the second metatarsal, and callosities form under the metatarsal head—especially if there is associated hammer toe deformity of the second toe. Ask the patient to move the great toe and see the extensor hallucis longus come into prominence;

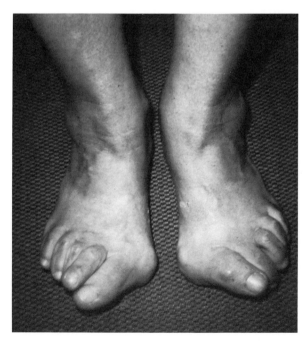

FIG 12–8. Severe bilateral hallux valgus.

note its relation to the long axis of the first metatarsal and the great toe. Despite significant deformity, the metatarsophalangeal joint usually has a good range of motion. Measure and record the dorsiflexion obtained.

Palpate the foot for localized tenderness over the medial prominence, under the metatarsal heads and on squeezing the forefoot. Palpate the second toe in cases of hammer toe to see if the deformity is flexible or rigid. Feel the dorsalis pedis and posterior tibial arteries before sending the patient for a roentgenogram. It is necessary to obtain standing anteroposterior, lateral, and oblique views of the foot, and sometimes axial views of the sesamoids.

Hallux Rigidus. This term literally means a rigid great toe and is a localized arthritic process involving the first metatarsophalangeal joint caused by trauma. The condition can sometimes be traced to a single specific episode of trauma; however, in most cases, the etiology is repeated episodes of mild trauma, such as stubbing of an overly long great toe in shoes that are too short. A flat or beaked first metatarsal head may be a contributing factor to this pathology. Secondary hallux rigidus may result from rheumatoid arthritis, gout, or other metabolic conditions. Decreased motion of the great toe interferes with the normal gait pattern. Each step normally requires dorsiflexion of the great toe, which is limited and painful in hallux rigidus. In extreme cases, all movements of the first metatarsophalangeal joint are abolished and the great toe may become relatively painless. The patient may then actually complain of pain elsewhere in the foot as weight-bearing is shifted to the lateral side. The foot is kept adducted and inverted to roll off the fifth metatarsal head. This may lead to pressure symptoms under the fifth metatarsal head.

In the more common, less-advanced cases, the patient, usually a young adult male, presents with pain in the great toe. Occasionally the condition is bilateral. On inspection, the great toe is straight, not in valgus. The metatarsophalangeal joint is enlarged and swollen circumferentially. Ambulation is usually painful. When seated, ask the patient to flex and extend the toe actively: only the interphalangeal joint of the great toe moves while the metatarsophalangeal motion is restricted. Passive dorsiflexion of the great toe is painful. Record the range. The interphalangeal joint may show hypermobility especially in dorsiflexion as a compensatory phenomenon. Palpate the metatarsophalangeal joint; irregular osteophytes can be palpated especially on the dorsal medial aspect of the first metatarsal head (hence the term "dorsal bunion"). Look for calluses along the medial side of the great toe and under the fifth metatarsal head. Roentgenograms should be obtained in three views to demonstrate the osteophytes and rule out other arthritic processes.

Hallux Varus. This is a medial deviation of the great toe that may be congenital, but in the majority of cases is the result of an overzealous correction of hallux valgus. The congenital variety is believed to result, at least in part, from an anatomical variation in the insertion of the abductor hallucis tendon. Congenital hallux varus may be the primary deformity or it may exist in conjunction with clubfeet, polydactyly, or supernumerary metatarsals. The more common iatrogenic variety (Fig 12–9) is a dreaded complication of McBride's bunionectomy in which the adductor hallucis has been released and the fibular sesamoid excised, thus weakening the flexor brevis. The resulting muscle imbalance pulls the great toe medially, hyperextends the metatarsophalangeal, and flexes the interphalangeal joints. This deformity is not only cosmetically unpleasant but also may be quite painful and disabling.

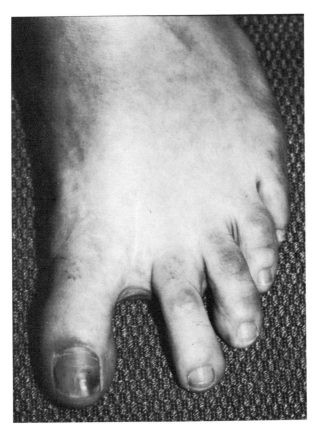

FIG 12–9. Iatrogenic hallux varus resulting from adductor hallucis tenotomy and removal of fibular sesamoid during a bunionectomy.

The Lesser Toes

Deformities of the lesser toes may be congenital or acquired. Usually associated with great toe problems, they can occur as individual unrelated problems. The second toe is most commonly affected by acquired postural conditions, especially when it is the longest digit in the foot. The little toe appears to be undergoing phylogenetic retrogression. Frequently, it has only two phalanges due to the absence of middle phalanx. It is a common site for congenital malformations.

Hammer Toe. This is a flexion deformity of the proximal interphalangeal joint with extension at the metatarsophalangeal articulation. When the toe is deformed, the head of the proximal phalanx is subjected to intermittent pressure from the shoe. A corn, and in some instances a bursa, may develop over the proximal interphalangeal joint. If the deformity is severe enough to produce a subluxation of the metatarsophalangeal joint, pressure transmitted through the plantarly displaced metatarsal head can cause a painful callus.

Hammer toe deformities can cause marked pain. The second toe is most frequently involved, especially in association with hallux valgus. These cases are usually bilateral although one side may be more severely affected than the other. The diagnosis is obvious on inspection. Try to passively straighten the toe to see if the deformity is flexible or fixed.

Mallet Toe. It is a flexion deformity involving the distal interphalangeal joint, which can cause a painful corn at the tip of the toe. In some cases the end corn will be obvious while the toe is straight. These patients have a dynamic contracture that becomes apparent when the patient takes a few steps. The mallet toe deformity most frequently involves the fourth toe.

Claw Toes. Hyperextension of the metatarsophalangeal joints with flexion at both interphalangeal joints indicates weakness of the intrinsic muscles of the foot. Sometimes the deformity may involve only one foot. If bilateral or associated with cavus of the hindfoot, neurologic evaluation is necessary to rule out neuropathic causes.

The deformity causes symptoms because of difficulty in shoe fitting. Evaluate the flexibility of toes by finger pressure under the second and third metatarsal heads, while the knee is kept in 90° flexion. Nearly complete extension of the toes should occur if the deformity is flexible.

Overlapping Fifth Toe. This is a common congenital anomaly with a strong familial tendency. The fifth metatarsophalangeal joint is held in a position of extension, adduction, and external rotation due to a contracture of the dorsal joint capsule and shortening of the long extensor tendon. Patients may complain of pain on the dorsum of the toe due to shoe pressure. Despite subluxation, the metatarsophalangeal joint is seldom painful.

Bunionette. When there is a wide angulation between the fourth and fifth metatarsals, medial angulation (not overlapping) of the little toe can cause the fifth metatarsal head to become prominent laterally. Intermittent pressure from the shoe will cause local hyperkeratosis or an adventitious bursa may develop.

The Toenails

Because they are appendages of the skin, besides local causes, nails can be affected by dermatologic disorders and constitutional conditions with skin manifestations. On close inspection nails may show: (1) onycholysis or separation of the free edge of the nail from the nail bed, which results in accumulation of debris under the nails. This can result from generalized endocrine disorders, collagen diseases, and mycotic infections of the nails; (2) onychodystrophy or poor nutrition of the nails, which causes ill-defined stippling, pitting, fraying, and ridging of the nails. This can result from systemic collagen diseases such as psoriasis, circulatory or trophic disorders in the extremity, and mycotic infections of the nails; and (3) onychauxis or thickening of the nail due to piling up of irregular layers of keratin on the nails and nail beds. This can result from local causes such as trauma or pressure from shoes, poor hygiene, and mycotic infections of the nails. Thus, the three different types of nail lesions can all be the result of fungal infections of the nails themselves. Therefore, scrapings of the nail should be taken for microscopic examination and fungal culture before deciding on treatment. Deformities of the nails that lead to local pressure and problems with shoe fitting may present difficult surgical challenges.

Onychogryphosis. This describes a massive overgrowth and hypertrophy of the nail, which actually folds over the tip of the toe in a claw-shaped manner (Fig 12–10). Picturesquely described as ram's horn nails, these seem to be the result of repeated local trauma, poor hygiene, and a congenital tendency. Mycotic infection does not seem to play any part in the development of these deformities.

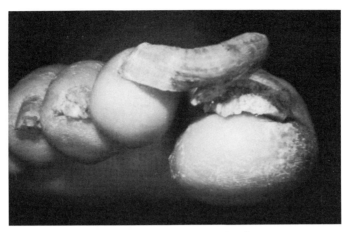

FIG 12–10. Onychogryphosis.

Ingrowing Toenail (Onychocryptosis). This is a misleading term that seems to imply that the side of the toenail grows into the nail fold, whereas the true pathology is a "hypertrophy of the ungualabia." The process is probably first invoked by cutting off the corners of the nail at an angle instead of straight across the free edge of the nail. As the nail grows, and the nail fold is pushed over the sharp edge of the nail by pressure from the shoe, it lacerates the nail fold. Chronic infection then establishes in the pocket thus formed causing purulent discharge or excrescences of granulation tissue. The course of this painful condition is punctuated by attacks of acute paronychia. Each attack leaves the nail fold with progressively greater hypertrophy.

On examination, the lesion is nearly always situated along the lateral edge of the big toenail. It is extremely tender on palpation during an acute exacerbation. Inspect the nail closely at the edges. Three types of ingrown toenails may be seen: (1) nails with a normal nail plate but with badly trimmed edges forming fish hooks that dig into the nail fold; (2) nails with a normal nail plate but with hypertrophied nail folds growing over the edges of the nails; and (3) nails with incurvated edges and distortion of the nail plate. This may be the result of bone spurs on the distal phalanx or thickening of the nail bed due to mycotic infections. Roentgenograms are required to rule out bony pathology.

Subungual Exostosis. This is a benign bony outgrowth from the dorsal surface of the distal phalanx, which is practically always confined to the great toe. This condition is not related to conventional exostoses (i.e., osteochondromas) but has been variously attributed to trauma, chronic infection, or an attempt on the part of the great toe to form another digit. The outgrowth usually presents itself along the medial half of the distal part of the big toenail (Fig. 12–11). Initially, it pushes the nail from its bed, causing discoloration and longitudinal splintering of the nail in several places. Later, the exostosis forces its way through the nail and reaches the surface covered by a mass of granulation tissue.

The condition is symptomless unless it is traumatized and becomes infected. In early stages, subungual exostosis may be mistaken for mycotic infection of the nail. In later stages, when ulceration occurs, it may be confused with an ingrown

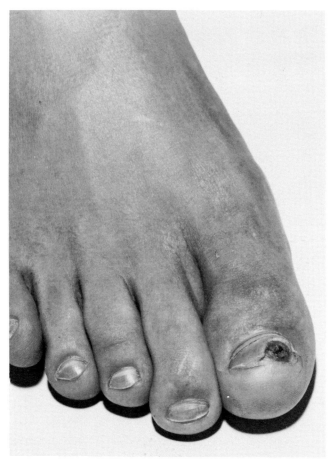

FIG 12–11. Subungual exostosis typically appearing from under the medial side of distal half of great toenail.

toenail. Examined carefully, an ingrown toenail usually involves the lateral half of the nail and is associated with hypertrophy of the nail fold. Occasional hyperpigmentation may necessitate differential diagnosis from melanoma of the nail bed. In any event, a lateral radiograph of the toe clinches the diagnosis of subungual exostosis.

The Forefoot

Metatarsalgia is a symptom that indicates pain in the forefoot, usually in the region of metatarsal heads on the plantar surface, which results from abnormal weight-bearing mechanics in the forefoot. The definition is somewhat imprecise and the term "metatarsalgia" is sometimes applied loosely to any painful condition in the forefoot. It is essential, therefore, to distinguish (1) primary metatarsalgia: due to a chronic disorder of weight-bearing in the forefoot; (2) secondary metatarsalgia: due to traumatic, inflammatory or neurogenic disorders involving the forefoot secondarily; and (3) other causes of forefoot pain such as Morton's neuroma, occasionally called Morton's metatarsalgia. All these conditions should be considered in differential diagnosis but the term metatarsalgia should probably be reserved for chronic disorders of weight-bearing across the metatarsophalangeal articulations.

Metatarsalgia usually presents as an aching pain in the plantar aspect of the forefoot. The patient frequently describes a sensation of "walking with a pebble in the shoe." Ask the patient to point to the area of greatest discomfort with a pencil rather than the finger. Look for the presence of a secondary callosity in the area. Localize the areas of tenderness by digital palpation. Next squeeze the forefoot, exerting transverse pressure on the metatarsal heads, and note if this causes pain. Repeat the maneuver, this time pushing up on the metatarsal heads to enhance the transverse arch and note if this maneuver relieves pain. Occasionally, the information may be volunteered that the patient uses this manipulation to obtain relief. Consider the various causes listed in Table 12–2 and work out the diagnosis repeating diagnostic maneuvers and collecting further information about the underlying pathology as the circumstances warrant.

Primary Metatarsalgia. This is most commonly seen in middle-aged individuals after weight gain caused by a sedentary life-style. The intrinsic muscles of the foot lose their tone and the transverse arch flattens. The patient has a splay foot and callosities develop under one or more metatarsal heads. Tenderness is noted under several metatarsal heads and pain is relieved by raising the transverse arch. Footprints should be obtained to localize areas of increased pressure under the metatarsal heads. Patients with hallux valgus or hallux rigidus frequently show increased pressure under the second metatarsal due to transfer of weight-bearing as the first metatarsophalangeal joint is deformed. Inadequate surgical procedures on the forefoot are another common cause of primary metatarsalgia.

Morton's syndrome consists of a congenitally short, hypermobile first metatarsal, proximal displacement of the sesamoids, and thickening of the second metatarsal shaft due to transfer of weight to the second ray. Calluses develop under the second and third metatarsal heads. Initially asymptomatic, the condition may become painful in later life when tenderness can be elicited at the base of the first

TABLE 12–2.

Causes of Metatarsalgia

Primary metatarsalgia
   Statis disorders of forefoot
   Iatrogenic after forefoot surgery
   Hallux valgus or rigidus
   Freiberg's disease
Secondary metatarsalgia
   Stress fracture of metatarsal bone
   Sesamoid pathology
   Rheumatoid arthritis
   Neurogenic disorders
Other forefoot pain
   Morton's metatarsalgia
   Tarsal tunnel syndrome
   Plantar warts
   Plantar fibromatosis

---

two metatarsals and the head of the second. Morton's syndrome in its full-blown form is probably very rare.

Freiberg's disease, which leads to deformity of the second metatarsal head and stiffness of the metatarsophalangeal joint, is another cause of primary metatarsalgia. The third metatarsal head may be occasionally involved. The condition starts as an osteochondritis dissecans in the metatarsal head and is initially quite painful. At that stage, there is edema over the dorsum of the involved bone. There is extreme tenderness on both dorsal and plantar palpation of the metatarsal head. As inflammation subsides the joint stiffens, tenderness decreases, and a bony lump becomes palpable.

Secondary Metatarsalgia. Although these patients give a typical history of metatarsalgia, have evidence of abnormal weight-bearing under a metatarsal head on footprint analysis, and exhibit secondary callosities with metatarsophalangeal joint pain that can be seen on clinical examination, the cause of their metatarsophalangeal imbalance lies at a site other than the forefoot joints themselves. Carefully look for causes listed in Table 12–2.

Stress fracture of a metatarsal bone should always be kept in mind when dealing with painful conditions of the forefoot. Usually it is an undisplaced fracture of the second or third metatarsal shaft in the distal third. The condition frequently presents as pain in the forefoot after a long march, and is therefore also known as a march fracture. However, it can occur in civilian life in individuals whose duties entail long periods of standing. In these cases, onset is often undramatic. There is no history of violent trauma. A cramplike pain is felt when the shoe is removed and edema is noted over the dorsum of the involved metatarsal. Movements of the toe corresponding to the metatarsal are painful. Palpate the shaft of the metatarsal along the dorsal surface and a point tenderness will be noted over the lesion. Roentgenograms are not necessary to make the diagnosis in an army recruit; however, in civilian cases, fracture is seldom suspected until periosteal reaction develops.

Morton's Metatarsalgia. Forefoot pain can result from many causes unrelated to imbalance in weight-bearing between the metatarsals and the toes. The term "metatarsalgia" should be avoided for such conditions; however, the eponym Morton's metatarsalgia is deeply entrenched in orthopedic literature. It refers to a fusiform fibrous thickening of the interdigital nerve between the third and fourth metatarsals, due to intermittent pressure from the metatarsal heads. Occasionally, the nerve between the second and third metatarsals may be so affected. The "neuroma" is usually located in the area where the nerve divides into its two contiguous digital branches. Common in middle-aged women, the neuritic pain radiates from the area near the metatarsal heads into the toes. The typical history is of pain during weight-bearing, which is relieved by rest. Characteristically, the desire to remove the shoes and massage the foot is more intense than mere need for relief from weight-bearing. Compression of metatarsal heads together causes pain. On digital palpation, tenderness is present between the metatarsal heads, whereas in cases without neuroma, tenderness is over the metatarsal heads. A large neuroma may occasionally be palpable.

The Dorsum of the Foot

The midfoot area, consisting of the tarsal bones excluding the talus and the calcaneus, is readily accessible to examination from the dorsal and the medial aspects. Swelling and pain in the midfoot area should bring to mind generalized conditions such as diabetes and chronic infections such as tuberculosis, but certain local conditions must be considered.

Ganglion of the Foot. This nearly always arises on the dorsolateral aspect of the foot in relation to an extensor tendon or one of the tarsal joints. Usually symptomless, it can cause difficulties with shoe wear or cause pain due to pressure. The diagnosis is obvious in most cases and should be confirmed by aspiration of clear gelatinous fluid under local anesthesia. A well-developed belly of the extensor digitorum brevis has occasionally been mistaken for a pathologic swelling. On the dorsomedial side, exostoses along the naviculo-cuneiform and cuneiform-metatarsal joints are frequently seen. These are hard bony swellings and the overlying tibialis anterior tendon sheath may be thickened. Symptoms result from shoe pressure. Oblique views of the foot will show the exostosis.

Accessory Navicular. Os tibialae externum is a common accessory bone in the foot (Fig 12–12). Located medially near the tuberosity of the navicular, it may

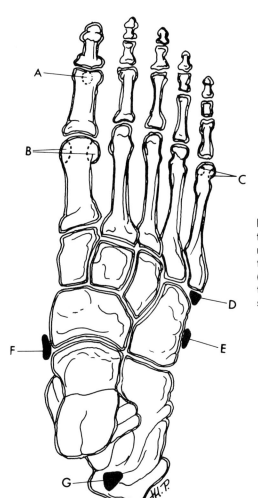

FIG 12–12. Common accessory bones of foot: interphalangeal accessory (*A*), sesamoids of great toe (*B*), sesamoids under fifth metatarsal head (*C*), os vesalianum (*D*), os peroneum in peroneus longus tendon (*E*), os tibiale externum or accessory navicular (*F*), and os trigonum (*G*).

sometimes be difficult to delineate as a separate structure. Symptomless in the majority, it may be the source of pain caused by shoe pressure in active adolescents. On inspection, the medial prominence gives the foot a pronated appearance. Accessory navicular can result in abnormal insertion of the tibialis posterior tendon and flatfeet in some cases. Weight-bearing lateral views of the foot should therefore be obtained to study the longitudinal arch when accessory navicular is noted.

Kohler's Disease. This is also known as osteochondritis of the navicular bone and is a rare condition affecting children between ages 4 and 8 years. Without history of preceding trauma, the patient starts limping and complains of vague pain over the dorsomedial aspect of the midfoot. On inspection, the child tends to bear weight on the lateral side of the foot. Inversion of the foot is limited due to pain. On palpation, tenderness can be localized over the navicular bone. Soft tissue swelling may or may not be present. Roentgenograms of the foot show characteristic pathology.

The Sole of the Foot

The skin of the sole of the foot carries a log of the weight-bearing history of the foot. A thickening of the skin or hyperkeratosis develops as a protective measure in areas of intermittent pressure on the plantar surface of the foot. A certain amount of callus formation is, therefore, normal in active individuals. Such callosity is diffuse, and the cornified skin blends into the normal skin at the periphery of the lesion. Usual sites for asymptomatic callus formation are beneath the forefoot area, around the heel, and along the inferomedial border of the great toe (pinch callus).

Plantar Callosities. When callus formation is localized underneath a single metatarsal head and becomes symptomatic it is referred to as an intractable plantar keratosis. Development of such lesions is preceded by abnormal weight-bearing because of forefoot deformities (such as hallux valgus and hammer toes), bony abnormalities (such as prominent condyles of metatarsal heads and enlarged tibial sesamoid), or faulty footwear. When examining a keratotic lesion on the plantar surface, carefully pare down the callus and examine the deeper layers. Plantar callosities show normal skin lines running throughout the deeper layers. If paring reveals a translucent area with small vessels that lie parallel (and not vertical) to the surface, you are dealing with a neurovascular corn that can be extremely painful. On the other hand, removal of keratotic skin from a wart will reveal distinct margins and a central mottled area with tips of vertically running capillaries that bleed readily. Small metal markers are taped to the areas of callus formation before obtaining roentgenograms to study the relationship to bony structures.

Plantar Warts. These are simple papillomas produced by an unidentified virus. Common in young adults, especially swimmers, warts are not confined to weight-bearing areas of the plantar surface. Three different types of lesions can be identified: (1) The solitary wart appears initially as a dark, sharply defined lesion in the skin. If it is present in a weight-bearing part it will soon get covered by keratotic skin and look like a plantar callosity. Palpate for tenderness by squeezing the lesion from side to side and by pressing it against the underlying bone. Warts are painful when squeezed from side to side, while callosities are more painful when pressed against underlying bone. Paring down of the keratotic skin will reveal the characteristic mottled lesion of a wart, that will bleed profusely on deeper probing. (2) The mother and daughter warts form characteristic constellations (Fig. 12–13). (3) The mosaic wart is formed by a tightly packed crop of warts which may form a large irregular granular lesion. The individual warts in this lesion show the characteristics of a solitary wart.

Corns.　As opposed to callosities, corns occur chiefly in areas where skin is normally thin on the dorsum of the foot. They result from more localized pressure over a bony prominence and rarely occur in a normal foot. Corns consist of a conical wedge of highly compressed keratotic tissue. The apex of the cone points to the underlying bony prominence and impinges on the nerve endings in the skin causing pain. Pare away the superficial layers of the lesions and a central hard core will be uncovered that can be removed and that leaves a concave surface with a narrow area of hyperkeratosis around it. When a corn occurs in a web space, it becomes macerated because of moisture or sweat, and is then called a soft corn. The keratotic skin looks whitish due to maceration. Such corns are common in the fifth web space where distal end of the proximal phalanx of the fifth toe impinges against the flare of the base of the proximal phalanx of the fourth toe.

Perforating or Neuropathic Ulcers.　Ulceration of the plantar skin occurs most commonly over the metatarsal heads in conditions that lead to loss of sensation

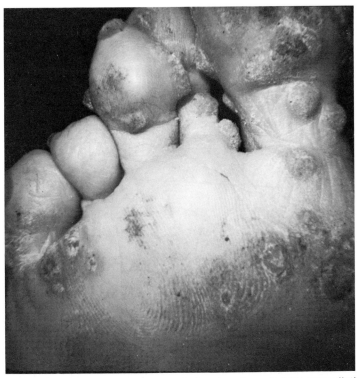

FIG 12–13.　Mother and daughter warts forming characteristic constellations.

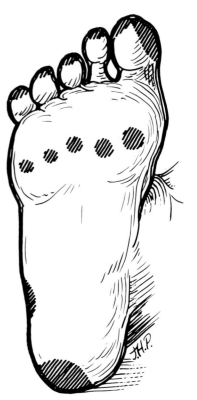

FIG 12–14. Common sites of neuropathic ulcers under foot.

in the foot. Peripheral neuropathy caused by diabetes accounts for more than half of these, followed by myelodysplasia and nerve injuries. Ulcers located over the metatarsal heads are usually covered by thick callosities that should be pared down to study the extent of the lesion. Other frequent sites of neuropathic ulcers are shown in Figure 12–14. A bounding pedal pulse will distinguish perforating ulcers of the toes from a pregangrenous condition due to ischaemia. Roentgenograms of the foot are obtained in three views to rule out osteomyelitis.

The Instep

Pain in the region of the instep is a common complaint in adults. The pain is usually bilateral, resulting mostly from the strain of excessive weight-bearing in pronated or flatfeet. Unilateral cases may be the result of injuries to the posterior tibial tendon or conditions affecting the plantar fascia.

Chronic Foot Strain. Mechanical strain on the longitudinal arch of the foot results in pain in the instep area in the adult. It may be the result of: (1) abnormal stress on a structurally normal foot; (2) normal stress on a structurally normal foot that is not accustomed to such a stress; or (3) normal stress on a structurally abnormal foot. Foot strain may be acute or chronic. Acute foot strain in a normal foot is a self-limited condition and seldom presents a clinical problem. On the other hand, chronic foot strain in a pronated flatfoot creates persistent foot pain at first, due to microscopic tears in the stretched ligaments; later, due to inflammation of stretched joint capsules because ligamentous support is lost; and finally, due to breakdown of articular cartilage, resulting in osteoarthritis.

A patient with foot strain usually complains of an aching pain in the sole of the foot, in the calf and occasionally in the anterior part of the leg at the end of a long day. The discomfort is not immediately relieved by rest. A weekend athlete suffering from acute foot strain in a structurally normal foot will, however, recover over the week. Chronic foot strain, conversely, gradually progresses to involve different areas of the foot in sequence. The stresses of weight-bearing tend to flatten the longitudinal arch and pronate the foot. The posterior tibial muscle, which opposes this eversion of the forefoot, is thus overworked and becomes inflamed and tender. As the forefoot pronation persists, the peroneii undergo an adaptive shortening and may become spastic and painful. In long-standing cases of pronated feet, the sinus tarsi deforms and the interosseous ligament between the talus and calcaneus becomes inflamed. The area over the lateral opening of the sinus tarsi, just anterior to the lateral malleolus, then becomes tender. Ultimately, the midtarsal joints sustain articular stress, and degenerative changes develop in the talonavicular and calcaneocuboid joints. These joints become tender to palpation as arthrosis develops.

On examination, the foot may be structurally normal but is more likely to show a slight heel valgus, a flattened longitudinal arch, and abnormal shoe wear along the inner side. Range of motion at the ankle is usually normal, but inversion is likely to be limited because of peroneal "spasm" in long-standing cases. Palpate for areas of tenderness along the instep, below the medial malleolus, and over the sinus tarsi on the lateral side.

Flatfoot in Adults. As in the child, flatfoot in adults can be flexible, rigid, or acquired. Flexible flatfoot has a good longitudinal arch that disappears on weight-bearing and is due to ligamentous laxity. Examine from behind and ask the patient to rise on tiptoes. The heels roll into inversion and the longitudinal arch reappears except in severe cases. The condition may have existed since childhood or it may arise in middle-aged persons who may have gained excessive weight, performed little exercise, or who have been employed in professions requiring prolonged standing. When it becomes symptomatic, flexible flatfoot manifests itself in the form of chronic foot strain, as discussed above. As midtarsal arthrosis develops, the foot may become rigid.

Rigid flatfoot is a pronated foot with an inflexible depressed longitudinal arch and peroneal spasm. Ask the patient to stand barefoot and roll onto the outer borders of the feet. The involved foot remains rigid, as inversion of the foot is limited in these cases. Rigid flatfoot may be the result of (1) tarsal coalitions, which although present from birth, usually become symptomatic only in adult life; (2) fibrous or bony ankylosis of subtalar joints due to fractures or dislocations; and (3) acute or chronic arthritis involving the midtarsal joints.

Acquired flatfoot in adults can result from spontaneous rupture of the posterior tibial tendon. Patients present with unilateral flatfoot and progressive heel valgus. The usual symptom is mild to moderate pain near the medial malleolus or medial arch following relatively trivial trauma.

Tibialis Posterior Tendon Disorders. Many individuals enter the middle life with moderate degree of planovalgus feet either partially treated or controlled by properly fitted shoes. The added insult of a relatively minor trauma such as

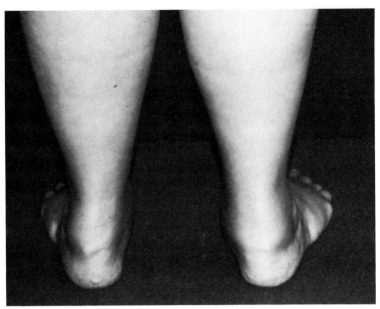

FIG 12–15. Too many toes sign: posterior tibial tendon rupture has resulted in pronation and external rotation of right foot so that when viewed from behind, "too many toes" are visible on outer side of right foot.

stepping off a curb or jumping off a ladder, which causes a valgus stress, can cause the posterior tibial tendon to be stretched, partially ruptured, or on occasion completely torn. This is followed by progressively increasing discomfort that is frequently not connected to the trauma by the patient. A profound flatfoot is the outstanding change when there is complete rupture. Examine the patient from behind; "too many toes" will be visible laterally because the foot is externally rotated (Fig 12–15). Ask the patient to rise on tiptoes; the heel fails to invert and weakness of plantar flexion is evident. The patient is unable to easily raise the heel from the floor when asked to rise on the tiptoes on the affected side. On further examination, active inversion is weak and usually limited. Passive subtalar motion may be somewhat painful. A bulging is noted on the medial aspect of the ankle and there is tenderness along the posterior tibial tendon sheath.

Plantar Fibromatosis. Fibrosis and contracture of the plantar fascia can lead to the formation of nodular swellings similar to Dupuytren's contracture of the hand. In fact, the hand should be examined in every patient with plantar fascial fibromatosis. When contracture of the plantar fascia occurs without Dupuytren's contracture of the hand, it is called Ledderhose's disease. The condition is usually symptomless and may regress spontaneously. Symptoms may develop if there is pressure over a nodule during weight-bearing. On examination, the nodules are confined to the plantar fascia, but may be tethered to the skin.

The Heel

Localization of heel pain to plantar, medial, lateral, or posterior aspects is important in differential diagnosis. Plantar heel pain is usually related to weight-bearing, while posterior heel pain is present both when weight-bearing and at rest. Medial and lateral heel pain is typically intermittent, occurring with certain types of motion.

Painful Heel Syndrome. This refers to plantar heel pain, typically occurring in middle-aged persons whose occupation entails much standing and walking. The pain is most noticeable when the patient takes the first few steps in the morning or gets up after sitting for a while. Gradually the pain may become more persistent, and sooner or later it involves the opposite foot also. On inspection, the general architecture of the foot is normal. Pain on ambulation varies in intensity. Ask the patient to rise on tiptoes and note if this causes pain. Palpate the foot for tenderness over the plantar surface of the calcaneus, along the medial tubercle of the bone, and by squeezing the fibrofatty subcutaneous tissue of the heel. In cases with plantar fasciitis, tenderness is localized to the medial tubercle where the dense central portion of the plantar fascia is attached. With the ankle in neutral position, push up on the great toe and palpate along the tight band of plantar fascia. Tenderness confirms the diagnosis of fasciitis. Subcalcaneal bursitis causes only local tenderness over the posterior aspect of the heel behind the medial tubercle. Generalized discomfort in the whole heel pad without localized tenderness indicates inflammation due to strain of the fibrofatty tissue covering the calcaneus. Lateral-view roentgenograms of both feet should be obtained to look for heel spurs, which are present in about 50% of cases, although no causal relationship to painful heel syndrome has been shown.

Tarsal Tunnel Syndrome. Pain along the medial side of the hindfoot has been better defined in recent years with identification of posterior tibial tendon disorders (discussed above) and tarsal tunnel syndrome. The tarsal tunnel syndrome results from entrapment of the posterior tibial nerve or one of its branches. Symptoms are gradual in onset, in some cases traceable to an injury such as an ankle or foot sprain. The pain radiates from the posterior aspect of the heel, along the medial side below the malleolus, and to the midtarsal area. The pain is usually burning in character, aggravated by activity, and diminished by rest. On occasion, the pain will be distributed along one of the three terminal branches of the posterior tibial nerve. On examination, the gait may be abnormal but the characteristic finding is a positive Tinel sign along the posterior tibial nerve or its branches (Fig 12–16). Actual numbness, loss of two-point discrimination, or weakness of intrinsic muscles should be tested for but is not usually demonstrable. The diagnosis is supported by electrodiagnostic studies.

Peroneal Tendon Disorders. Pain along the lateral aspect of the heel can sometimes be traced to peroneal tendon pathology. The peroneal tubercle, situated on the lateral aspect of the calcaneus about a finger's breadth below the lateral malleolus, separates the tendons of peroneus longus and brevis. The tubercle may be large, resulting in irritation due to pressure from the footwear. In cases of fracture calcaneus, the peroneal tubercle may be distorted, leading to irritation or subluxation of the peroneal tendons. The peroneal tendons may also slip out of the shallow groove behind the lateral malleolus if the anchoring ligament is torn or incompetent. The patient complains of "clicking" and pain on the lateral side of the heel or ankle. Ask the patient to dorsiflex and evert the foot actively: one or both peroneal tendons may subluxate anteriorly. This subluxation is sometimes very painful and accompanied by an audible click. Palpate along the peroneal tendon sheath for tenderness and look for prominence of the

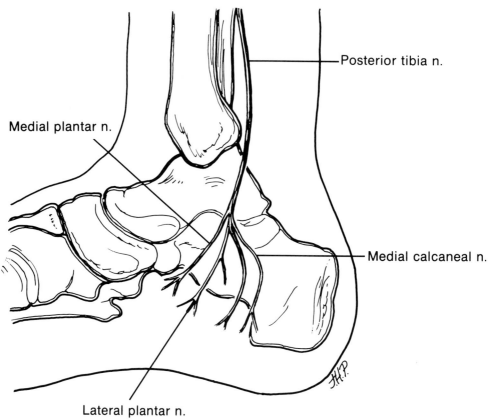

FIG 12–16. Posterior tibial nerve and its branches: Percuss along course of the nerve and its three branches for Tinel's sign.

peroneal tubercle. A chronic stenosing tenosynovitis of the peroneal tendons is sometimes seen. Passive inversion of the foot is painful in such cases.

Calcaneal Exostosis and Bursitis. These can be the cause of posterior heel pain resulting from tight-fitting or high-heel shoes. Anatomically, the posterior surface of the calcaneus is divided into two parts by an irregular horizontal ridge that gives attachment to the heel cord. A bursa (the retrocalcaneal) separates the superior facet from the tendo Achillis, while another bursa (the calcaneal) lies subcutaneously, posterior to the tendon (Fig 12–17). In rare cases, the two bursae may coalesce together to form a true sheath for the tendo Achillis. Inflammation of these bursae can be the result of mechanical irritation from the counter of the shoe, especially if the underlying bone is enlarged. The bony protuberance of the posterior superior facet of the calcaneus is known as a "pump bump." Except for its ugly appearance, due to thickening and pigmentation of the overlying skin, the condition is usually asymptomatic. Occasionally, a patient may complain of disabling pain. On examination, distention of the retrocalcaneal bursa will present with swelling on either side of the tendo Achillis, while swelling due to calcaneal bursitis is situated over the tendon and not to one side. Palpate the skin behind the tendon for thickening and tenderness. Pinch the soft tissues in front of the tendo Achillis for the retrocalcaneal bursa and any bony prominence of the calcaneus. Passive stretching of the heel cord does not cause pain in these cases. Lateral-view roentgenograms of the calcaneus are studied for any abnormality of bony contours.

Sever's Disease. Posterior heel pain due to the traction apophysitis of the calcaneus occurs most often in active adolescent boys between the ages of 10 and 13 years. Without any preceding trauma, the child starts to limp. This progresses to a complaint of dull ache in the heel. Pain is aggravated by running and shoe wear is painful. The condition is usually bilateral. On examination, the child may be able to walk normally. Ask him to walk on his tiptoes; this will cause pain. A slight swelling may be noticeable over the heel. Palpate for localized tenderness; it will be located below the insertion of tendo Achillis. Roentgenograms of the feet in lateral projection may be helpful in unilateral cases.

Achillis Tendinitis. In considering inflammatory conditions of tendons, it is useful to distinguish between (1) peritendinitis or inflammation of the tendon sheath; (2) tendinitis or inflammation of the tendon itself, usually near its inser-

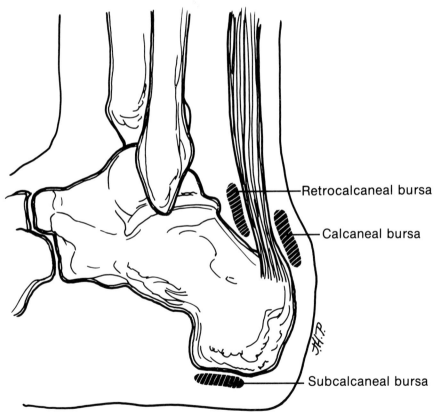

FIG 12–17. Bursae around calcaneus: inflammation will cause tenderness localized to area of involved bursa.

tion; and (3) tendinosis that is mucoid or calcific degeneration of the tendon involved. Painful inflammation of the tendo Achillis is encountered most frequently in young athletes or new joggers. Since tendo Achillis does not normally possess a tendon sheath, the condition is either a tendinitis or tendinosis. On inspection, obvious nodular swelling is only rarely encountered. Patients may have pain on attempts at walking on tiptoes. Palpate for tenderness localized at the insertion of the tendon and pain on forced dorsiflexion at the ankle. It is not known if tendinosis is a precursor of attrition ruptures of the tendo Achillis. Roentgenograms of the ankle in three projections are taken to rule out calcification; soft tissue views may help in excluding xanthomatous deposits if localized swelling is encountered in the tendon.

The Ankle

Painful conditions around the ankle joint may be traumatic, inflammatory, or degenerative. Examination is directed at first establishing the tissue layer involved and then judging the pathology. Involvement of the ankle joint itself leads to effusion. When distended with fluid, the ankle assumes a position of inversion and slight dorsiflexion. As pressure builds up, the joint first develops fullness underneath the extensor tendons and anterior to the malleoli; next a bulge develops posteriorly filling up the hollows on either side of the tendo Achillis. Place a finger on either side of the tendon and palpate for fluctuation from one side to the other. Effusion in the ankle can be the result of injury, infection, or arthritis.

Ankle Sprain. The ligaments on the lateral aspect of the ankle are most frequently involved in inversion injuries of the ankle commonly sustained in the relatively benign activity of stepping off the curb without looking. The anterior talofibular ligament (Fig 12–18), which is taut in plantar flexion, is therefore the first and the most common ligament to be injured. The calcaneofibular ligament, which becomes taut as the foot goes into dorsiflexion, is next to be injured. The posterior talofibular ligament is injured only in extreme cases. Clinical assessment of the extent of injury is extremely important. First-degree sprains in which the ligament is merely stretched cause localized tenderness but little swelling. Second-degree sprains in which some of the ligamentous fibers are torn cause tenderness, local edema, and sometimes joint effusion. Third-degree sprains with complete rupture of the ligament lead to instability, which should be tested for even in recent injuries. Local infiltration with lidocaine may be helpful before the following two maneuvers are performed: (1) For the anterior drawer test place the foot in slight inversion, stabilize the tibia with one hand, and grab the heel with the palm of the other hand, pulling it forward with gradual pressure. Forward movement of the talus in the ankle mortice indicates a tear of the anterior talofibular ligament. (2) For the inversion test place the foot near neutral position, stabilize the tibia, and push the heel into inversion using steady, gentle force. Abnormal motion indicates a rupture of the calcaneofibular ligament.

Tears of the ligaments holding the ankle mortice result from a twisting, external rotation injury of the supinated foot. Usually such injuries progress to fractures of the malleoli. If there are no fractures, palpate anteriorly between the

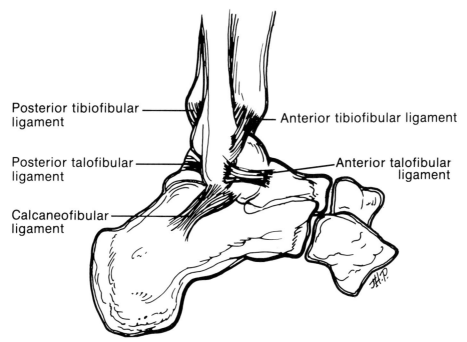

FIG 12–18. Ligaments around ankle: On lateral side anterior talofibular ligament is injured most commonly.

lateral malleolus and the extensor digitorum tendons. Look for ecchymoses, edema and effusion in the ankle joint.

Rupture of the Tendo Achillis. This is a common tendon to rupture spontaneously in the ankle region. The injury occurs frequently in middle-aged persons when they are engaged in an unaccustomed physical activity. There is a sudden sharp pain, occasionally with an audible snap, and the patient feels that he has been kicked on the back of the ankle. The diagnosis is frequently missed. On examination, the patient lacks a normal heel-toe gait and is unable to rise on the toes on the affected side. With the patient lying prone on the table and the feet dangling over the edge, note that the foot is held in less equinus than the opposite side. Despite complete rupture, the patient may be able to actively plantar flex the foot using deep flexors. Diagnosis is therefore made using Thompson's squeeze test. Squeeze the belly of the calf muscles transversely; if the tendo Achillis is ruptured completely the foot does not plantar flex. On careful palpation, a gap may be palpable if the tendon has ruptured through its substance.

Chronic Stenosing Tenosynovitis. This is similar to de Quervain's stenosing tenosynovitis at the wrist, and can involve the posterior tibial tendon medially and peroneal tendons laterally at the ankle, and cause localized pain in these regions.

Generalized Conditions

Injuries of the Foot

Discussion of the various fractures and dislocations in the foot and ankle areas is beyond the scope of this chapter. However, some general principles of physical examination in cases of foot and ankle trauma are reiterated. Fractures in the forefoot area are common and usually present no problems in diagnosis. Injuries of the midfoot and hindfoot, on the contrary, require careful evaluation. In fact, in many instances a search for specific soft tissue and ligamentous injuries must be carried out even after a roentgenologic examination has revealed the presence of a fracture.

Elicit the exact mode of injury from the patient or observers. Inspect the foot for color, skin lacerations, and bony contours. Presence of gross deformity of the ankle indicates significant displacement of the talus. Widening of the heel should arouse suspicion of a calcaneal fracture. Grossly swollen and bruised midfoot area dictates a search for dislocation of metatarsal bases. Ask the patient to actively move the joints of the foot and ankle. Severe pain limits the range of motion in cases of fractures.

Palpation of the foot in cases of injury must begin with a search for the dorsalis pedis and posterior tibial arteries. The pulses must be dutifully compared with the opposite side. Palpate the swollen areas for tenderness and bony crepitus. Routine roentgenograms are then obtained. The clinical examination is repeated after the roentgenograms have been reviewed. Look for the well-known association of conditions such as deltoid ligament injury in lateral malleolar fractures and proximal fibular tenderness in cases of medial malleolar fractures.

Infections of the Foot

Infections of the foot may be (1) superficial soft tissue infections; (2) deep infections involving and spreading along tissue planes; and (3) bone or joint infections. These may result from acute bacterial, tubercular or fungal organisms.

Superficial Foreign Bodies and Infections. The sole of the foot is particularly vulnerable to foreign bodies such as thorns, nails, needles, glass pieces, and toothpicks. Depending on the area of penetration the infection may be confined to one of the following spaces: (1) web space between the toes—infections in this space cause tenderness on dorsal as well as plantar aspects of the web; (2) interdigital subcutaneous space—these infections result in extreme tenderness between two metatarsals; and (3) heel space where septae in the fat impede spreading, but also cause increased pressure, resulting in throbbing pain that is severe enough to interfere with sleep. The heel is untouchable, there is swelling on both sides of the heel, and the ankle becomes edematous.

Deep Fascial Space Infections. The thick central part of the plantar fascia covers four layers of muscles of the sole of the foot. Infections deep to the plantar fascia can arise from direct penetration but most commonly start as an extension from the interdigital subcutaneous space. Pus can spread rapidly along the long flexor tendons of the toes to the back of the leg, particularly in persons with diabetes. On inspection, the most reliable sign of infection deep in the sole is edema on the dorsum of the foot. Palpate along the instep; it is exquisitely tender and bulges to obliterate the normal concavity. Infection of the deep fascial space is a diagnosis of such serious consequence that in cases of doubt it is better to explore than to wait.

Osteomyelitis and Septic Arthritis. Acute hematogenous osteomyelitis of the foot is rare. Chronic tuberculous and fungal infections leading to multiple draining sinuses are mostly seen in tropical countries. Differential diagnosis in such cases includes tuberculosis, Madura foot, and Kaposi's sarcoma.

Tumors of the Foot

The majority of tumors arising in the foot are of soft tissue origin and benign. Although they are not true neoplasms, ganglia arising in the midfoot area top the list that includes giant cell tumors of the tendon sheath, hemangiomas, fibromas, and plantar fascial fibromatosis. Malignant soft tissue tumors are for all practical purposes limited to melanoma and squamous cell carcinoma. Soft tissue sarcomas are exceedingly rare.

Melanoma. The foot is a fairly common site for malignant melanomas. They may start anywhere in the foot, but usually arise in a benign mole in the instep area. In the early stages of malignant degeneration there is mottling due to different shades of color, or fuzziness of the edges may occur. Unfortunately, the lesion is asymptomatic at this stage. By the time pain, ulceration and bleeding develop in the tumor, deep invasion has already occurred. Palpate the regional lymph nodes and the liver.

Subungual melanoma deserves to be considered as a separate clinical entity. The lesion starts as a deeply pigmented spot in the nail bed, frequently in the great toe. Initially it is mistaken for a subungual hematoma or fungal infection. Advancing slowly it lifts the nail out of its bed, ulcerates and becomes infected. Any pigmented lesion of the nail in a patient older than 50 years must be viewed suspiciously. Remember that a subungual hematoma will advance with the nail growth but melanoma will not.

Bone Tumors of the Foot. Benign or malignant, primary or secondary bone tumors of the foot are rare. Osteoblastoma, chondroblastoma, and chondromyxoid fibroma are the most common benign tumors of the foot and should be considered in the tarsal lesions. Ewing's sarcoma is the most commonly reported malignant bone tumor to involve the foot. Metastatic lesions are exceedingly rare in the foot.

The Foot in Diabetes

The foot problems associated with diabetes can be classified into three categories: septic, neuropathic, and ischaemic. The interplay of these three components determines the outcome when a diabetic patient is seen with an ulcerative lesion on the foot.

Septic Changes. The incidence of infection in diabetics is probably no greater than in the general population, but its effects in combination with neuropathy and ischaemia are devastating.

Neuropathic Changes. The initial manifestation of peripheral neuropathy in diabetes is usually a loss of ankle reflexes, frequently accompanied by loss of vibration sense. Sense of joint position, appreciation of superficial pain, and light

TABLE 12–3.

Grading the Dysvascular Foot

GRADE	LESION
0	No open lesion, healed scars
1	Superficial ulcer
2	Deep ulcer up to tendon sheath
3	Deep abscess, osteomyelitis
4	Gangrene in forefoot
5	Gangrene in entire foot

Adapted from Wagner FW Jr: The dysvascular foot: A system for diagnosis and treatment. *Foot Ankle* 1981; 2:64–122.

touch are lost later. In long-standing cases, trophic changes develop with lack of sweating, hyperkeratosis, and fissuring of the skin. Charcot-type changes in the midtarsal joints can develop very rapidly following a minor injury.

Ischaemic Changes. Atherosclerosis frequently accompanies diabetes. Although the pathology is no different than in non-diabetic patients, arterial occlusion below the knee is more common in persons with diabetes. Using the diabetic foot as the prototype, a grading system has been devised for the dysvascular foot (Table 12–3).

The Foot in Neurologic Disorders

Generalized neurologic disorders can produce various types of acquired foot deformities depending on the neurologic deficit. However, a foot deformity that begs for a neurologic examination is the cavus foot with claw toes. The percentage of so-called "idiopathic" cavus has declined with the advent of measures such as electrodiagnostic studies, myelography, and computed tomography for examination of the spine. On inspection, the cavus deformity may be plantar flexion of the forefoot (cavus), elevation of the midfoot with hindfoot varus (cavovarus), or calcaneus of the hindfoot (calcaneocavus). The cavovarus deformity with claw toes due to intrinsic paralysis usually occurs in Charcot-Marie-Tooth disease and Friedreich's ataxia. Calcaneocavus deformity due to weakness of the triceps surae, on the other hand, is more commonly seen with Guillain-Barré syndrome and myelodysplasia.

Cerebral Palsy. The classic deformity in cerebral palsy is equinus. Varus or valgus may develop in spastic hemiplegia due to an overactive or paralyzed tibialis posterior muscle. The equinus deformity in spastic diplegia must be assessed carefully; it may be compensating for hip and knee flexion contractures.

Spinal Dysraphism. This refers to all deformities occurring in the midline of the back. Spina bifida aperta or neural arch defects with herniation of the meninges or neural elements causes gross foot deformities such as severe calcaneovalgus or equinovarus. The two feet may actually have different deformities, which may be present at birth. Tethering of the spinal cord in spina bifida occulta or diastematomyelia, on the contrary, causes more subtle progressive changes with growth. Such patients present with a peculiarity of gait, asymmetrical wearing out of one shoe, or poor posture. Pain is not a symptom in this condition that starts around 4 to 6 years of age. On examination, the child has a cavovarus foot, which may be slightly smaller than the other and associated with a short leg. No detectable loss of power may be seen. Examine the lumbar spine area; you may be rewarded by finding a dimple, desired sinus, sacral lipoma, pigmented nevus or a tuft of hair. Thorough evaluation, including myelography, is essential.

Hemiplegia in Adults. When the acute phase is over, hemiplegia leaves behind two patterns of deformity: a flexor synergy with hip flexion, knee flexion, and ankle dorsiflexion during swing phase; or an extensor synergy with hip extension, plantar flexion, and inversion of the foot with curling of the toes during the swing phase.

Poliomyelitis. In developed countries, it is now rare. The foot deformities in polio vary depending on which muscles are paralyzed and progress in severity as the bone grows and weak muscles are further stretched. Valgus deformity is probably the commonest since tibialis anterior is frequently involved and the valgus position of the foot is made worse by weight-bearing. Varus due to paralysis of peroneii is less common. Equinus develops due to weak dorsiflexors and is aggravated by gravity. Calcaneocavus deformity results from weak triceps surae.

The Foot in Rheumatic Disorders

The foot is a common target for many generalized rheumatic disorders. Involvement of the foot may be late, when the diagnosis is already known; or the foot may be the site for presenting symptoms. In the latter case, the type of involvement in the foot can point to the underlying disease process.

Gout. Acute gouty arthritis most commonly presents with foot involvement, selecting the metatarsophalangeal joint of the great toe for its initial attack. The patient, usually an elderly man, wakes up in the early hours of the morning with pain in the great toe. The pain is worse on weight-bearing and soon becomes excruciating as the skin over the metatarsophalangeal joint becomes swollen, red and shiny. There is extreme tenderness and the toe looks infected. Suppuration, however, never develops, and even if untreated the attack subsides in two or three days. In the chronic stage, a vague aching sensation may be present or the recovery may be complete between attacks. Gout should always be considered in the differential diagnosis of vague aches in the forefoot. Roentgenograms of the foot may or may not be useful. Long-standing untreated cases may develop large tophaceous deposits.

Rheumatoid Arthritis. Synovium of the joints and tendon sheaths are the major targets of rheumatoid process. Bilaterally symmetrical synovitis of multiple joints in the forefoot is a frequent presenting complaint in rheumatoid arthritis. Palpate each metatarsophalangeal joint for localized tenderness and look for the swelling of an inflamed bursa under the metatarsal heads (Fig 12–19). In late cases, hallux valgus and lateral subluxation of the lesser toes are frequently seen; there is splaying of the forefoot due to weakening of ligamentous structures. Late changes in the hindfoot include synovitis of the ankle and subtalar joints and tenosynovitis of adjacent tendons. With continued weight-bearing, progressive valgus deformity of the hindfoot develops, leading to flattening of the longitudinal arch and tenderness over the sinus tarsi.

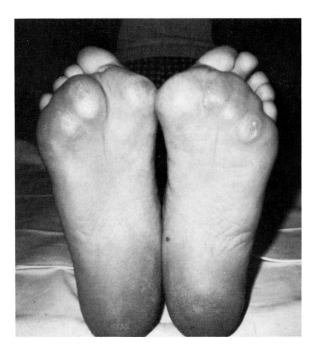

FIG 12–19. Rheumatoid arthritis involving feet: Note prominent inflamed bursae under metatarsal heads on plantar surface.

Rheumatoid Variants. These are also known as the so-called seronegative spondyloarthropathies and they differ from rheumatoid arthritis in that the inflammatory process involves not only the synovium but also the fibrous joint capsule, ligamentous insertions, and the joint cartilage itself. Involvement of the foot in these processes is also different: involvement of the hindfoot is most frequent. Reiter's syndrome frequently presents as synovitis and capsulitis of the joints around the talus. Pain and tenderness over the medial tubercle of the calcaneus, with plantar fasciitis and spur formation is the characteristic lesion of all rheumatoid variants. In Reiter's syndrome, it may be the presenting complaint. In ankylosing spondylitis, it develops after spinal disease is well established. In psoriatic arthritis, the skin lesions nearly always predate the plantar fasciitis.

Osteoarthritis. Along with other weight-bearing joints, the metatarsophalangeal joint of the great toe is a common site for primary osteoarthritis. Involvement of the ankle joint in the osteoarthritic process is usually due to previous trauma. Multiple joint pathology in the midfoot area should arouse suspicion of neuropathic involvement (Charcot's joint) in processes such as diabetes or neurosyphilis.

Reflex Sympathetic Dystrophy

The term "algodystrophy" has been coined to consolidate under one heading a group of related disorders in which there is an inappropriate hyperactivity of the autonomic nervous system following a relatively minor insult to an extremity. Prolonged persistent pain, hyperesthesia, and vasomotor disturbances delay recovery of function and trophic changes ensue.

Following a relatively simple injury, such as an ankle sprain or a metatarsal fracture, reflex sympathetic dystrophy develops in three distinct stages. Stage 1 starts within three to six weeks. Clinically, there is pain out of proportion to the injury or insult. There is localized edema, muscle spasm, and tenderness with hyperesthesia and dysesthesia. The skin is warm, dry, and red to begin with and later becomes cold, clammy, and cyanotic. The clinical course is spontaneous resolution or progression to stage 2. Stage 2 develops within three to six months. The pain decreases, but edema becomes brawny, joints thicken, and muscles become wasted. Skin becomes thin and glazed and trophic changes develop if the condition is not treated. Roentgenograms at this stage will show spotty osteopenia. Stage 3 becomes established as edema decreases and skin becomes smooth and shiny. Nails become brittle and ridged, fat pads of the foot become atrophic and muscles waste away as joints stiffen. Roentgenograms will show diffuse atrophy of bones at this stage.

Suggested Reading

1. Cailliet R: *Foot and Ankle Pain*. Philadelphia, FA Davis Co, 1979.
2. Inman VT: *The Joints of the Ankle*. Baltimore, Williams & Wilkins Co, 1976.
3. Klenerman L: *The Foot and Its Disorders*, ed 2. Boston, Blackwell Scientific Publications, 1982.
4. Mann RA: *Surgery of the Foot*. St Louis, CV Mosby Co, 1986.
5. Tachdjian MO: *The Child's Foot*. Philadelphia, WB Saunders Co, 1985.
6. Wagner FW Jr: The dysvascular foot: A system for diagnosis and treatment. *Foot Ankle* 1981; 2:64–122.

Index